NUCLEAR CARDIOLOGY, THE BASICS

CONTEMPORARY CARDIOLOGY

CHRISTOPHER P. CANNON, MD
SERIES EDITOR
ANNEMARIE ARMANI, MD
EXECUTIVE EDITOR

Nuclear Cardiology, The Basics

How to Set Up and Maintain a Laboratory

Second Edition

by

Frans J. Th. Wackers, MD, PhD
Yale University School of Medicine, New Haven, CT

Wendy Bruni, BS, CNMT
Yale–New Haven Hospital, New Haven, CT

and

Barry L. Zaret, MD
Yale University School of Medicine, New Haven, CT

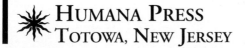 Humana Press
Totowa, New Jersey

Cover illustrations provided by Dr. Frans J. Th. Wackers.

Background image: Chapter 11, Fig. 1. Thumbnail images: Chapter 10, Figs. 20, 34, 40, 42, and 42; Chapter 11, Figs. 6 and 20.

Cover design by Karen Schulz

Printed in the United States of America. 10 9 8 7 6 5 4 3 2 1

eISBN 978-1-59745-262-5

Library of Congress Control Number: 2007929352

PREFACE

In the USA, the performance of nuclear cardiology studies increased dramatically over the past 5 to 10 years. In 2001, the number of patient visits for myocardial perfusion imaging was 7.9 million. In 2005, the number of patient visits increased to 9.3 million. Roughly 96% of these studies used ECG-gated single-photon emission computed tomography (SPECT) imaging. Roughly half (47%) of these studies were performed in nonhospital settings (1).

The growth of nuclear cardiology as an expanded outpatient laboratory enterprise is readily apparent. In the USA, as well as in other parts of the world, this growth has been linked to the recognition of the ability of cardiologists to perform these studies.

Certification examination in nuclear cardiology is now an established cardiology phenomenon in the USA. Certification by one of several mechanisms is now generally required for hospital privileges in reading studies and is also often required to obtain reimbursement for study performance and interpretation.

Accreditation of laboratories is also well established. Indeed, at the time of this writing, we have learned that one large payor, responsible for 70 million lives, will require laboratory accreditation for reimbursement by March 2008.

Over the years, some of the most frequent questions asked of us by our former trainees after leaving the program relate to practical issues involved in the establishment of a nuclear cardiology laboratory. In view of the growth of the field, this is certainly not surprising.

There are a number of excellent texts on general nuclear cardiology available (2–5). These books generally deal with the overall concepts of the field, its scientific basis, techniques, clinical applications, and clinical value. However, to our knowledge, there does not presently exist a volume designed to provide the nuclear cardiologist with a manual dedicated specifically to how to establish and run a well organized and state-of-the-art nuclear cardiology laboratory.

Consequently, the purpose of this book is to provide the outline for the "nuts and bolts" establishment and operation of a nuclear cardiology laboratory. In so doing, we have attempted to deal with the relevant issues that a laboratory director must address in either setting up the laboratory or maintaining its competitive edge and clinical competence over time. We primarily attempt to identify issues related to outpatient imaging facilities. However, where appropriate, issues related to in-patients in hospital-based laboratories are also discussed.

This book is aimed at cardiology fellows, nuclear cardiology fellows, and nuclear medicine and radiology residents completing training as well as established cardiologists, radiologists, or nuclear physicians who want to establish a nuclear cardiology laboratory. The book should also be of value to nuclear cardiology technologists, laboratory managers, and health maintenance organizations. Attention has also been paid to those factors relevant for laboratory accreditation.

The book is organized in what we feel is a logical progression. In this new edition, we have kept the basic format established in the first edition. In addition to reviewing, modifying, and updating each chapter in the first edition, we have added entirely new chapters on positron emission tomography (PET) imaging, hybrid imaging, and the clinical appropriateness of nuclear cardiology procedures.

The initial chapter addresses what is required to establish the laboratory in terms of equipment, availability of radiopharmaceuticals, and staff qualifications. A chapter is devoted to the types of information patients should be provided with, prior to arriving in the laboratory. Chapters are devoted to laboratory logistics and appropriate clinical protocols for stress studies. Several chapters deal with the technical aspects of performance of studies, such as those acquisition parameters relevant for high-quality studies, processing parameters, and quantification and display options. Sections on attenuation correction have been expanded. Examples are given of commonly encountered artifacts. We deal with issues relating to networking, both within one laboratory and linking several laboratories. Issues relating to dictation and reporting, coding and reimbursement, and quality assurance are also separately addressed. Finally, we address key policy issues that are relevant to high-quality clinical performance and conclude with a chapter addressing issues relevant to laboratory accreditation. The new chapter on PET imaging and hybrid imaging reflects new clinical advances in the field since the first edition. It is likely that these technologies will have an increasing clinical utilization in the immediate and near future. The new chapter on appropriateness guidelines reflects the recent joint attempt of ACC/ASNC to establish clinical criteria for technology utilization. It is important for practioners of nuclear cardiology to perform studies only when appropriate. It is not enough to run a highly capable technologic enterprise; it must be clinically relevant as well.

We are hopeful that this second edition will continue to fill an important clinical need within the cardiology and imaging communities. The book has been designed to be straightforward and to deal directly with the issues at hand and to build on the strengths established in the first edition. In many instances, we present several sides of a particular issue. The final decision on which approach to take will depend on local circumstances.

Finally, in conclusion, it is very important to acknowledge the multiple lessons we have learned from the many technologists and trainees, both in cardiology and nuclear medicine who have passed through our laboratory over the past two decades. Their input, as well as the opportunity to take part in their training, has helped us enormously in the conception and writing of this book. Some of the useful websites are http://www.asnc.org, http://www.cbnc.org, and http://www.icanl.org.

Frans J. Th. Wackers, MD, PhD
Wendy Bruni, BS, CNMT
Barry L. Zaret, MD

REFERENCES

1. IMV Medical Information Division (2006). *2005 Nuclear Medicine Census Summary Report.* Available at http://www.imvlimited.com/mid/.
2. Zaret BL, Beller GA (eds) (2005). *Clinical Nuclear Cardiology, State of the Art and Future Directions,* 3rd Edition. Elsevier Mosby, Philadelphia, PA.
3. Iskandrian AE, Verani MS (eds) (2003). *Nuclear Cardiac Imaging, Principles and Applications,* 3rd Edition. Oxford University Press, New York, NY.
4. Gerson MC (ed.) (1997). *Cardiac Nuclear Medicine,* 3rd Edition. McGraw-Hill, New York, NY.
5. Sandler MP, Coleman RE, Patton JA, Wackers FJTh, Gottschalk A (eds) (2003). *Diagnostic Nuclear Medicine,* 4th Edition. Lippincott Williams & Wilkins, Philadelphia, PA.

CONTENTS

Acknowledgments

We are grateful for the invaluable work done by Vera Tsatkin, CNMT, Donna Natale, CNMT, Mary Jo Zito, CNMT, Chris Weyman, CNMT, and Ramesch Chettiar, CNMT, by providing help and expertise with the collection and formatting of the illustrations in this book. We also acknowledge Suman Tandon, MD, Matt Al-Shaer, MD, Yi-Hwa Liu, PhD, Patricia Aaronson, Stefanie L. Margulies, CNMT, and Chris Gallagher for reviewing selected portions of the manuscript and providing valuable input. We also thank Ernest V. Garcia, PhD, Guido Germano, PhD, and Edward Ficaro, PhD, for providing us with illustrations of their proprietary software.

About the Authors

Frans J. Th. Wackers, MD, PhD

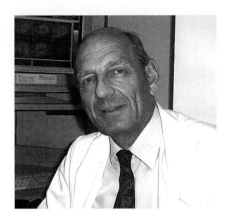

Frans J. Th. Wackers, MD, is Professor of Diagnostic Radiology and Medicine and served as Director of the Cardiovascular Nuclear Imaging Laboratory at Yale University School of Medicine for 22 years.

Born in Echt, The Netherlands, Dr. Wackers received both his MD and PhD degrees from the University of Amsterdam School of Medicine in 1970. He completed training in Internal Medicine and Cardiology in the former Wilhelmina Gasthuis, Amsterdam in 1977. Dr. Wackers moved to the USA in 1977, where he was on the faculty of the Section of Cardiovascular Medicine at Yale University School of Medicine (1977–1981), the University of Vermont College of Medicine (1981–1984), and since 1984 at Yale University School of Medicine.

Dr. Wackers is a Fellow of the American College of Cardiology; a Fellow of the American Heart Association, Council on Clinical Cardiology; a member of the Society of Nuclear Medicine; and a member and Fellow of the American Society of Nuclear Cardiology. He is also a Diploma European Cardiologist of European Society of Cardiology. He is on the Editorial Board of the *Journal of the American College of Cardiology*, the *American Journal of Cardiology*, and the *Journal of Nuclear Cardiology*. He was President of the Cardiovascular Council of The Society of Nuclear Medicine (1992–1993), President of the American

Society of Nuclear Cardiology (1994–1995), President of the Certification Council of Nuclear Cardiology (1996–1997), and President of
the Intersocietal Commission for Accreditation of Nuclear Laboratories
(1997–2005). He is the recipient of the Rescar Award of the University
of Maastricht, The Netherlands (1988), the Herrman Blumgart Award of
the Society of Nuclear Medicine, New England Chapter (1995), the Homi
Baba Award of the Indian Nuclear Cardiological Society (1997), the
Eugene Drake Award of the American Heart Association, New England
Affiliate (1999), the Distinguished Service Award of the Society of
Nuclear Cardiology (1999), the third Mario Verani Memorial Lecturer
of the American Society of Nuclear Cardiology (2004), the Wenckebach
Lecturer of the Dutch Society of Cardiology (2005), and the Mario Verani
Lecturer of Methodist Hospital, Houston, Texas (2006).

Dr. Wackers is considered a pioneer in Nuclear Cardiology. He is
the founder of the American Society of Nuclear Cardiology (1993),
the Certification Board of Nuclear Cardiology (1996), and the Intersocietal Commission for Accreditation of Nuclear laboratories (1997). He
was Co-Chair of the 6th and 7th International Conference of Nuclear
Cardiology (2003 and 2005, repectively).

Dr. Wackers has published more than 300 articles on nuclear cardiology and clinical cardiology.

Dr. Wackers is presently the Principal Investigator and Chairman
of the multicenter Detection of Ischemia in Asymptomatic Diabetics
(DIAD) study. The study began in September 2000, recruitment was
completed in August 2002, and continued until September 2007.

Dr. Wackers is also the director of the Yale University Radionuclide Core laboratory. The laboratory has been involved in numerous
multicenter clinical studies utilizing cardiac nuclear imaging since its
inception in 1984.

Wendi Bruni, BS, CNMT

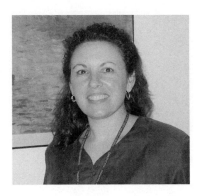

Wendy Bruni is manager of the Nuclear Cardiology and Nuclear Medicine laboratories of the Department of Diagnostic Radiology at Yale-New Haven Hospital, New Haven, CT. She served as chief technologist of the Cardiovascular Nuclear Imaging Laboratory for 10 years. Ms. Bruni received her BS in nuclear medicine from the Rochester Institute of Technology, Rochester, NY, in 1986. She worked in the nuclear medicine department at the Community General Hospital, Syracuse, NY, from 1986 to 1992. In 1992, she moved to Yale-New Haven Hospital. In 1995, she became Chief Technologist of the Yale Nuclear Cardiology Department. In 2004, she became the administrative manager of Yale-New Haven Hospital Nuclear Cardiology and Nuclear Medicine laboratories.

Ms. Bruni is an active member of the American Society of Nuclear Cardiology, participating in the technologist, newsletter, and program committees. She was secretary of the New England Chapter of the Society of Nuclear Medicine (1999) and Chair of the Nuclear Cardiology Council of the Society of Nuclear Medicine Technologist Section. Ms. Bruni was selected to be on the panel of nuclear cardiology technologists who helped the NMTCB evaluate the Nuclear Cardiology Specialty Exam for technologists. She was one of the first to obtain the specialty certification of Nuclear Cardiology (NCT) in June 2001.

Barry L. Zaret, MD

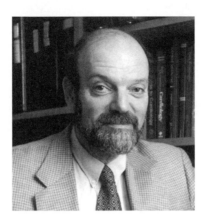

Barry L. Zaret, MD, is Robert W. Berliner Professor of Medicine (Cardiovascular Medicine) and Professor of Diagnosis Radiology. He served as Chief of Cardiovascular Medicine at Yale University for 26 years.

Dr. Zaret received his BS degree from Queens College, City University of New York, and MD degree from New York University School of Medicine.

He completed training in cardiology in 1971 at The Johns Hopkins University School of Medicine. He became Chief of Cardiology at Yale University School of Medicine in 1978.

He is a Fellow of the American College of Cardiology; Fellow of the American Heart Association; and a Founding member of the American Society of Nuclear Cardiology. He is founding Editor-in-Chief of the *Journal of Nuclear Cardiology* and is on the Editorial Board of the *Circulation*, the *Journal of the American College of Cardiology*, the *American Journal of Cardiology*, and the *Journal of Nuclear Cardiology*. He was president of the Association of Professors of Cardiology (1992–1993).

He has received numerous awards and recognitions, including the Herrman Blumgart Award of the Society of Nuclear Medicine, New England Chapter (1978), the Louis Sudler Lecturer and Medalist, Rush-Presbyterian Mediacl College (1993), the Award for Contribution and Leadership in Noninvasive Cardiology, 4th International Conference on Noninvasive Cardiology, Cyprus (1993), the 29th Nathan J. Kiven Orator award, Providence RI (1996), The Solomon A. Berson Medical Alumni Achievement Award in Clinical Science, New York University

School of Medicine (1998), Co-Chair of the 1st and 2nd International Conference of Nuclear Cardiology (1993 and 1995, respectively), Co-Director of the 2nd, 3rd, and 4th Wintergreen Conference on Nuclear Cardiology (1994, 1996, 1998, respectively), First Samuel and Patsy Paine Lecturer, University of Texas (2001), 2nd Annual Mario Verani Lecture, American Society of Nuclear Cardiology (2003), the Ellis Island Medal of Honor (2003), and the American Society of Nuclear Cardiology Distinguished Service Award (2006).

Dr. Zaret is considered one of the founders and present leaders of the subspecialty of Nuclear Cardiology. He has made numerous contributions to cardiology literature on myocardial perfusion imaging and assessment of cardiac function using radionuclide imaging methodology.

Using This Book
and the Companion CD

All illustrations and movies in this book can be found in digital format on the accompanying CD. The images are best viewed on a high-resolution (1280 × 1280) color (24-bit or higher true color) computer monitor. The movies are best viewed at a display of 8–10 frames per second.

1 Getting Started

Whether planning a new nuclear cardiology imaging facility or renovating an existing laboratory, there are many factors to be considered and many decisions to be made. This chapter will highlight and discuss many of these practical decisions. The following issues will be considered:

- Physical space
- Equipment
- Radiopharmacy
- Additional miscellaneous supplies
- Staffing
- Radiation safety officer (RSO)
- Laboratory license

Key Words: Physical laboratory space, Imaging rooms, Stress rooms, Equipment (imaging and non imaging), Computer hardware and software, Supplies, Staffing (medical and technical), Training requirements staff, Radiation safety officer (RSO), Nuclear Regulatory Commission, Radiopharmacy, Radiopharmaceutical unit doses or kits, Laboratory license.

PHYSICAL SPACE

Imaging Rooms

Imaging rooms should be spacious enough to accommodate gamma camera systems. Currently, a typical imaging room should be at the minimum 14 × 14 ft (4.3 × 4.3 m) (**Fig. 1-1**). Cameras of different vendors differ in space requirements. It is important to know the footprint of the imaging system selected and that all equipment can be accommodated in the available space. "Hybrid" systems [e.g., single photon emission computed tomography (SPECT)–CT, positron emission tomography (PET)–CT] require more space. Typically, they require at least a 20 × 16 ft (6.1 × 4.9 m) room plus a 12 × 4 ft (3.6 × 1.2 m) control room. If CT is used, lead shielding of the walls, floor, and ceiling may be necessary.

From: *Contemporary Cardiology: Nuclear Cardiology, The Basics*
By: F. J. Th. Wackers, W. Bruni, and B. L. Zaret © Humana Press Inc., Totowa, NJ

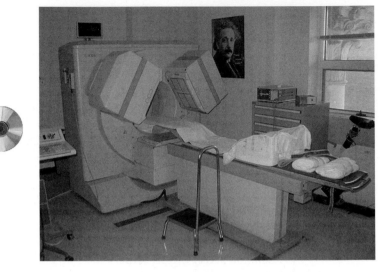

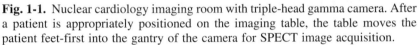

Fig. 1-1. Nuclear cardiology imaging room with triple-head gamma camera. After a patient is appropriately positioned on the imaging table, the table moves the patient feet-first into the gantry of the camera for SPECT image acquisition.

Stress Rooms

Stress rooms must be in close proximity to imaging rooms. A typical stress room requires at a minimum 8 × 8 ft (2.5 × 2.5 m) (**Fig. 1-2**).

Injection Room

The injection room is useful for the injection of radiopharmaceuticals at rest. The minimal size required is 6 × 6 ft (1.8 × 1.8 m).

Patient Preparation Area

This area is optional but will facilitate the flow of patients. A minimum size is 8 × 8 ft (2.5 × 2.5 m). This area can also be used to monitor patients after stress testing when necessary.

Reception/Waiting Rooms and Toilet Facilities

These areas should be large enough to accommodate the expected patient volume and should be accessible to handicapped persons. A patient bathroom should be in close proximity of the waiting area.

Bathroom(s)

There should be separate bathrooms for patients (including handicapped-accessible) and for staff in the imaging area.

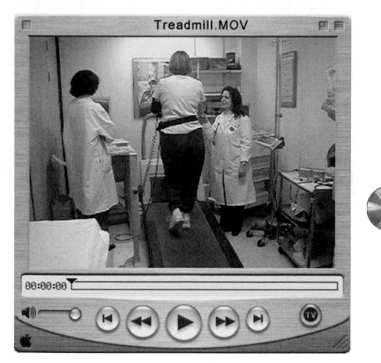

Fig. 1-2. Treadmill exercise testing *(movie)*. It is good medical practice to have two people present during an exercise test. One person, a physician or experienced nurse supervises the test and observes the ECG during exercise and operates the controls of the treadmill. Another person is present for taking and recording vital signs.

Radiopharmacy

This area is a necessity whether one plans for a fully operational "hot lab" or merely for the storage of "unit doses." Minimum required space is 6 × 6 ft (1.8 × 1.8 m) (**Fig. 1-3**).

Reading/Interpretation Area

A separate and quiet area for interpretation of studies is very convenient. In compliance with Health Insurance Portability and Accountability Act (HIPAA) regulations, patient's protected health information (PHI) must be viewed and discussed with consideration of patient confidentiality. This space also serves to preserve patient privacy and confidentiality.

Storage Area

To store supplies, patient files, and digital image data.

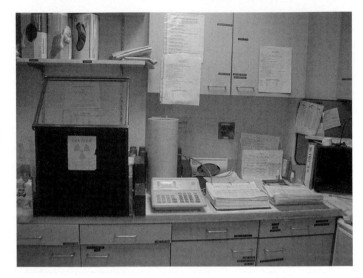

Fig. 1-3. Interior of the radiopharmacy, also known as hot lab. On the left is the lead-shielded work area. In the middle is the dose calibrator. On the right are the logbooks for recording the use of radioisotopes.

Staff Area

Area for storage of personal items and for lunch breaks and staff meetings.

Office Space

Offices for medical and technical directors.

EQUIPMENT

Acquiring a Gamma Camera

Before one begins to explore the options of different gamma cameras on the market, one should decide on a number of important issues that may narrow down the search.

- Will the camera be a *dedicated* cardiac gamma camera, or will general nuclear medicine imaging procedures be performed as well?
  For dedicated cardiac cameras, one can purchase cameras with smaller detector heads and smaller field of view (FOV).
- How much physical space is available?
  Does the gamma camera fit in the room? Is there enough workspace around the camera? Vendors usually provide help with planning and the design of a floor plan.
- Will attenuation-corrected imaging be performed on the gamma camera?

Hardware Considerations

Size Field of View

If a camera will be used for other organ imaging in addition to cardiac imaging, a large FOV is needed. If the camera will be used only for nuclear cardiology imaging, a smaller FOV is appropriate.

Number of Heads

Triple-head or dual-head gamma camera? Dual heads are better for general nuclear medicine imaging. They are also cheaper.

Collimator Options

One should choose a collimator that will be adequate for different acquisition needs anticipated. Cardiac SPECT studies are acquired with parallel-hole collimators. For technetium-99m (Tc-99m) agents, usually parallel-hole low-energy high-resolution (LEHR) collimators are used, and for thallium-201 (Tl-201), parallel-hole low-energy all-purpose (LEAP) collimators are used.

SPECT/CT, PET/CT Option

These hybrid cameras require larger imaging space to accommodate the X-ray gantry. Consideration should be given to appropriate lead-shielded area for the technologist or a separate shielded monitoring room.

Attenuation Correction

One should make a choice between sealed sources and X-ray CT-based attenuation correction devices. Additional hardware and software are necessary for attenuation correction.

Automatic Collimator Changer

This feature is an excellent choice if collimators are to be changed frequently. However, close attention must be paid to floor leveling.

Patient Table: Manual or Automatic

The imaging table needs to be movable; this can be done by hand or with a motor. Manual tables are difficult to move when obese patients are on the table and require exact floor leveling.

Table Weight Limits

The maximal patient weight that the table can support is identified. The average weight of patients in one's practice is considered. Maximal acceptable patient weight for imaging tables generally 350–400 lb (160–180 kg).

Gantry Size and Weight

Prior to committing to purchase of a camera, one should consult with an engineer concerning whether the floor of the imaging room has the capacity to support the camera's weight. Reinforcement of the floor may be necessary, which adds to the overall cost of one's purchase and increases installation time.

Power Requirements

Many gamma camera systems have special electrical power needs. This has to be checked with the manufacturer.

Universal Power Supply

If electrical power from the outlet fluctuates, one may need a universal power supply (UPS) to maintain power to the gantry and prevent system failures. Even if power supply is stable, it is a good optional feature.

Computer Speed

If quantitative processing is performed routinely, or if 16-bin ECG-gated studies are acquired, a fast(er) computer is required. Typical required speed is at least 2 GHz.

Computer Memory

It is preferred to acquire ECG-gated SPECT images with 16 rather 8 frames per cardiac cycle. Extra computer memory may be needed, particularly if both stress and rest images are acquired in ECG-gated mode. The typical amount of required computer storage space and RAM memory is 2 GB. For the storage and access of prior studies at 500 GB, disk memory space is needed.

Networking Capabilities

Can the new system be networked to existing systems in the laboratory, and can image data be transferred back and forth? Does the system allow for remote access and/or web home reading? (see Chapter 18).

Acquisition Terminal

Is the acquisition terminal separate from the processing computer? Is there space in the imaging room for the extra computer?

Service Issues

Is there local service for the equipment? What is their average service response time? What is their backup or support? Talk to an area hospital or other area users who have the same service and ask about the average downtime of the camera, the service response times, and the service technician's capabilities. Negotiate prior to purchase for guaranteed minimal downtime.

Quality Control Requirements

How often is quality control (QC) required and how easy can QC be performed? What are acceptable limits? We recommend that new equipment be tested for uniformity and resolution by a physicist using the Jaszczack three-dimensional (3-D) phantom.

Display Computer

Cardiac SPECT imaging must be interpreted from a high-resolution (1280 × 1024 pixels) color monitor (24 bit or higher true color). Multiple color scales, including a linear gray scale, should be available. Flat panel monitors are currently of sufficient high quality that they can be used for diagnostic reading.

Storage of Digital Data

Computer memory and storage media are presently relatively cheap. Depending on volume of patient studies and ECG-gating parameters, one may need sufficient on-computer memory space, at least 500 GB. Raw image data can be stored on 2.3–4.2 GB optical disks or, if a large amount of data is to be stored, a 1.7 TB RAID (redundant array of independent drives) archiving system. Processed data, gif and tiff files, may be kept on 700 MB CDs. Unprocessed and processed imaging data should be kept for at least 3 years or as regulated by state laws. This is required also by Intersocietal Commission for Accreditation of Nuclear Laboratories (ICANL) for laboratory accreditation. Storage is also of clinical importance: when interpreting a current study of a patient, it is considered good practice to compare the current study with previous ones. Therefore, long-term storage is important.

Software Considerations

Quantitative Software

Does the system provide adequate quantitative software programs? What are the choices? Are the programs validated in the literature? How much extra do they cost?

Display Options

Are the display options easy to use and can they be modified to specific needs? Is the display of images in compliance with American Society of Nuclear Cardiology (ASNC) standardized display?

Transfer of Images

Is it possible to take screen captures (jpeg, gif, or tiff) of reconstructed slices and of movies (mpeg)? To apply for ICANL accreditation, it is required that one submits processed images with the application package.

Ease of Learning

Is the software user-friendly and easy to learn by the technical staff?

Applications

Can a staff member attend classes to learn about the equipment and use of software? Does the vendor provide application specialists who come on-site to teach the technical staff how to use the equipment and software? If so, for how many days? These are very important questions to have answered clearly.

Software Flexibility

Is the software flexible? Can the software easily be manipulated to perform nonstandard tasks? Some software is written in a way that processing steps are strung together in "macros," which make it virtually impossible, or at least very difficult, to deviate from routine protocol. One should also consider whether software is in compliance with new HIPAA regulations (see Chapter 18).

Additional Ancillary Equipment

Printer

Networking Capabilities. In a laboratory with multiple camera systems, it important to purchase a printer that can be integrated into the local area network (LAN) and is capable of printing from all imaging equipment. However, because printing is rather expensive, many laboratories have elected in recent years to become "film-less." At the present time, it is feasible to provide referring physicians with online access to patient image data through a secure network.

Quality. Some laboratories send hard copies of images with the reports to referring physicians. Glossy paper prints are expensive. For archiving and for documentation in the patient's chart, less expensive plain printing paper is also available.

Paper and Ink Cost. Calculate the cost-per-print when comparing different systems.

Scanner. The storage and archiving of large volumes of hard copy patient records has become an increasing practical problem. Patient records, reports, ECGs, etc. can be scanned for digital archiving as jpeg, tiff, or gif files. The use of scanners and the uploading of digitized patient information also greatly facilitates remote web-based image interpretation.

Treadmill and ECG monitor

Software Options. Can the treadmill/ECG software easily be modified? Can laboratory-specific protocols be inserted in the program? Examples include printing ECGs at predetermined time intervals and the printing of selected exercise data in the final report.

Archiving. Some ECG machines have the option of digital storage of ECG tracings. Digital archiving of stress ECGs will be useful in an environment where other patient information also is stored electronically.

Test Setup. Is the setup of a patient, i.e., entering patient information in computer, placement of electrodes, and arrangement of ECG cables, easily performed?

Bicycle Compatibility. Can the ECG computer, if needed, also operate in conjunction with upright bicycle exercise?

Cardiopulmonary Exercise Testing Compatibility. With increasing numbers of patients with congestive heart failure, cardiopulmonary exercise testing with measurements of oxygen consumption has become a more common procedure. Is ECG computer compatible with cardiopulmonary testing equipment?

Stress Protocol Options. Are all required exercise and pharmacological stress protocol options available?

Treadmill Speed. Can the motorized treadmill start slowly enough so that the patient can easily step onto the belt? What is the maximal speed of the treadmill? The recommended range of speed is 1–8 mph (1.6–12.8 km/h).

Weight Limit. Is the weight limit of the treadmill adequate for the majority of patients who will come for testing?

Infusion Pump for Pharmacological Stress

Ease of Use.   Make sure that the setup of the pump is easy and that infusion rates can be adjusted. This is especially important if dobutamine pharmacological stress is performed.

Infusion Rates.   The pump must have the ability to infuse over a wide range of infusion rates, so that patients of all body weights receive the appropriate doses. Smaller pumps may have pre-set infusion rates and are not adjustable. Although these in general are very easy to use, they cannot be adequately adjusted for obese patients.

Syringe Compatibility.   Make sure the pump works with the brand of syringes used in the laboratory. Syringes of different brands have slightly different diameters. The pump must be adjustable for each particular brand of syringe.

Exercise Bicycle

Compatibility.   Is the bicycle compatible with the ECG computer equipment?

Ease of Use.   Can the bicycle seat be adjusted easily for patients of different heights? Is it easy to monitor and to change the Watts during stress?

Camera Compatibility.   If the bicycle is to be used in conjunction with exercise first-pass imaging, the handlebars must be removable so that the patient can be positioned with the chest close to camera head.

Emergency Equipment

The following are required emergency equipment and drugs:

- Oxygen tank and regulator
- Nasal cannula and extension tubing
- Mouth piece
- Ambu bag
- Code cart and defibrillator
- Portable ECG monitor(s)
- Nitroglycerin tablets
- Aminophylline
- Lidocaine
- Atropine
- Metoprolol
- Adenosine

- Aspirin
- Diltiazem
- Nebulizers
- Albuterol inhalers

Optional Emergency Drugs

- Furosemide
- Intravenous (IV) nitroglycerin
- Heparin

RADIOPHARMACY

Setting up the Hot Lab

Whether one decides to purchase Tc-99m generators and prepare radiopharmaceuticals on-site in the laboratory, or to buy "unit doses" from a local commercial radiopharmacy, one needs to make sure that there is a separate and dedicated area for radiopharmaceutical preparation and storage, the "hot lab." The area is set aside from the usual work areas, has limited access, and therefore does not expose staff and patients to unnecessary radiation.

This area must be large enough to provide storage of isotopes received, to provide storage of radioactive trash, and to allow for preparation and calibration of radiotracers. The minimal size of a hot lab with a generator is approximately 6 × 6 ft (1.8 × 1.8 m). For the handling of unit doses, one needs to reserve an area of at least 4 × 4 ft (1.2 × 1.2 m).

It is prudent to plan this component of the imaging facility with an RSO and have him/her involved in the design of the facility from the very beginning. At least one cabinet, in which radioisotopes and radioactive trash are stored, needs walls with lead shielding. Whether or not the door and walls of the hot lab need lead shielding depends on what is being stored, where the hot lab is located, and the assessment by the RSO.

Supplies Needed for Radiopharmacy (Whether One Uses a Generator or Unit Doses)

Radiation Caution Sign

The door of the radiopharmacy, or area set aside as radiopharmacy, must be marked with the standard radiation warning decal "Caution Radioactive Materials" (**Fig. 1-4**). Containers of radioactive material (lead pigs, syringes) must be marked with the same radiation warning labels (**Fig. 1-5**).

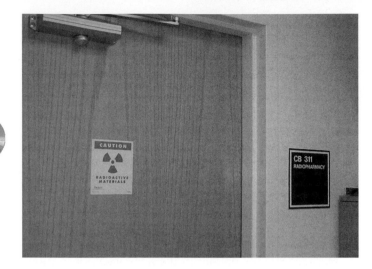

Fig. 1-4. Entrance door to the radiopharmacy must be locked at all times and show a caution sign for radioactive materials.

Dose Calibrator

Some of the newer models come with "Radiopharmacy manager" computers. This program *requires* QC data to be entered prior to use on each working day. This eliminates forgotten QC. This ensures that QC is always up to date, which is crucial for the Nuclear Regulatory Commission (NRC) inspections.

Cesium-137 Source

Needed for daily QC of the dose calibrator (see Chapter 19).

Lead Molybdenum Coddle

Necessary for QC of Tc-99m from generators.

Dose Calibrator Dippers

Multiple dippers should be available. A second or extra dipper is recommended in case the first dipper was contaminated.

Lead Shield with Glass

Necessary for visual control when drawing up doses.

Lead Bricks

Used for additional shielding. Necessary for use with molybdenum-99 (Mo-99) generators **(Fig. 1-6)**.

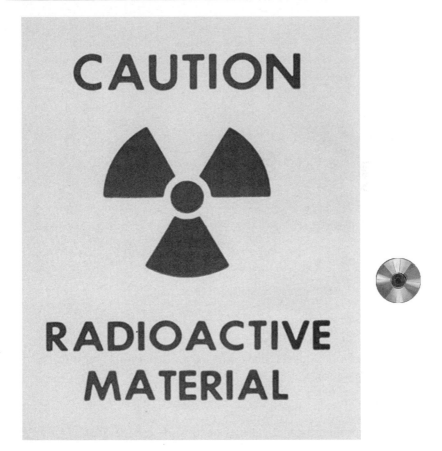

Fig. 1-5. Caution sign for radioactive materials. This sign must be posted at the entrance of all areas where radioactive materials are being used.

Lead Vials

Necessary if preparing radiopharmaceuticals.

Lead Pigs and Carrying Cases

Necessary to reduce radiation exposure to personnel when carrying doses to different rooms.

Lead Syringe Shields

Necessary to reduce technologist radiation exposure.

Lead-Lined Trash Containers

Necessary to store radioactive trash. It is necessary to have a separate container for sharps/needles as well as one for all other waste.

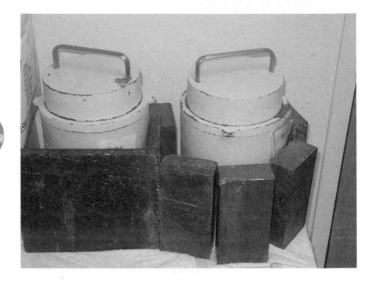

Fig. 1-6. Technetium generators and lead brick wall.

Heat Block or Microwave

Some radiopharmaceuticals kits, e.g., sestamibi, require heating during preparation.

Refrigerator

Some radiopharmaceutical kits need to be refrigerated.

Long-Handled Tongs

These are used to minimize radiation exposure when handling radiopharmaceutical kits.

Survey Meter

This is mandatory for detecting spills and for performing daily room and trash surveys.

Syringes

Various sizes may be needed depending on the type of radiopharmaceutical kits to be prepared.

Alcohol Pads

These are necessary for drawing up doses and for preparation of radiopharmaceutical kits under aseptic conditions.

Gloves

All radiopharmaceuticals must be handled with proper protective equipment.

Absorbent Pads

Useful to line counters and work area to absorb spills and make decontamination and spill containment easier.

Logbooks

A logbook is needed for each isotope or radiotracer used. A logbook is also needed for dose calibrator QC, daily room surveys, Mo QC, package survey/receipt, wipe tests, and hot trash disposal (see Chapters 3 and 20).

Labels

All radiopharmaceutical vials and pre-drawn doses should be labeled.

Calculator

This is necessary to calculate radiopharmaceutical decay, concentrations, and doses.

Additional Supplies for Radiopharmaceutical Kit Quality Control

Beakers

To hold chemicals for chromatography.

Chemicals

The type of chemical needed will vary depending on the radiopharmaceutical being prepared. Refer to the package insert for a list of chemicals needed.

Chromatography Paper

Often used for QC of radiopharmaceutical kits. Refer to the package insert for specific instructions.

Ruler

Used to mark chromatography paper for origin and cutting points.

An Important Choice: Making Your Own Kits or Purchasing Unit Doses

For freestanding imaging facilities, a practical arrangement to ensure a regular supply of radiopharmaceuticals is through a contract with a regional commercial radiopharmacy. Radiopharmacies deliver pre-calibrated vials of quality-controlled radiopharmaceuticals, also known as "unit doses." The unit dose approach is generally more expensive than the use of an on-site generator.

It may be useful to compare the pros and cons of receiving unit doses versus preparing radiopharmaceuticals on-site in an imaging facility. Cost and staffing are probably the two most important issues to consider.

The price of Mo-99 generators and of radiopharmaceutical kits depend on whether or not the imaging facility has a contract with a pharmaceutical vendor and also on the volume of patient studies. If the imaging facility has a contract with a pharmaceutical vendor, one may be entitled to discount pricing. In addition, the greater the patient volume, the better the price can be negotiated. This is also true for unit dosing: the more doses one orders, the cheaper each dose will be. If price is a major factor, one should meet with local sales representatives and obtain quotes for the products.

Staff availability is also an important consideration. To elute the generator, to perform the QC, and to prepare the kits, a technologist has to come to the laboratory earlier in the morning than the rest of the technical staff. Depending on the number of kits to be made, this can take from 30 min to over 1 h. This technologist will be entitled to leave earlier at the end of the day than the rest of the staff. Therefore, one needs to have sufficient staff to be able to stagger shifts and to accommodate these hot lab duties.

Table 1-1 lists some other issues to consider when deciding to order unit doses or to prepare radiopharmaceuticals on the premises.

Preparing Radiopharmaceutical Kits On-Site

If the decision is made to prepare radiopharmaceuticals on-site in the imaging facility, written protocols must be in place that describe the procedures in detail. These detailed procedure protocols are required for accreditation by the ICANL. For each specific brand of radiopharmaceutical, separate protocols should exist. Kits from different vendors have different procedural steps and criteria. The protocol should meet the manufacturers' recommendations that can be found in the package insert. The protocol should also detail radiation safety equipment and techniques to be used for the preparation of kits.

Table 1-1
Considerations for Using Unit Doses or Making Kits

Consideration	Unit doses	Making kits
Staff time	Fast, no quality control needed, except for logging in delivery container	Time consuming
Lead brick shielding	Minimum needed, each dose comes individually shielded	Need lead bricks and lead glass shield
Lead waste containers	Few needed, syringes are usually returned to vendor. Small container may be needed for non-sharps waste	Sharps and non-sharps containers will be needed as well as long-term storage space for longer lived radioisotopes
Supplies	Intravenous (IV) supplies needed	IV supplies, syringes, needles, and above-mentioned hot lab supplies needed
Flexibility	Less flexible. Set delivery times and sometimes additional delivery charges for doses delivered	More flexible. Make kits and draw up doses as needed
Changes	Doses are ordered the day before scheduled use. Sometimes, a charge is applied for unused doses if there is patient cancellation. Doses cannot be adjusted for unexpected obese patients	Changes in schedule and add-ons easily accommodated. Doses can be adjusted when necessary
Cost	Need large volume of patients to get cheapest price. Generally more expensive than making own kits	Often cheaper than unit dosing

ADDITIONAL MISCELLANEOUS SUPPLIES

Caution Signs

Door of areas in which radioactive materials are stored, handled, or imaging is performed must be marked with the standard NRC radiation caution sign: "Caution Radioactive Material" (**Fig. 1-4**).

Dosimeters

Staff exposed to >10% of occupational limits for radiation exposure must wear personal dosimeters, such as X-ray film badges and optically stimulated luminescent (OSL) or thermoluminescent dosimeters (TLDs). These dosimeters should be read and changed on a monthly basis.

Table and Pillow Covering

Compare cost and ease of use of paper versus linen.

Gowns

Necessary for patients who wear clothing with metal buttons.

Blankets/Sheets

Imaging room may be cold. Patients will be more comfortable (and still) when covered with a blanket or linen sheet.

Intravenous Supplies

Every patient who undergoes a stress test *must* have IV access and a running IV during the test. This is needed for the injection of the radiopharmaceutical at peak stress but also for IV injection of pharmaceuticals in case of emergency. Patients who have rest imaging also need IV access for radiopharmaceutical administration.

Glucose Meter

Useful for quick assessment of blood glucose level of patients with diabetes. Also required to monitor glucose levels during glucose loading for PET viability studies.

ECG Leads

Radiolucent chest leads are preferred for patients who will have subsequent imaging.

ECG Paper

Sufficient amounts of ECG paper must be in stock.

Worksheets

Worksheets are very useful for documentation of details and events by technologists and nurses during procedures. A separate worksheet may not be needed during treadmill exercise if the ECG computer generates a complete printable report. For pharmacological stress procedures, a chart is necessary on which one can record heart rate, blood pressure and ECG response, patient symptoms, and given medication. A worksheet that documents the dose administered and time of administration, time imaging started and finished, camera used, and other imaging parameters are important for QC. Additional notes by the technologist for the interpreting physician on patient height, weight, chest circumference, and bra size are also very useful. Sample stress worksheets can be found at the end of Chapter 5 and sample imaging worksheets are provided at the end of Chapter 6.

Charts/Scanner

Hard copy charts are still used for archiving purposes of recorded stress test parameters, ECGs, and images. Many laboratories are planning for digital archiving in the near future. A scanner that converts hard copy documents to electronic files is needed for this purpose.

LABORATORY STAFF

The staff of a nuclear cardiology imaging facility typically consists of a medical director, a technical director, medical staff, technical staff, an RSO, stress testing personnel, and clerical staff. In smaller laboratories, several functions may be fulfilled by one person.

Qualifications

Nuclear Medicine Technologists

Technical Director (Chief Technologist). The technical director must have the following:

1. Appropriate and current credentials in nuclear medicine, i.e., either American Registry of Radiologic Technologists-Nuclear Medicine [ARRT(N)] or Certified Nuclear Medicine Technologist (CNMT) and/or State license.
2. At least 3 years of clinical experience in nuclear medicine.
3. Current Basic Life Support (BLS) certification.
4. At least 15 h of Verification of Involvement in Continuing Education (VOICE) credits over 3 years.

The Technical Director is responsible for the day-to-day operations of the laboratory, verification/documentation of proper training of technical staff, and up-to-date laboratory policies and procedures protocols.

Staff Nuclear Medicine Technologists. All nuclear medicine technologists must have also appropriate credentials in nuclear medicine, either ARRT(N) or CNMT (NCT: nuclear cardiology technologist), or/and State license. In addition, they must have at least 15 h of continuing education over 3 years. Furthermore, it is recommended that all technical staff be certified in BLS.

ECG/Stress Technologists

Ideally, stress technologists should be trained in exercise physiology. Unfortunately, these highly trained people are difficult to find. With additional on-site training in recording ECGs and administering stress tests, nuclear medicine technologists, emergency room technicians, or other medical technicians can be utilized as stress technologists. It is recommended that all technical staff be certified in BLS.

Monitoring Stress Tests

Physicians (cardiologists) usually monitor stress tests and interpret exercise ECGs. However, personal physician supervision of all stress tests may be difficult to realize in some laboratories. To facilitate the coverage of stress tests, physician-assistants and registered nurses with extensive cardiology experience, especially intensive care, can be trained to monitor stress tests and to interpret stress ECGs. Thus, whereas the type of personnel available in each laboratory may vary, it is important that adequate physician support is assured in case of emergencies. A physician should always be nearby the stress testing area. For Medicare reimbursement for the performance of stress test, "direct supervision" is required. That is, the physician must be in the immediate vicinity when the test is performed. The staff supervising stress testing should be Advanced Cardiac Life Support (ACLS) certified. The ICANL requires, since January 2004, ACLS-certified personnel on-site during all cardiac stress procedures.

In our laboratory, stress testing routinely is administered by two persons (at least one with extensive training and experience in stress

---

Required Training and Experience for the Medical Director (ICANL Standards)

The medical director must meet one or more of the following criteria:

1. Certification in nuclear cardiology by the CBNC (see http://www. cbnc.org), or
2. Board certified or Board eligible within 2 years of finishing training in cardiology and completion of a minimum of a 4-month formal training program in nuclear cardiology (Level 2 training according to the 2002 ACC/ASNC Revised COCATSTraining Guidelines, see http://www.acc.org/clinical/training/cocats2.pdf). This is mandatory for cardiologists who began their cardiology training in July 1995 or later, or

3. Board certification in cardiology and training equivalent to Level 2 training, or at least 1 year of nuclear cardiology practice experience with independent interpretation of at least 600 nuclear cardiology studies. This requirement applies only to cardiologists who began their cardiology training before July 1995, or

4. Board certified or Board eligible within 2 years of finishing training in nuclear medicine, or

5. Board certified or Board eligible within 2 years of finishing training in radiology with at least 4 months of nuclear cardiology training, or

6. Board certification in radiology and at least 1 year of nuclear cardiology practice experience with independent interpretation of at least 600 nuclear cardiology studies.

7. Ten years of nuclear cardiology practice experience with independent interpretation of at least 600 nuclear cardiology procedures.

testing), one for operating the treadmill, watching the ECG, and communicating with the patient and another person for recording vital signs.

Medical Staff Interpreting Studies

All nuclear cardiology studies should be interpreted by a physician with special training in nuclear cardiology. The ICANL has defined the required training and credentials for nuclear cardiologists (see http://www.icanl.org). The medical director should have a current state medical license, meeting the training and experience requirements outlined below, and be an authorized user of radioisotopes. All interpreting medical staff should have current state medical licenses and preferably also be authorized users of radioisotopes, as well as Certification Board of Nuclear Cardiology (CBNC)-certified. It is also recommended that all medical staff be certified in BLS and/or ACLS.

Furthermore, the medical director and interpreting medical staff should obtain at least 15 h of American Medical Association (AMA) Category 1 continuing medical education (CME) credits relevant to nuclear cardiology, every 3 years. Yearly accumulated CME credits should be kept on file and available for inspection.

The medical director is responsible for all clinical services provided and for the quality and appropriateness of care provided. The medical director may supervise the entire operation of the laboratory or delegate specific operations.

The interpreting medical staff members preferably are CBNC-certified and have training and/or experience in nuclear cardiology as defined for the medical director. The interpreting medical staff should meet the same CME criteria as the medical director.

Physician Supervision of Diagnostic Tests

Medicare regulation defines three levels of physician supervision:

General Supervision

A procedure is performed under the physician's overall direction and control, but the physician's presence is not required during the performance of the procedure. The physician is responsible for protocols, policies, and training of personnel who actually perform the test. Nuclear cardiology imaging procedures are performed under general supervision.

Direct Supervision

The physician must be present in the office and must be immediately available for assistance and direction throughout the performance of the procedure. It does not mean that the physician must be present in the room when the procedure is performed. Stress testing is performed under direct supervision.

Personal Supervision

The physician must be present in the room during performance of the procedure.

RADIATION SAFETY OFFICER (RSO)

An imaging facility that uses radiopharmaceuticals must have a designated person who assumes the role of RSO and is responsible that the imaging facility operates within Federal or State regulations for radiation safety (see also Chapter 3).

The RSO can be either an authorized user according to NRC or State regulation, or a qualified health physicist.

Authorized User

The NRC (http://www.nrc.gov) has regulated the medical use of byproduct material. Authorized user means a physician who has fulfilled training or certification requirements as outlined in NRC Regulations 10 CFR Part 35.290: Training for imaging and localization studies.

How Does One Become an Authorized User?

Since October 2002, new NRC training and experience requirements are in effect. In the 15 NRC or non-agreement states (see **Fig. 1-7**), there are two pathways:

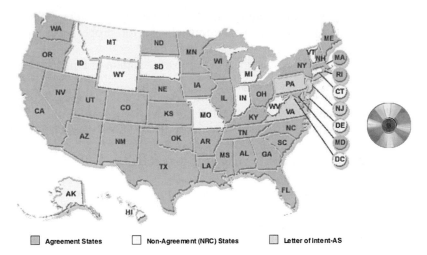

☐ Agreement States   ☐ Non-Agreement (NRC) States   ☐ Letter of Intent-AS

Fig. 1-7. There are fifteen NRC States. Through the "Agreement State Program", thirty-four other states have signed formal agreements with the NRC, by which those states have assumed regulatory responsibility over certain byproduct, source, and small quantities of special nuclear material. Three states have filed a letter of intent to become Agreement States. NRC States, agreement states and states with letter of intent to become agreement states are depicted in map (source: http://www.hsrd.ornl.gov/NRC/asdirectr.htm).

1. Completion of a total of 700 h of training and experience in specified subject areas and supervised work experience in areas specified in 10 CFR Part 35.290. More specifically, the 700 h must include 80 h of classroom and laboratory training. See also ASNC website (http://www.asnc.org) for details.
2. CBNC board certification is recognized by the NRC as an alternative pathway (retroactive to October 22, 1996). See also CBNC website (http://www.cbnc.org).

Radiation Safety Work Experience

This experience is important for individuals with clinical cardiology training background and should be acquired during the at least 4 months' training in the clinical environment where radioactive materials are being used and under the supervision of an authorized user who meets the NRC requirements of Part 35.290 or Part 35.290(c)(ii)(G) and Part 35.390 or the equivalent Agreement State requirements. The training experience must total a minimum of 620 h and include the following:

1. Ordering, receiving, and unpacking radioactive materials safely and performing the related radiation surveys;

2. Performing QC procedures on instruments used to determine the activity of dosages and performing checks for proper operation of survey meters;
3. Calculating, measuring, and safely preparing patient or human research subject dosages;
4. Using administrative controls to prevent a medical event involving the use of unsealed byproduct material;
5. Using procedures to safely contain spilled radioactive material and using proper decontamination procedures;
6. Administering dosages of radioactive material to patients or human research subjects; and
7. Eluting generator systems appropriate for preparation of radioactive drugs for imaging and localization studies, measuring and testing the eluate for radionuclide purity, and processing the eluate with reagent kits to prepare labeled radioactive drugs.

In the 34 Agreement States, one can become an authorized user by completing 200 h of didactic training in radiation safety, 500 h of clinical experience, and 500 h of supervised work experience in radiation safety procedures. The states of Florida, Georgia, and Colorado require authorized user status to interpret nuclear medicine studies. In other states, authorized user status has (as yet) no connection with reading nuclear studies and reimbursement.

A list of NRC Agreement States can be found at http://www.hsrd. ornl.gov/NRC/asdirectr.htm.

Agreement States have until April 29, 2008 to adopt regulations that are "essentially identical" (language from the Code of Federal Regulations 10 CFR Part 35) to the training and experience requirements in 10 CFR Part 35.290.

LABORATORY LICENSE

Before a nuclear cardiology facility can begin to perform clinical imaging and procedures in patients, the necessary NRC and State licenses must be obtained. Licenses to use radioactive materials are granted to laboratories that are in compliance with federal and state regulations governing the medical use of byproduct material. The NRC license assures that the facility has a radiation protection program to protect both the patients and the staff. In addition, the staff must meet certain standards of training and experience before they are allowed to administer radioactive material to patients. Each state also has one or more radiation programs that ensure safe use of radioactive materials. One needs to submit a state "Ionizing Radiation Registration and Compliance Form." To apply for an NRC license in diagnostic nuclear medicine, the applicant must file one original and one copy of NRC form 313, Application for Material License, which includes a facility diagram, equipment, and training and experience of the RSO and authorized user. This form may be downloaded from http://www.nrc.gov/reading-rm/doc-collections/forms/nrc313info.html (accessed January 19,2007).

The First Steps of Planning a New Laboratory

We recommend that one of first things to do when one is planning a new imaging facility is to seek assistance of a health physicist with experience in practical nuclear medicine. A physicist will be very helpful in surveying the physical space of the future imaging facility, particularly from the point of view of radiation safety, and choosing a location for storage of radioactive material and/or hot lab. He or she may assist with the purchase of imaging and nonimaging equipment. The physicist would file applications for material licenses with NRC and State on behalf of the medical director. Finally, the physicist might be engaged to serve as the RSO and perform periodical inspections and quality assurance (QA) of the laboratory to ensure compliance with NRC and State regulations.

2   Laboratory Logistics

The operation of a nuclear cardiology imaging facility requires planning, scheduling, and modifications that depend on the types of procedures and the number and type of patients referred for imaging. In most imaging facilities, two types of cardiac studies are performed:

- Radionuclide myocardial perfusion imaging and
- Radionuclide angiocardiography

Key Words: Radionuclide myocardial perfusion imaging, Stress procedures, Imaging protocols, Radiation exposure, Laboratory schedule, Equilibrium radionuclide angio-cardiography.

MYOCARDIAL PERFUSION IMAGING

The majority of myocardial perfusion imaging procedures are performed in conjunction with either physical or pharmacological stress. The imaging procedure itself consists of two parts: post-stress imaging and rest imaging.

Standard imaging protocols are described in detail in the ASNC *Imaging Guidelines for Nuclear Cardiology Procedures (1)*. We refer also to the Society of Nuclear Medicine (SNM) *Procedure Guidelines for Myocardial Perfusion Imaging (2)* and are discussed in detail in chapter 6.

The efficiency of a laboratory and its daily schedule are affected by the choice of stress procedures and imaging protocols.

Tables 2-1 and 2-2 list typical stress and imaging procedures that may be performed in a cardiac imaging facility as well as the advantages and disadvantages of various imaging protocols. The availability of physicians or other medical staff to monitor stress tests may also influence the choice of protocols.

Time Requirements

The time requirements for stress procedures and imaging procedures are to be considered when making the daily laboratory schedule.

From: *Contemporary Cardiology: Nuclear Cardiology, The Basics*
By: F. J. Th. Wackers, W. Bruni, and B. L. Zaret © Humana Press Inc., Totowa, NJ

Table 2-1
Type of Stress Procedures

Physical exercise
  Treadmill exercise
    Bruce protocol
    Modified Bruce protocol
    Naughton protocol
  Supine or upright bicycle exercise
  Cardiopulmonary exercise testing
Pharmacological stress
  Dipyridamole vasodilation stress
  Adenosine vasodilation stress
  Dobutamine adrenergic stress

Table 2-2
Type of Imaging Protocols

Tl-201 perfusion imaging
One-day
  Exercise–redistribution
  Pharmacologic stress–redistribution
  Rest (or reinjection)–redistribution
Tc-99m agents (sestamibi or tetrofosmin) perfusion imaging
Two-day
  Rest only
  Stress (exercise or pharmacologic) only
One-day (low dose–high dose)
  Exercise–rest
  Pharmacologic stress–rest
  Rest–exercise
  Rest–pharmacologic stress
Dual isotope perfusion imaging
One-day
  Rest Tl-201/stress Tc-99m agent

Table 2-3 summarizes the time slots required for the various myocardial perfusion imaging protocols as well as the approximate total time required to perform each protocol.

From Table 2-3, it should be clear that the 1-day imaging protocols with Tc-99m-labeled agents may be the most difficult protocols to

Table 2-3
Myocardial Perfusion Imaging

One-day Tl-201 protocols

Protocol									Total time
Tl-201 Ex–Red	Ex 30 min	Ex Inj/Int 10 min	Ex SPECT 30 min	Red Int 150 min	Red SPECT 30 min				250 min
Tl-201 PhStr–Red	PhSt 30 min	PhSt Inj/Int 10 min	PhSt SPECT 30 min	Red Int 150 min	Red SPECT 30 min				250 min
Tl-201 Rest–Red	R Inj 10 min	R Inj/Int 10 min	R SPECT 30 min	Red Int 240 min	Red SPECT 30 min				320 min

One-day Tc-99m protocols

Protocol									Total time
Tc-99m 1 day Ex–R	Ex 30 min	Ex Inj/Int 15 min	Ex SPECT 30 min	Int 60 min	R Inj 10 min	R Inj/Int 30 min	R SPECT 30 min		205 min
Tc-99m 1 day R–Ex	R Inj 10 min	R Inj/Int 30 min	R SPECT 30 min	Int 60 min	Ex 30 min	Ex Inj/Int 15 min	Ex SPECT 30 min		205 min
Tc-99m 1 day PhSt–R	PhSt 30 min	PhSt Inj/Int 30 min	PhSt SPECT 30 min	Int 60 min	R Inj 10 min	R Inj/Int 30 min	R SPECT 30 min		220 min
Tc-99m 1 day R–PhSt	R Inj 10 min	R Inj/Int 30 min	R SPECT 30 min	Int 60 min	PhSt 30 min	PhSt Inj/Int 30 min	PhSt SPECT 30 min		220 min

(Continued)

Table 2-3
(Continued)

Two-day Tc-99m protocols

								Total time
Tc-99m Ex[a]	Ex 30 min	Ex Inj/Int 15 min	Ex SPECT 30 min					75 min
Tc-99m PhSt[a]	PhSt 30 min	PhSt Inj/Int 30 min	PhSt SPECT 30 min					90 min
Tc-99m R[a]	R Inj 10 min	R Inj/Int 30 min	R SPECT 30 min					70 min
Dual isotope protocols								
Dual Isot 1 day R–Ex	R Inj 10 min	R Inj/Int 30 min	R SPECT 30 min	Int 10 min	Ex 30 min	Ex Inj/Int 15 min	Ex SPECT 30 min	155 min
Dual Isot 1 day R–PhSt	R Inj 10 min	R Inj/Int 30 min	R SP 30 min	Int 10 min	PhSt 30 min	PhSt Inj/Int 30 min	PhSt SPECT 30 min	170 min

Ex, exercise; PhSt, pharmacological stress; R, rest, Red, redistribution; SP, SPECT imaging; Inj, injection; Int, interval; Isot, isotope.
[a]Ex performed on one day and R performed on a different day.

fit into a daily schedule. However, if the stress study of a 1-day protocol is unequivocally normal, a rest study is generally not needed (see below under "advantages Tc-99m agent 1-day stress first.").

Logistical Advantages and Disadvantages of Various Myocardial Perfusion Imaging Protocols

TL-201 1-DAY STRESS–REDISTRIBUTION

Advantages

- Widely used.
- Cost is less than Tc-99m-labeled agents.
- High myocardial extraction fraction.
- Good linearity of myocardial uptake versus blood flow.
- Compared with Tc-99m-labeled agents less gastrointestinal uptake after pharmacological stress.
- Delayed rest uptake reflects myocardial viability.

Disadvantages

- Relatively long half-life limits maximal dose to 4.5 mCi.
- Substantial portions of photons in image are scattered photons.
- Low-energy photons are easily attenuated and cause artifacts especially in obese patients and women with large breasts.
- Long protocol: approximately 4 h.

TC-99M AGENT 2-DAY STRESS–REST

Advantages

- Relatively high dose (20–30 mCi) administered; good count statistics and good quality.
- Efficient protocol; if stress images are completely normal, and clinical and exercise parameters do not suggest coronary artery disease, no rest study may be needed. Thus, this is the shortest protocol: <1.5 h.
- Good-quality ECG-gated study due to high dose.

Disadvantages

- Takes 2 days to get final results.
- Inconvenient; patient needs to come to the laboratory on 2 separate days.
- Relatively high sub-diaphragmatic activity after pharmacological stress.

TC-99M AGENT 1-DAY STRESS FIRST–REST SECOND

Advantages

- All stress testing is done in the morning. This may be more convenient depending on physicians' practice patterns (e.g., physicians seeing patients in the afternoon).

- Efficient protocol; if stress images are completely normal, and clinical and exercise parameters do not suggest coronary artery disease, no rest study may be needed.

Disadvantages

- Relatively low-count-density stress images (first injection is low dose).
- Low-count-density ECG-gated stress images.
- Not feasible in obese patients.
- Long time required to complete stress–rest study ($\sim$3.5 h).

TC-99M AGENT 1-DAY REST FIRST–STRESS SECOND

Advantages

- High-count-density stress images (second injection is high dose).
- Good-quality ECG-gated images.
- All stress testing is done in the afternoon. This may be more convenient depending on physicians' practice patterns (e.g., physicians seeing patients in the morning).

Disadvantages

- Stress coverage needed in the afternoon.
- Long time required to complete rest–stress study ($\sim$3.5 h)

DUAL ISOTOPE TL-201 REST/TC-99M STRESS

Advantages

- Fast protocol; < 3 h for complete study.
- High-count stress study.
- Good-quality ECG-gated stress study.

Disadvantages

- Comparison of myocardial distribution of two different radioisotopes with different physical characteristics which may affect image pattern.
- Relatively high radiation exposure compared with Tc-99m agent protocols (Table 2-4).

Daily Schedule for Stress Testing and Imaging

The time slots that are given in Table 2-3 should be considered when making a daily work schedule. Creating an efficient patient schedule can be a substantial challenge, particularly because certain time intervals are required between the two myocardial perfusion imaging sessions.

Table 2-4
Radiation Exposure of Various Cardiac Imaging Procedures

Procedure	Total body effective dose[a]
Tl-201 stress redistribution (4 mCi)	25.1 mSv (2.5 Rem)
Dual isotope (3 mCi Tl-201 + 30 mCi Tc-99m)	26.3 mSv (2.6 Rem)
Tc-99m tetro rest–stress (10 + 30 mCi)	11.2 mSv (1.1 Rem)
Tc-99m sestamibi rest–stress (10 + 30 mCi)	12 mSv (1.2 Rem)
Tc-99m sestamibi 2-day stress rest (30 + 30 mCi)	17 mSv (1.7 Rem)
Rb-82 rest–stress (45 + 45 mCi)	11.3 mSv (1.1 Rem)
Gd-153 transmission SPECT	0.05 mSv (0.005 Rem)
Ge-68 transmission PET	0.08 mSv (0.008 Rem)
CT transmission SPECT	1 mSv (0.1 Rem)
CT transmission PET	0.8 mSv (0.08 Rem)
F-18DG for viability (10 mCi)	7 mSv (0.07 Rem)
Tc-99m ERNA (20 mCi)	5.2 mSv (0.52 Rem)
EBCT calcium scoring	1.3 mSv (0.13 Rem)
16-slice MDCT angiography	7.0 mSv (0.70 Rem)
64-slice MDCT angiography	12 mSv (1.2 Rem)
Invasive X-ray coronary angiography	4.60–15.80 mSv (0.46–1.58 Rem)
Percutaneous coronary intervention	7.50–57.00 mSv (0.75–5.7 Rem)

ERNA, equilibrium radionuclide angiocardiography.
[a]http://www.doseinfo-radar.com/radardoseriskcalc.html (Radar Medical Procedure Radiation Dose Calculator).
For dosage abbreviation see table 6-1.
EBCT = electron beam computed tomography.
MDCT = multidetector computed tomography.

The schedule for cardiac nuclear imaging is unique in that it does not consist of just a series of consecutive patient exams; each patient often requires two imaging sessions (stress and rest), separated by a time interval of a number of hours. In order to use the time intervals between the two imaging sessions efficiently, patients should be staggered.

The following examples are provided for an imaging facility with one exercise treadmill and one gamma camera.

Depending on patient volume, for increased efficiency, it may be better to have one technologist perform imaging and another person (e.g., exercise physiologist, technologist, or physician) perform the injections of radiopharmaceuticals (during stress and at rest).

With increasing numbers of treadmills and gamma cameras, the schedules are more complicated. In addition, a schedule depends on the type of stress and imaging protocols performed.

The Simplest Patient Imaging Schedule is a 2-Day Schedule for a One Gamma Camera Imaging Facility

The schedules below are for a laboratory that uses a Tc-99m-labeled radiopharmaceutical for both rest and stress imaging.

It should be noted that in these examples it is assumed that the patient arrives at the appointment time and that it takes 30 min to prepare and stress the patient. The patient is injected 30 min after arrival and imaged 30 min after injection. The rest images are acquired 45 min after injection of the radiopharmaceutical. Patients A, B, C, and D are patients who have their stress tests and stress imaging on this day. Patients 1, 2, 3, and 4 had a stress test the previous day and return on this day for rest imaging.

Example of 2-Day Imaging Schedule

8:00 am	Stress patient A	9:00 am	Image patient A
8:45 am	Stress patient B	9:45 am	Image patient B
9:30 am	Stress patient C	10:30 am	Image patient C
10:15 am	Stress patient D	11:15 am	Image patient D
11:00 am	Stress patient E	12:00 pm	Image patient E
Lunch			
12:30 pm	Inject rest patient 1	1:15 pm	Image patient 1
1:00 pm	Inject rest patient 2	1:45 pm	Image patient 2
1:30 pm	Inject rest patient 3	2:15 pm	Image patient 3
2:00 pm	Inject rest patient 4	2:45 pm	Image patient 4
2:30 pm	Inject rest patient 5	3:15 pm	Image patient 5

The following is an example of the schedule for the same laboratory for a 1-day imaging schedule.

The same assumptions as shown above for the 2-day schedule, i.e., time required for patient preparation, time intervals after injections and for imaging, are taken into account. Patients 1, 2, 3, 4 and 5 all have a same day imaging protocol. Patients 1 and 2 have rest imaging first, whereas patients 3, 4 and 5 have the stress portion first.

Example of 1-Day Imaging Schedule

7:30 am	Inject rest patient 1	8:15 am	Image (rest) patient 1
8:00 am	Inject rest patient 2	8:45 am	Image (rest) patient 2
8:15 am	Stress patient 3	9:15 am	Image (stress) patient 3
9:00 am	Stress patient 4	10:00 am	Image (stress) patient 4
9:45 am	Stress patient 5	10:45 am	Image (stress) patient 5
10:30 am	Stress patient 1	11:30 am	Image (stress) patient 1
11:15 am	Stress patient 2	12:15 pm	Image (stress) patient 2

Lunch

12:45 pm	Inject rest patient 3	1:30 pm	Image (rest) patient 3
1:30 pm	Inject rest patient 4	2:15 pm	Image (rest) patient 4
2:15 pm	Inject rest patient 5	3:00 pm	Image (rest) patient 5

Example of 1-Day Imaging Schedule (Rest Studies First in the Morning)

8:00 am	Inject rest patient 1	8:45 am	Image (rest) patient 1
8:30 am	Inject rest patient 2	9:15 am	Image (rest) patient 2
9:00 am	Inject rest patient 3	9:45 am	Image (rest) patient 3
9:30 am	Inject rest patient 4	10:15 am	Image (rest) patient 4
10:00 am	Inject rest patient 5	10:45 am	Image (rest) patient 5
10:30 am	Inject rest patient 6	11:15 am	Image (rest) patient 6

Lunch

11:15 pm	Stress patient 1	12:15 pm	Image (stress) patient 1
12:00 pm	Stress patient 2	1:00 pm	Image (stress) patient 2
12:45 pm	Stress patient 3	1:45 pm	Image (stress) patient 3
1:30 pm	Stress patient 4	2:30 pm	Image (stress) patient 4
2:15 pm	Stress patient 5	3:15 pm	Image (stress) patient 5
3:00 pm	Stress patient 6	4:00 pm	Image (stress) patient 6

The details of a daily schedule of procedures and tests differ from laboratory to laboratory because they depend on the radiopharmaceuticals and protocols used. In addition, they depend on the availability of physicians to monitor stress tests.

For example, if physicians have office hours in the morning, it may be practical and convenient to perform rest imaging in the morning and stress testing in the afternoon (example 3).

EQUILIBRIUM RADIONUCLIDE ANGIOCARDIOGRAPHY

Although radionuclide myocardial perfusion imaging is the most frequently performed imaging modality, in many laboratories equilibrium radionuclide angiocardiographies (ERNAs) are performed to assess left ventricular function in a variety of clinical circumstances. In our laboratory, ERNAs are frequently requested for oncology patients before and during the course of therapy with potentially cardiotoxic drugs, for evaluation of patients with cardiomyopathy or recent infarction, and to follow the effect of therapy in patients with abnormal left ventricular function.

Time Requirements

The following tables summarize the time slots required for rest and rest–exercise ERNA protocols as well as the approximate total time required to perform the protocols. We usually acquire SPECT ERNA plus one planar left anterior oblique (LAO) view. It is assumed that in vitro kits are used for labeling of the patient's red blood cells. (Refer to Chapters 8 and 9 for complete discussion of ERNA imaging procedures.)

Rest Equilibrium Radionuclide Angiocardiography

Rest ERNA	IV line	Draw blood	Label blood	Reinject blood	Imaging	Total time
Planar	10 min	1 min	20 min	1 min	30 min	62 min
SPECT	10 min	1 min	20 min	1 min	40 min	72 min

Rest–Exercise Equilibrium Radionuclide Angiography

Rest–exercise ERNA	Blood labeling	Rest ERNA	Stress setup	Exercise ERNA stage 1	Exercise ERNA stage 2	Exercise ERNA stage "n"	Rest ERNA	Total time
Planar	30 min	30 min	30 min	3 min	3 min	$3 \times n$ min	3 min	102+ min

Note: Rest–exercise ERNA is shown for completeness. In actual practice, exercise ERNAs are currently infrequently performed in most laboratories.

Fitting ERNAs into the Daily Schedule

Fitting ERNAs into the daily laboratory schedule is usually relatively easy if the ERNA volume is small. If the gamma camera used for myocardial perfusion imaging is also used for ERNAs, the most practical approach is to schedule ERNAs either at the beginning or at the end of the working day.

It is generally not practical attempting to "squeeze" ERNAs between two myocardial perfusion studies in the course of the day. A complex schedule has the unavoidable tendency to run behind in time. A schedule that is too tight also causes problems and undesirable delays.

Obviously, if the laboratory has a dedicated gamma camera for ERNAs, there is no interference with the general daily schedule.

NOVEL ITERATIVE RECONSTRUCTION ALGORITHMS

At the time of this writing considerable effort is directed towards the clinical validation of novel iterative reconstruction algorithms, that may radically shorten the time required for the acquisition of radionuclide images.

If future clinical and peer-reviewed validation of these novel reconstruction methods demonstrate equivalency with conventional filtered back projection reconstruction methods, acquisition times may be considerable shortened and the time and scheduling considerations discussed in this chapter may become obsolete.

REFERENCES

1. DePuey GE (2006). *Imaging Guidelines for Nuclear Cardiology Procedures*, available at http://www.asnc.org—Menu: "Manage Your Practice": "Guidelines and Standards" (accessed May 2007).
2. Siegel JA (2002). *Guide for Diagnostic Nuclear Medicine*, Society of Nuclear Medicine (http://www.snm.org). This publication also can be downloaded free as a PDF-file from http://www.nrc.gov—Menu: "Nuclear Materials": "Med, Academic & Ind Uses": "Medical Uses": "Medical Licensee Toolkit": "Other Guidance" (accessed May 2007).

3   Radiation Safety

Radiation safety is an extremely important issue for nuclear cardiology laboratories. It is mandatory that imaging facilities operate in compliance with NRC regulations (http://www.nrc.gov) and/or those imposed by the state and local agencies in states not directly under NRC supervision ("agreement states," see **Fig. 1-7**). Each laboratory must have detailed written radiation safety and radioactive materials handling protocols. The content and implementation of these protocols are the responsibility of the technical director and RSO.

Key Words: Radiation safety officer (RSO), Radiation safety protocols, Occupational and public exposure limits.

RADIATION SAFETY OFFICER

It is the responsibility of an RSO to ensure that the daily operation of a nuclear cardiology imaging facility is in compliance with radiation safety regulations. An RSO should help in developing policies and procedure protocols for radiation safety. The RSO should provide input with the setup of the hot-lab area and should ensure that all necessary areas are adequately lead-shielded. Furthermore, the RSO will make sure that all necessary equipment for handling and monitoring radioactive materials is available. The RSO will also help in monitoring the radiation exposure of patients, staff, and environment such that exposure levels are as low as reasonably achievable (ALARA). The RSO also may help in setting up guidelines for patient dosing. Written protocols and policies should be in place to ensure compliance with regulations. The protocols should be reviewed and updated *at least yearly*. Records of this review should include program changes, noted deficiencies, and actions taken.

For compliance with the NRC or similar regulations regarding medical use of byproduct materials, the *Guide for Diagnostic Nuclear*

From: *Contemporary Cardiology: Nuclear Cardiology, The Basics*
By: F. J. Th. Wackers, W. Bruni, and B. L. Zaret © Humana Press Inc., Totowa, NJ

Table 3-1
The Responsibilities of an RSO

Instruction and training of personnel in radiation safety
Maintain list of authorized user(s), individuals trained to handle
   radionuclides
Monitoring personnel radiation exposure
Radiation safety of facility and equipment
Incident response (overexposure, spills, etc.)
Security of licensed material
Radiation surveys
Radioactive material inventory records
Radioactive waste management
Maintenance of appropriate records and reports concerning radiation
   safety

Medicine published by the SNM *(1)* is a good reference source.
Responsibilities of an RSO are listed in Table 3-1.

How to Find an RSO for a New Imaging Facility?

An RSO can be either a physician who is an authorized user
according to NRC or state regulations, or a health physicist with special
radiation safety training. Health physicists are often willing to serve
as part-time consultants to freestanding imaging facilities.

Information can be obtained by contacting the following:

- RSOs in local hospitals,
- State Health Agencies,
- American Association of Physicists in Medicine (http://www.aapm.
  org), or
- Health Physics Society (http://www.hps.org).

A list of recommended radiation safety policies that are required
in any nuclear cardiology laboratory is given in Table 3-2. These
policies are also an absolute requirement for laboratory accreditation
as outlined in the ICANL "Standards" *(3)* and Chapter 22.

General Radioactive Materials Handling and Radiation Safety

An extensive review of radiation safety policies is beyond
the scope of this book. We refer to the "ICANL Standards"
(http://www.icanl.org) for the required content of radiation safety
policies *(3)* and to *Guide for Diagnostic Nuclear Medicine (1)*.

Table 3-2
Recommended written Policies for Radiation Safety

General radioactive materials handling and radiation safety
Mo-99 check (only in laboratories that elute Tc-99m generators)
Dose calibrator daily constancy check
Radioactive package receipt
Daily survey of trash and work areas
Weekly wipe test of all work areas
Radioactive spill containment and decontamination
Disposal and storage of radioactive hot trash
Accuracy and linearity testing of dose calibrator
Calibration of survey meter
Leak testing sealed source
Misadministration

Molybdenum-99 Check

After eluting a generator, the Tc-99m eluant must be checked for contamination with Mo-99. The limit of µCi of Mo-99 per mCi of Tc-99m is set by the RSO. If the limit is exceeded, the Tc-99m eluant should not be used. The NRC-recommended limit for Mo-99 contamination is 0.15 µCi of Mo-99 per mCi of Tc-99m, not to exceed 5 µCi of Mo-99 per dose.

Dose Calibrator Daily Constancy Check

This quality assurance measure should be performed daily prior to using the dose calibrator. Normally, a cesium-137 (Cs-137) source is measured in the dose calibrator and the amount of activity is recorded. This measurement will alert the user if there is a calibration problem. The RSO can set the limits for acceptable measurements.

Radioactive Package Receipt

All radioactive packages must be surveyed and undergo wipe tests prior to opening to ensure that the package is not contaminated. It is also a good idea to do a wipe test of the lead container inside the package to make sure it is not contaminated either. The written policy should state what to do in the event the package is contaminated. Activity should not exceed 0 mRem/h at 1 m distance and 0.5 mRem/h (5 µSv/h) at the package surface. The RSO and NRC must be notified if activity exceeds 200 mRem/h (2 mSv/h) at the package surface or 10 mRem/h (0.1 mSv/h) at 1 m distance (1).

Leak Testing Sealed Sources

The NRC requires that all sealed sources in use be leak tested every 6 months. The measurable activity must be <0.005 µCi.

Daily Survey of Trash and Work Areas

At the end of each day all trash, linen carts, and work areas should be surveyed to detect any radioactive spills that may have occurred. Any work surfaces found to be contaminated should be cleaned following the radioactive spill policy and then resurveyed. If the area is still contaminated, it may need to be sealed off and resurveyed in the morning prior to use. Any trash or linen found to be contaminated should be held for decay following local hot trash policy. A log of the daily surveys should be kept on hand.

Weekly Wipe Test of All Work Areas

Each week, all work areas (i.e., counters and adjacent floor where radiotracers are placed or used, treadmills, etc.) where contamination is possible should be wipe tested. Any areas found to be contaminated should be cleaned following your radioactive spill policy and then rewiped. If the area is still contaminated, it may need to be sealed off and rewiped in the morning prior to use.

Radioactive Spill Containment and Decontamination

This written policy should describe how to protect personnel, confine the area, and decontaminate a radioactive spill using the proper radiation safety equipment. It should also specify the limits that would indicate that the area is usable or that the area needs to be sealed off until contamination has decayed to the proper level. The policy should also list whom to contact in the event of a radioactive spill.

Misadministration

All misadministrations of radiopharmaceuticals must be reported in detail to the medical director and the RSO. The circumstances of misadministration should be investigated and measures must be taken to prevent recurrence. According to NRC regulatory requirements, a misadministration must be reported by telephone no later than the next calendar day if the administered activity is given to the wrong patient and the effective dose equivalent exceeds 5 Rem.

Disposal and Storage of Radioactive Hot Trash

All radioactive trash must be held for decay before it can be discarded. The policy should discuss where the trash is stored, how it is to be labeled, the acceptable level at which it can be discarded safely, and where to discard it. Radioactive waste must be held for a minimum of 10 half-lives and be indistinguishable from background activity before disposal.

Accuracy and Linearity Testing of Dose Calibrator

Depending on the regulations in your area or on the RSO's requirements, this testing is done either quarterly or yearly. This QC test helps to ensure that the dose calibrator is working properly.

Calibration of Survey Meter

This test is usually done by the RSO or can be done by an independent company annually. It is important to determine that the survey meter is functioning properly.

Personnel Dosimeter

Individuals who receive more than 10% of the quarterly limits of radiation exposure for occupational workers must wear dosimeters. These may consist of X-ray film badges, OLS dosimeters, or TLD rings. The dosimeters allow the RSO to maintain a permanent record of individual dose equivalent to skin. The most effective means for limiting radiation exposure are time, distance (inverse square law), and shielding (half-value layers).

If a member of the technical staff becomes pregnant, she must declare her pregnancy in writing to the employer and RSO. The radiation exposure of pregnant personnel must be monitored and is limited to 50 mRem/month during the pregnancy. No other special protection is required. Occupational and public radiation exposure limits are listed in Table 3-3. In order to place radiation exposure

Table 3-3
Occupational and Public Exposure Limits

Occupational dose limits	
Total	5 Rem/year (5000 mRem/year)
ALARA 10%	0.5 Rem/year (500 mRem/year)
Organ limit (hands, feet, skin)	50 Rem/year
Lens of eye	15 Rem/year
Declared pregnant occupational worker	0.5 Rem/9 months
General public dose limits	0.5 Rem/year ($\sim$1 mSv/year)

ALARA, as low as reasonably achievable.

Table 3-4
Radiation Exposure and Acute Effect

Natural background radiation
Cosmic (sun, stars)	27 mRem/year
Terrestrial (uranium, thorium, etc.)	28 mRem/year
Internal (K-40, C-14, H-3, etc.)	40 mRem/year
Radon	200 mRem/year
Total, natural background	~300 mRem/year

Man-made radiation
Medical X-ray	39 mRem/year
Nuclear medicine	14 mRem/year
Consumer products	7 mRem/year
Other (nuclear fuel cycle, fallout, etc.)	<1 mRem/year

Acute radiation effect
No effect	<25 Rem
Slight blood changes	50 Rem
Nausea, fatigue	100 Rem
First death	250 Rem
Lethal Dose (LD) 50/30	500 Rem
Lethal dose	700 Rem

in appropriate perspective, Table 3-4. lists natural and man-made radiation and levels causing clinical symptoms.

REFERENCES

1. Siegel JA (2001). *Guide for Diagnostic Nuclear Medicine 2001*, published by the Society of Nuclear Medicine (http://www.snm.org). This publication also can be downloaded free as a PDF-file from http://www.nrc.gov—Menu: "Nuclear Materials": "Med, Academic & Ind Uses": "Medical Uses": "Medical Licensee Toolkit": "Other Guidance" (accessed February 5, 2007).
2. Bushberg JT, Leidholdt EM (2003). Radiation protection. In Sandler MP, Coleman RE, Patton JA, Wackers FJTh, Gottschalk A (eds), *Diagnostic Nuclear Medicine*, 4th Edition, Lippincott Williams & Wilkins, Philadelphia, PA.
3. ICANL, available at http://www.icanl.org "The Standards" (download as PDF).

4   Patient Preparation

Patients should be well informed about what to expect during the nuclear cardiology procedure. In order to keep the number of rescheduled and canceled appointments to a minimum, it is important to make sure patients are not only properly prepared for the procedure but also that they are well informed about the examination. They should be informed about all aspects, including the duration of the procedure, before they arrive in the laboratory. This chapter discusses the following:

- Patient preparation
- Preparation for stress protocols

Key Words: Patient preparation, Consent stress testing.

The following is the minimum information to be communicated to a patient:

1. Date and time of test
2. Directions and parking information
3. Location of imaging facility

Preparation for procedure:

4. Light meal or fasting on morning of test
5. Possible discontinuation of medication in consultation with referring physician
6. Notify patients not to drink coffee or caffeine-containing beverages on morning of test
7. Wear comfortable clothing and rubber-soled shoes or sneakers

Very important:

8. Information about total duration of stress and imaging test
9. Notify male patients that some chest hair may be shaved for ECG electrode placement
10. Advise that IV line will be inserted in forearm
11. Explain purpose and endpoint(s) of stress test

From: *Contemporary Cardiology: Nuclear Cardiology, The Basics*
By: F. J. Th. Wackers, W. Bruni, and B. L. Zaret © Humana Press Inc., Totowa, NJ

12. Provide information when the referring physician can be expected to have the results of the test. Emphasize that results will be reported quickly to the physician

Additional relevant information for patients can be found on the ASNC website: http://www.asnc.org—Menu: "Patients": "About Nuclear Cardiology" and "Patient & Professional Information." Patient brochures in PDF format are available for download and distribution to patients.

PATIENT PREPARATION

The preparation of patients for stress procedures is different depending on the stress modality, i.e., physical exercise or pharmacological stress. For both stresses, it is recommended that the patient is fasting and has an empty stomach. For pharmacological stress, the patient is asked to abstain from caffeine-containing beverages of food at least 12 h before the procedure.

> There is a practical advantage to give *identical preparatory instructions* to every patient regardless whether they are scheduled for physical exercise or for pharmacological stress. Frequently, a patient's ability to exercise is overestimated, and an adequate exercise endpoint cannot be attained. A patient scheduled for an exercise test can be switched readily to pharmacological stress if he/she received the same instructions as a patient scheduled for pharmacological stress.

Discontinuation of Medication

Depending on the indication for stress testing and the clinical question to be answered, it may be advisable to discontinue medication such as β-blocking medication, calcium-blocking medication, and long- and short-acting nitrates before the procedure.

For example, if a patient is referred for the *diagnosis* of coronary artery disease, medication probably can be stopped. However, if a patient has known coronary artery disease, the purpose of the test may be to evaluate the patient on his/her daily medical regimen. The decision to temporarily stop medication should always been done in consultation with the referring physician.

If the test is performed for diagnostic purposes, β-blocking and calcium-blocking medication should preferably be stopped 24 h before, or at the least on the day of the procedure. Nitrates should not be taken on the day of the procedure.

Patients with Diabetes

Diabetic patients on oral agents and no insulin may also fast on the morning of the physical stress test and hold their medications until after the completion stress test.

For those diabetic patients taking insulin, we advise taking a modestly (−25 to −50%) reduced dose with a light breakfast; the balance of the insulin may be taken after the completion of the physical stress test. A capillary glucose should be obtained with the glucose meter prior to the test. If glucose is <100 mg/dL, approximately 15 g of liquid carbohydrate should be administered, such as 4 oz of juice, to prevent exercise-induced hypoglycemia. Specific instructions from the patient's diabetologist may also be helpful in individual patients, particularly those with labile control.

Pregnancy

All female patients under 50 years of age must be asked if they are, or might be, pregnant. If the patient does not know, or might be pregnant, a urine pregnancy test must be performed.

If a patient states that she is pregnant or that she is breast-feeding, a radionuclide study can only be performed after consulting with the RSO and medical director. All benefits and risks must be weighed and discussed with the patient before proceeding with the procedure. The discussion with the patient and RSO must be documented in writing.

Breast-Feeding Mothers

At times, it may be medically indicated to perform radionuclide imaging in breast-feeding mothers. Radioisotopes are excreted in breast milk and expose the infant to radiation. The radiation safety approach is to either pump the breasts before the injection of radioisotope and store the milk or, if this is not feasible, collect milk and allow for appropriate radioisotope decay before giving the milk to the infant. Breast milk can be stored in the refrigerator for 5 days or frozen for up to 6 months. The physician or RSO should determine how long (e.g., 48 h for Tc-99m agents) the milk should be stored for adequate decay. There is no need to discard the milk. For exams that are scheduled ahead of time, the policy and method should be explained to nursing mother. It is not always possible to pump ahead of time so it is important to discuss the storage and time required for decay with the mother prior to performing the imaging procedure.

Example of Patient Appointment Information Sheet that Can Be Mailed to a Patient Before the Procedure

APPOINTMENT(S):

DATE: _____   TIME: _____
DATE: _____   TIME: _____

Please arrive 15 min prior to your scheduled appointment for registration and insurance purposes.

PLACE:

- (address of imaging facility)
- Take the "C"elevators to the xth floor, room XXXX (directly across from the elevator).
  Park in the parkinggarage and bring your parking ticket with you to be validated.

HOW LONG WILL IT TAKE?

The test consists of two parts: each portion takes approximately 2 h with a 1.5–3 h break between the two parts depending on the exam scheduled.

PREPARATION:

- Absolutely no caffeine or decaffeinated beverages 12 h before the test (including coffees, teas, sodas, and chocolates). You may eat a light breakfast up to 2 h before your test (e.g., small bowl of cereal OR toast and juice). We may have to cancel your test if you have taken caffeine.
- If you have diabetes and take only diabetes pills, you may eat the same light breakfast and hold your medication until after the exercise test is finished.
- If you take insulin, we recommend that you take a light breakfast with a reduced (one-quarter to one-half) dose of insulin. The rest of your insulin dose you will take after the stress test is finished. You may wish to discuss this with your doctor.
- Wear comfortable clothing and rubber sole shoes.

PRECAUTIONS:

If you think you may be pregnant or if you are breast-feeding, please tell your doctor immediately. If you might be pregnant, we will perform a urine pregnancy test.

MEDICATIONS:

Unless instructed by your doctor, continue to take your medication(s).

If you are taking theophylline or any other asthma or emphysema medication, please contact your doctor as it may need to be discontinued 48 h before the test.

If you have diabetes, see instructions above.

WHAT CAN YOU EXPECT:

- The two parts of the test consist of a stress study and a rest study. The stress OR the rest study can be done first and will depend on the type of exam you have been scheduled for.

- The stress test will require that ECG leads be placed on your chest to monitor your heart rate. A small dose of a radioactive tracer will be injected through an IV in your arm and images of your heart will be taken for approximately 45 min.

    There are no side effects to the injection. However, if you think you are pregnant please inform the technologist immediately.

- The rest study will consist of another injection of the radioactive tracer through the IV and a second set of images to be taken of your heart.

- There will be a break between the stress and rest portions of the test. The break ranges from 1.5–3 h depending on the type of study you are having. The technologist will tell you when you need to return and what restrictions, if any, there are for eating.

- The test may be completed in 1 day OR over 2 days. If you are scheduled to have the test over 2 days, the stress is done on one day and the rest is done on the other. It does not matter which is done first.

    Please refer to the appointment section to see when you are scheduled to have your test.

HOW DO YOU GET TEST RESULTS?

A nuclear cardiologist will study all the images and ECGs, prepare a report, and send it to your physician. This may take 1 or 2 days. Your personal physician will discuss the results with you and what they mean for your health. If your study is abnormal, the laboratory may call your physician immediately.

If you have any concerns or questions about your appointment, you can call the Cardiology Stress Laboratory at 999-999-9999.

CONSENT FOR STRESS TESTING

Although the risk for adverse effects due to stress testing is low (death or acute infarction may occur in less than 1:10,000), it is not nonexistent. In many facilities, the patient is asked to sign a consent form prior to the procedure. A sample consent form for stress is shown in the accompanying box. Others examples can be found in the AHA Guidelines for Clinical Exercise Laboratories (1).

**Cardiovascular Nuclear Imaging
and Exercise Laboratory**

99 Main St., City, CT 9999   ph: (999) 999-9999

Consent for Stress Testing

I am scheduled to undergo a cardiac stress test.

I understand that this test involves walking or running on a treadmill

I understand that this test involves the infusion of a medication that stresses the heart

During the test I will be watched for symptoms and monitored by an electrocardiogram. In addition heart rate and blood pressure measurements will be taken.

I understand that certain complications may occur including, but not limited to, heart attack, heart rhythm abnormality, stroke and death. I also understand that physical trauma may be incurred during the performance of the test.

The general purpose, potential benefits, possible hazards and inconveniences of stress testing have been explained to my satisfaction and I have been given the opportunity to ask any questions that I have concerning the test.

I hereby consent to the performance of the test.

_____   _____

Patient signature   Patient print name

_____   _____

Responsible physician   Responsible physician print
signature   name

PREPARATION FOR EXERCISE/STRESS PROTOCOLS

Stress Tc-99m Agent (Tc-99m Sestamibi or Tc-99m Tetrofosmin) First

The patient should be nil per os (NPO) 4 h prior to stress.

They are allowed to drink fruit juices, white milk, or water.

Patients with diabetes may eat a light meal (but no chocolate) and take their medications.

Patients should continue their medications unless directed otherwise by their physician.

The patient should not ingest coffee or caffeine-containing drinks (Table 4-1) during the 12 h prior to the test.

The reason for the latter instructions is that caffeine is a specific blocker of adenosine A2a receptor sites and that caffeine may attenuate the vasodilatory effect of dipyridamole or adenosine infusion and

Table 4-1
Caffeine-Containing Beverages, Food, and Medications that
Compete with Adenosine A2a Receptor Sites

Beverages
 Coffee (including "decaffeinated" coffee)
 Tea
 Sodas (including regular diet and "caffeine free" beverages)
 Chocolate drinks and chocolate products
Medications (partial list)
 Anacin®
 Exedrin®
 Cold combination medication (Kolephrin)
 Goody's headache powder
 Keep Alert
 Midol®
 Amaphen
 Cafergot®
 Darvon®
 Fiorinal®
 Theophylline
 Theo-Dur®
 Oxtriphylline (Choledyl®)
 Aminophylline®

theoretically cause false-negative tests. However, recently a clinical study in a limited number of patients showed that one single cup of coffee (8 oz, 100 mg of caffeine, taken 1 h before test, blood level 3.1 ± 1.6 mg/L) had no noticeable effect on the presence and magnitude of perfusion abnormalities (2). Although it appears prudent to continue to recommend that patients abstain from caffeine usage prior to the test, a single cup or a sip of coffee may not be a valid reason for cancellation of a vasodilator stress test.

It is not rare that a patient's exercise capacity is overestimated and they need to be switched to pharmacological stress. Therefore, it is advisable to give the same instruction about abstinence of caffeine-containing beverages and food to all patients.

Patients also should be off theophylline-based medications for 48 h prior to the test. This should be done in consultation with the referring physicians.

Rest Tc-99m Agent (Tc-99m Sestamibi or Tc-99m Tetrofosmin) First

The instructions are the same as for the "stress first" procedure. However, the patients may eat a light breakfast or a light lunch if time permits before rest study. Patients should be NPO 4 h prior to stress.

The patient should not ingest coffee or caffeine-containing drinks (Table 4-1) during the 12 h prior to the test.

Patients should be off theophylline-based medications for 48 h following their physicians advice.

Stress/Redistribution Tl-201

Prior to the test, the instructions are the same as for the "stress first" procedure.

Between the stress and redistribution part of the procedure, the patient may only take liquids but no meal. Caffeine is allowed after the stress portion. Diabetics may eat a light meal if needed.

The reason for this instruction is that ingestion of food after stress inhibits redistribution of Tl-201 and defects may appear falsely fixed.

Dual-Isotope Rest-Tl Stress-Tc-99m Agent (Tc-99m Sestamibi or Tc-99m Tetrofosmin) Imaging

The instructions are the same as for the "rest first" procedure. The patients may eat a light breakfast or a light lunch if time permits before rest study. Patients should be NPO 4 h prior to stress.

The patient should not ingest coffee or caffeine-containing drinks (Table 4-1) during the 12 h prior to the test.

Patients should be off theophylline-based medications for 48 h following their physician's advice.

REFERENCES

1. Pina IL, Balady GJ, Hanson P, Labovitz, Madonna DW, Myers J (1995). Guidelines for Clinical Exercise Testing 1995. A statement for healthcare professionals from the committee on exercise and cardiac rehabilitation, American Heart Association. *Circulation* 91:912–921.
2. Zoghbi GJ, Htay T, Aqel R, Blackmon L, Heo J, Iskandrian AE (2006). Effect of caffeine on ischemia detection by adenosine single-photon emission computed tomography perfusion imaging. *J Am Coll Cardiol* 47:2296–2302.

5   Stress Procedures

In a well-run facility, details of all procedures and policies are described in written protocols to ensure standardization and consistency of daily operations. Because no imaging facility operates under identical circumstances, protocols must be modified to meet specific needs. In order to meet standards for accreditation by the ICANL, well-detailed "laboratory-specific protocols" play an important role (see Chapter 22 and http://www.icanl.org). The protocols must be reviewed yearly and updated when and where necessary. This chapter discusses the following topics:

- Indications and methodology
- Physical exercise testing
- Pharmacological stress testing

Key Words: Stress procedures indications, Stress protocols, Treadmill testing, Pharmacologic testing, Adenosine testing, Dipyridamole testing, Dobutamine testing, ECG leads placement, End points stress testing, Contraindications stress testing, Worksheets, Interpretation stress test, Duke treadmill score.

PURPOSE OF STRESS PROCEDURES

Most stress procedures are performed in patients with symptoms of suspected or known ischemic heart disease. Patients must have stable symptoms or have been stabilized by therapy. The purpose of stress procedures is to provoke symptoms in a controlled and safe environment and thus aid in establishing the etiology of symptoms. Stress procedures must be performed under direct supervision by a physician.

Indications

Appropriate clinical indications for stress testing are discussed in the "AHA/ACC 2002 Guideline Update for Exercise Testing" *(1)* (see

From: *Contemporary Cardiology: Nuclear Cardiology, The Basics*
By: F. J. Th. Wackers, W. Bruni, and B. L. Zaret © Humana Press Inc., Totowa, NJ

http://www.acc.org—Menu: "Quality and Services": "Clinical State-
ments/Guidelines": "Exercise Testing"). More recently, the ASNC and
American College of Cardiology (ACC) established appropriateness
guidelines (see http://www.ascn.org [Menu: "Manage Your Practice":
"Guidelines and Standards": "Appropriateness Criteria for SPECT
MPI"] and Chapter 24).

In brief, indications for stress myocardial perfusion imaging include
the following:

1. Diagnosis of obstructive coronary artery disease.
2. Risk assessment and prognosis in patients with symptoms or known
   coronary artery disease.

EXERCISE TESTING

Standard stress protocols are described in detail in ref. *1* and online:
http://www.asnc.org—Menu: "Manage Your Practice"; "Guidelines &
Standards."

Before exercise testing, patient's history must be obtained to identify
any contraindications such as

- Recent acute myocardial infarction in the last 4 days,
- Unstable angina,
- Critical aortic stenosis,
- Congestive heart failure,
- Uncontrolled arrhythmias,
- Uncontrolled hypertension,
- Acute myocarditis/pericarditis,
- Aortic dissection,
- Fever, or other co-morbidities.

It is important that the patient understands the purpose and nature
of the stress procedure. For example, in many instances, the patient
must understand that the purpose of the test is to *reproduce symptoms*
and that he/she must give his/her best effort; otherwise the test may
be inconclusive.

A stress procedure, even an exercise ECG test, should never be
performed without an IV in place. Cardiac emergencies may occur in
apparently low-risk patients. Precious time may be lost if one has to
establish IV access during cardiac resuscitation

Perform a short and focused physical exam, which includes pulse,
blood pressure, assessment of jugular vein distension, presence of edema,
auscultation of the heart for gallops and heart murmur, and lung auscultation. Measure blood pressure with the patient in standing position.

Trunk Leads

A good-quality ECG is extremely important for diagnostic quality exercise testing.

To ensure optimal quality ECG recordings during exercise without artifacts and without interference, it is necessary to move the ECG electrodes from the conventional position on the extremities of the limbs to the patient's trunk (see **Fig. 5-1**). The right and left leads are moved close to the sternum, whereas the lower extremity leads are moved to above the navel in the axillary line just below the rib cage. It should be appreciated that the modified placement of the ECG extremity leads to the trunk for exercise testing may in some patients result in a right axis shift and ST-segment changes. The exercise ECG should be compared with the rest trunk ECG and not the rest limb ECG.

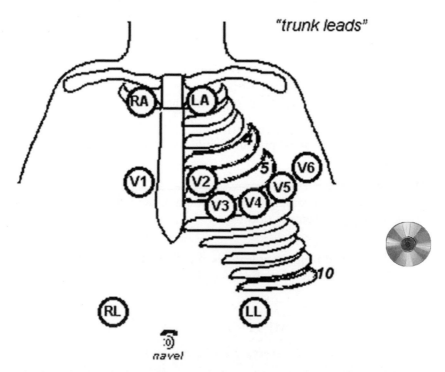

Fig. 5-1. Diagram of correct placement of ECG electrodes during exercise. In order to reduce motion artifacts the extremity leads are moved from the limbs to the trunk.

Measures that Ensure Optimal Quality Stress ECG Tracings

Proper Skin Preparation and Lead Placement

Preparation of Skin

- Cleanse skin with alcohol, especially oily skin.
- Shave areas where electrodes are to be placed.
- Lightly abrade skin with scrub pads.
- Place electrode with the patient standing or sitting.

Position Electrodes Correctly (See Diagram in Figure 5-1.)

- Position right arm and left arm electrodes close to the sternum.

Connect Wires Appropriately

- Double check that right and left are not reversed.

Causes for Artifacts and Noise on ECG and Corrections

Inadequate Skin Preparation
- Repeat preparation of skin and replace electrodes.

Patient Motion/Tight Grip on Handlebar
- No excessive arm movements.
- Hands should rest lightly on top of the handlebar.

Inflation of Blood Pressure Cuff
- Do not measure blood pressure while the ECG machine is printing.

Lead Reversal
- Replace leads according to color coding of the wires and according to schematic drawing.

Trunk Leads
- ECG obtained from trunk leads is slightly different compared with the conventional limb lead ECG.

METHODOLOGY

Exercise ECG Protocol

Although there are numerous graded exercise protocols, the Bruce protocol is the basis and most widely used method. For other protocols, we refer to specialized texts on stress testing *(2,3)*.

Bruce Exercise Protocol				
Stage	*Speed (mph)*	*Incline (%)*	*METs*	*Time (min)*
Stage 1	1.7	10	4.6	3
Stage 2	2.5	12	7.0	6
Stage 3	3.4	14	10.1	9
Stage 4	4.2	16	12.9	12
Stage 5	5.0	18	15.0	15
Stage 6	5.5	20	16.9	18

MET, metabolic equivalent

The treadmill should have a front rail. The patient may have the hands on top of the rail but should not grip it too tightly. The patient should walk upright looking forward. An emergency stop button should be readily reached.

The motorized treadmill is most commonly used in the USA because American patients are more familiar with walking than with bicycling. However, in many other countries, the upright stationary bicycle is used routinely for physical stress testing. There are no real practical differences between the two forms of exercise for the purpose of diagnostic testing. The treadmill should have an adequate range of speed: 1–8 mph (1.6–12.8 km/h).

In older individuals and in those who have limited exercise capacity, the Bruce protocol can be modified by two 3-min warm-up stages at 1.7 mph and 0 percent grade and 1.7 mph and 5 percent grade.

During the exercise procedure, the patient should be monitored as follows:

- Record ECG, blood pressure, and heart rate at least at the end of every 3-min stage.
- Continue to monitor ECG for changes and interrogate patients for symptoms (chest pain, lightheadedness, etc.).
- Consider using the Borg scale (see Table 5-1) as a reference to determine the patient's ability to continue physical exercise.
- Continue exercise until testing endpoint is reached. Optimally, the patient will achieve the stage at which he/she perceives the work load as "17" or "18" on the Borg scale.

Table 5-1
Borg Scale of Perceived Exertion or Pain

6	
7	Very, very light
8	
9	Very light
10	
11	Fairly light
12	
13	Somewhat hard
14	
15	Hard
16	
17	Very hard
18	
19	Very, very hard
20	

The Borg scale was developed based on the observation that young men can estimate their exercise heart rate in bpm by aligning a perceived level of exertion with a scale ranging from 6 to 20.

Endpoints of exercise

1. Reproduction of symptoms, angina
2. Marked fatigue and shortness of breath or wheezing
3. Achievement of at least 85% of age-predicted maximal heart rate (220-age). If the patient is not symptomatic at this point, the stress test could continue.
4. ≥2.5 mm asymptomatic horizontal/downsloping ST-segment depression
5. Leg cramps, claudication

Absolute indications for terminating exercise test

1. ST-segment elevation >1 mmHg in leads without Q-waves
2. Severe angina
3. Decrease of blood pressure (≥10 mmHg) with symptoms
4. Signs of poor peripheral perfusion, pallor, clammy skin, cyanosis
5. Central nervous system symptoms, such as ataxia, vertigo, confusion, gait problems

6. Serious arrhythmia: ventricular tachycardia, i.e., run ≥3 beats
7. Development of second or third degree atrioventricular (AV) block
8. Systolic blood pressure >220 mmHg or diastolic pressure >110 mmHg
9. Technical problems with monitoring vital parameters, including ECG
10. Patient's request

The most important and relevant clinical diagnostic endpoint is the *reproduction of symptoms.* If no symptoms occur, the attainment of target heart rate is only a general indication of the patient's effort. One should always attempt to achieve maximal effort with at least target heart rate.

If the patient is unable to reach an adequate exercise endpoint, i.e., cannot complete stage 2 or does not achieve at least 7 METs workload, consider switching to vasodilator stress.

- Inject radiopharmaceutical when an exercise endpoint is attained.
- The patient should continue to walk for at least 2 more minutes.

Mark clock time of the injection of radiopharmaceutical relative to the start and end of exercise effort.

The precise timing of the injection of radiopharmaceutical is very important. It takes at least 4 min after the injection of radiopharmaceutical for the blood level to decrease to about 50% of injected dose *(4).* Thus, the longer a patient continues to exercise after injection, the better the uptake in the heart reflects the exercise endpoint. However, in practice, it is usually not be feasible to continue exercise for longer than 2 min after injection. The best approach is then that the patient continues to exercise at the same maximal level for 1 min after injection, then to decrease the incline of the treadmill and speed as tolerated during the second minute.

After exercise, the following procedures should be followed:

- Monitor blood pressure, heart rate, and ECG for 5 min.
- Continue monitoring if chest pain or significant ECG changes persist.
- Start imaging 15–30 min after termination of exercise.
- Obtain follow-up 12-lead ECG after SPECT imaging is completed in patients who had ECG changes during stress.

PHARMACOLOGICAL VASODILATION STRESS

Exercise stress is always the preferred stress modality for evaluating patients with known or suspected coronary artery disease. Pharmacological stress is indicated in patients who are unable to perform adequate physical stress due to the following conditions:

- Musculoskeletal conditions
- Peripheral vascular disease
- Pulmonary disease
- Left bundle branch block or paced rhythm
- Treatment with medications that blunt heart rate response (β-blockers, calcium channel blockers)
- Recent acute myocardial infarction, i.e., 3–5 days
- Deconditioning

Many obese, de-conditioned, and frail elderly patients may not be able to complete stage 2 of the Bruce protocol (<7 METs) without clear cardiac symptoms. It is then advisable to switch to pharmacological vasodilation stress.

Standard stress protocols are described in detail in ref. *1*.

Dipyridamole

Patients with chronic obstructive pulmonary disease but without bronchospasm (wheezing) usually tolerate infusion of dipyridamole well. However, if active wheezing is present, the test should be switched to dobutamine infusion (see below).

One should be prepared for the development of high-degree AV block. Patients with baseline first-degree AV block are at higher risk. In the latter patients, one may consider to switch to adenosine (relatively safer because of the short half-life) or dobutamine.

Before dipyridamole vasodilator stress, the following steps should be obtained:

- Obtain short history of the patient.
- Perform focused physical examination to identify contraindications:
  - Recent acute myocardial infarction, <2 days
  - Unstable angina
  - Congestive heart failure
  - Severe asthma and active wheezing
  - Recent (<12 h) use of caffeine-containing products (Table 4-1).
    The reason for the latter instructions is that caffeine is a specific blocker of adenosine A2a receptor sites and that caffeine may attenuate the vasodilatory effect of dipyridamole or adenosine infusion and theoretically cause false-negative tests. However,

recently a clinical study *(5)* in a limited number of patients showed that one single cup of coffee (8 oz, 100 mg of caffeine, taken 1 h before test, blood level 3.1 ± 1.6 mg/L) had no noticeable effect on the presence and magnitude of perfusion abnormalities. Although it appears prudent to continue to recommend that patients abstain from caffeine usage prior to the test, a single cup or a sip of coffee may not be a valid reason for cancellation of a vasodilator stress test.
- Recent use (48 h) of theophylline-based medication
- Known hypersensitivity to dipyridamole
- Explanation of procedure and possible side effects.
- It is important that the patient is warned about the side effects of dipyridamole infusion (Table 5-2).
- Obtain IV access (for dipyridamole vasodilation, one IV line is sufficient).

Table 5-2
Frequent Side Effects of Dipyridamole and Adenosine Infusion (% of Patients)

	Dipyridamole (10)	*Adenosine (11)*
Cardiac		
Fatal myocardial infarction	0.05	0
Nonfatal myocardial infarction	0.05	0
Chest pain	19.7	57
ST-T changes on ECG	7.5	12
Ventricular ectopy	5.2	?
Tachycardia	3.2	?
Hypotension	4.6	?
Blood pressure instability	1.6	?
Hypertension	1.5	?
Atrioventricular block	0	10
Non-cardiac		
Headache	12.2	35
Dizziness	11.8	?
Nausea	4.6	?
Flushing	3.4	29
Pain (nonspecific)	2.6	?
Dyspnea	2.6	15
Paresthesia	1.3	?
Fatigue	1.2	?
Dyspepsia	1.0	?
Acute bronchospasm	0.15	0[a]

?, not reported for adenosine.
[a]Patients with history of bronchospasm were excluded.

- Record baseline 12-lead ECG, heart rate, and blood pressure.
- The total dose of dipyridamole (a vial contains 5 mg/mL) is dependent on the patient's weight.
- Dipyridamole dose is diluted with normal saline to 40 mL.

$$\frac{Wt(kg) \times 0.57mg/kg}{5mg/mL} = mL \text{ of dipyridamole to be drawn up}$$

- Because of the long-acting effect of dipyridamole, the maximal dose generally administered is 60 mg.
- Dipyridamole can be infused intravenously either by hand push over 4 min or by a motorized infusion pump. The infusion rate is 0.142 mg/kg/min or total of 0.568 mg/kg.

During vasodilator stress (**Fig. 5-2**), the following procedures are important:

- Record blood pressure, heart rate, and 12-lead ECG every minute.
  If the patient is able to walk, begin at slowest treadmill speed (modified Bruce protocol stage 1: 1.7 mph and 0 percent grade) at 4 min after start of dipyridamole infusion.
- Inject isotope at 7–8 min after start of infusion.
  The patient should continue walking for 2 min after radiopharmaceutical injection if at all feasible.
- At 10 min, stop walking and monitor vital signs 4–5 min into recovery.
- If side effects persist, administer aminophylline 75–125 mg IV over 2 min. Avoid (if clinically safe) injecting aminophylline earlier than

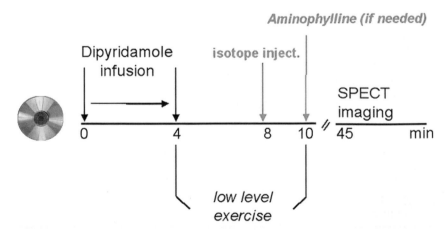

Fig. 5-2. Schematic representation of dipyridamole infusion protocol. After the infusion of dipyridamole is finished, the patient may perform low level exercise.

2 min after injection of radiopharmaceutical as it may adversely affect the diagnostic yield of the test.

Aminophylline is a specific blocker of adenosine A2a receptor sites. It is often needed to control symptoms caused by dipyridamole infusion. One should realize that the half-life of aminophylline is shorter than that of dipyridamole (40 min). Thus adverse effects may re-occur after approximately 15 min and require another dose of aminophylline.

- Start imaging at 30–60 min after radiopharmaceutical injection if low level of exercise was performed, 45–60 min after radiopharmaceutical injection if no low-level exercise was performed.
- In patients with severe symptoms or ECG changes, continue monitoring of vital signs and 12-lead ECG during imaging and after if necessary.

EXERCISE AUGMENTATION

The performance of low-level exercise in combination with vasodilation has been shown to reduce unpleasant side effects, to decrease subdiaphragmatic radiotracer accumulation, and to increase heart rate moderately due to the minimal workload *(6,7)*.

Adenosine

Before vasodilator stress, similar to the assessment prior to dipyridamole vasodilator stress, the following steps should be obtained:

- Obtain short history of the patient.
- Perform focused physical examination. Identify contraindications:
  - Recent acute myocardial infarction, i.e.,<2 days
  - Unstable angina
  - Congestive heart failure
  - Severe asthma and active wheezing
  - Greater than first-degree heart block or sick sinus node syndrome without pacemaker
  - Use of caffeine-containing products (Table 4-1). Note: recently a clinical study *(5)*, in a limited number of patients, suggested that one cup of coffee has no noticeable effect on the detection of myocardial ischemia using vasodilator stress with adenosine.
- Explain procedure and possible side effects to the patient (Table 5-2).
  - Obtain IV access.
  - Record baseline 12-lead ECG, heart rate, and blood pressure.

- Patients must have two separate IV lines or a short Y-connector attachment to prevent additional adenosine from being injected as a bolus during the injection of the radiopharmaceutical.
- Adenosine must be infused using a pump to ensure consistent dose administration at a rate of 140 mcg/kg/min.

The dose of adenosine needed (a vial contains 3 mg/mL) is dependent on the patient's weight:

$$\frac{\mathrm{Wt(kg)} \times 0.140\mathrm{mg/kg/min} \times 6\mathrm{min}}{3\mathrm{mg}} = \mathrm{mL\ of\ adenosine\ to\ be\ drawn\ up}$$

- Because of the short-acting effect of adenosine, there is no maximal dose limit.
- If the patient is able to walk, begin low-level exercise on treadmill without grade and at slowest speed (1.7 mph).
- When the patient is comfortably walking, begin infusion of adenosine using a motorized infusion pump.

Adenosine should not be injected by hand. It is impossible to mimic the steady slow flow of a motorized infusion pump. Because of the rapid action of adenosine, adverse effects are more likely to occur using hand push.

There are two commonly used adenosine infusion protocols: the *conventional long* protocol and the *short* protocol (**Figs. 5-3 and 5-4**). The conventional protocol is as follows:

- Adenosine is infused over a 6-min period.
- The radiopharmaceutical is injected during the third minute of infusion. Infusion is then continued for an additional 3 min.

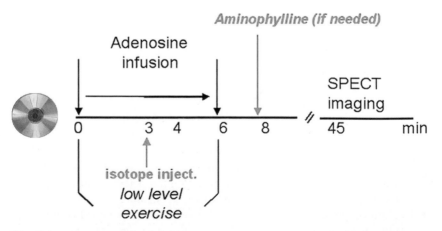

Fig. 5-3. Schematic representation of the long adenosine infusion protocol. During the infusion of adenosine the patient may perform low level exercise.

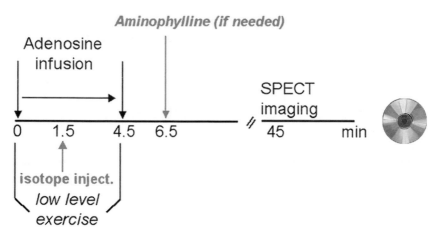

Fig. 5-4. Schematic representation of the short adenosine infusion protocol. During the infusion of adenosine the patient may perform low level exercise.

Because of the rapid onset of vasodilation by adenosine, a shortened protocol has become popular *(8,9)*. The radiopharmaceutical is injected at 1.5 min into infusion. The infusion is then continued for an additional 3 min (i.e., a total 4.5-min infusion).

Procedures Followed During Vasodilator Stress

- Record blood pressure, heart rate, and 12-lead ECG every minute.
- Record occurrence of symptoms (chest pain, lightheadedness, shortness of breath, nausea, etc.)
- Mark clock time of the injection of radiopharmaceutical relative to the start and end of dipyridamole or adenosine infusion.

After injection of the radiopharmaceutical, the infusion continues for 3 min and the patient continues to walk. The patient stops walking when the infusion is stopped.

Procedures Followed After Vasodilator Stress

- Monitor blood pressure, heart rate, and ECG for 5 min after the completion of infusion.
- Continue clinical monitoring if chest pain or significant ECG changes persist.
- Give aminophylline (75–125 mg IV over 2–3 min) when indicated for symptoms. If at all clinically possible, this should be delayed until at least 2 min after radiopharmaceutical injection.
- Start imaging 30–60 min after radiopharmaceutical injection.

If necessary (in patients with symptoms or ECG changes), continue monitoring vital signs and 12-lead ECG during and after completion of imaging.

PHARMACOLOGIC ADRENERGIC STRESS

Indication

Pharmacological adrenergic stress (with dobutamine) is indicated in patients who cannot perform physical exercise stress and have contraindications to pharmacological vasodilator stress. Dobutamine infusion stimulates β1 and β2 receptors and increases heart rate, blood pressure, and myocardial contraction. Although regional myocardial blood increases secondarily, this increase is less than with dipyridamole or adenosine.

Standard stress protocols are described in detail in ref. *1* and online: http://www.asnc.org—Menu: "Manage Your Practice"; "Guidelines and Standards."

Dobutamine

In general, the patient population that requires dobutamine stress is a more selected and sicker population. It is important that the patient is warned about possible side effects of dobutamine infusion. The increase in heart rate and palpitations are often experienced as unpleasant (see Table 5-3).

Before adrenergic stress, similar to the assessment prior to exercise testing, the following steps should be followed:

- Obtain short history of the patient.
- Perform focused physical examination to identify contraindications:

  - Recent acute myocardial infarction within prior 5 days
  - Unstable angina
  - Congestive heart failure
  - Critical aortic stenosis
  - Known supraventricular or ventricular tachycardia
  - Uncontrolled hypertension (>200/110 mmHg)
  - β-Blocking medication because of attenuation of heart rate response

- Explain procedure and possible side effects to the patient (Table 5-3).

Table 5-3
Frequent Side Effects of Intravenous Dobutamine *(12)*

	% of patients
Cardiac	
Fatal myocardial infarction	0
Nonfatal myocardial infarction	0
Chest pain	31
ST-T changes on ECG	50
Ventricular ectopy	43
Tachycardia	1.4
Hypotension	0
Hypertension	1.4
AV block	0.6
Non-cardiac	
Headache	14
Dizziness	4
Nausea	9
Flushing	14
Pain (nonspecific)	7
Dyspnea	14
Paresthesia	12

- Provide the patient with two separate IV lines, a short Y-connector attachment, or a dual-port connector to prevent additional dobutamine from being injected as a bolus during the radiopharmaceutical injection.
- Record baseline 12-lead ECG, heart rate, and blood pressure.

Procedures Followed During Adrenergic Stress

- The dose of dobutamine is dependent on the patient's weight and the time into the protocol.
- Dobutamine must be infused using a motorized pump to allow for variable infusion rates (**Fig. 5-5**).
- Dobutamine is infused starting at 10 mcg/kg/min, increasing the dose every 3 min: 20 mcg/kg/min, 30 mcg/kg/min, up to a maximum of 40 mcg/kg/min.
- Record blood pressure, heart rate, and 12-lead ECG every minute.
- Monitor occurrence of symptoms (chest pain, lightheadedness, shortness of breath, nausea, etc.) and arrhythmias.
- Monitor vital signs for 4–5 min into recovery:
    Side effects should subside within 5 min of completion of infusion.
    Continue monitoring or obtain 12-lead ECG post imaging if necessary.

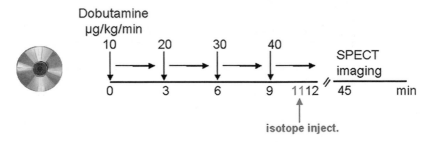

Fig. 5-5. Schematic representation of dobutamine infusion protocol.

- Atropine (0.5–2 mg IV) should be given if the target heart rate has not been attained at maximal dobutamine dose.
- Inject radiopharmaceutical at 11 min of protocol or at target heart rate. Dobutamine infusion should be continued for 2 min after injection of radiopharmaceutical.
- Mark clock time of the injection of radiopharmaceutical relative to the start and end of dobutamine infusion.
- Start imaging 30–45 min after radiopharmaceutical injection.

If necessary (in patients with symptoms or ECG changes) continue monitoring vital signs and 12-lead ECG during and after completion of imaging.

Procedures Followed After Adrenergic Stress

- Monitor blood pressure, heart rate, and ECG for 5 min after the completion of infusion.
- Continue clinical monitoring if chest pain or significant ECG changes persist.
- Give metoprolol (5–15 mg IV over 2–3 min) when indicated for symptoms. If at all clinically possible, this should be delayed until at least 2 min after radiopharmaceutical injection.
- Obtain, if necessary, a follow-up 12-lead ECG after SPECT imaging is completed.

STRESS PROTOCOL WORKSHEETS

Worksheets are useful for documentation of the details of a stress test, the patient's symptoms, drug given, etc. Below are sample worksheets for pharmacological vasodilator stress used in our laboratory.

CARDIAC EXERCISE LABORATORY DIPYRIDAMOLE
PROTOCOL/WORKSHEET

Date: _____

Name: _____   Unit Number: _____

Wt _____ kg

Ht _____ cm

Dipyridamole (Persantine®) contains 5 mg/mL
Dipyridamole infused at 0.142 mg/kg/min for 4 min, for a total of 0.57 mg/kg

1. _____ kg × 0.57 mg/kg = _____ total mg infused
2. _____ total mg infused/4 min = _____ mg/min infused
3. _____ total mg infused/5 min = _____ ml of dipyridamole to be drawn up in a 60 mL syringe
4. Reconstitute Dipyridamole with NaCl = 40 mL
5. Manually push 10 mL/min over the next 4 min
6. Isotope injected at 8 min
7. BP and 12-lead ECG every minute

Baseline   H.R. ___ bpm B.P. ___ mmHg

Time from start of infusion	Heart rate	Blood pressure	Comments/side effects
1			
2			
3			
4			
5			
6			
7			
Isotope inject. 8			
9			
10			

Side Effects:
     Onset _____ min   Duration _____ min
     Aminophylline amount _____ mg   Time inj. _____ min

CARDIAC EXERCISE LABORATORY 6-MINUTE ADENOSINE
PROTOCOL/WORKSHEET

Date: _____

1. Two IVs or Y-connector required
2. Infusion over 6 min via pump
3. Radioisotope injected at 3 min
4. Blood pressure and 12-lead ECG every min

Name: _____   Unit Number: _____
Wt _____ kg

Ht _____ cm
Adenosine (Adenoscan®) contains 3 mg/mL

Adenosine infused: _____ kg × at 0.140 mg/kg/min/3 mg = infusion
rate/min of Adenosine

1. _____ mL/min (infusion rate) × 6 min = _____ total mL infused
over 6 min(#1)
2. _____ total mL infused + 3 mL for tubing dead space = _____ total
adenosine to be drawn up (#2)
3. Place the total mL obtained from #2 in a 30 mL syringe
(If this number >30mL, use a 60 mL syringe)
4. DO NOT DILUTE USING GRAESBY PUMP.
5. If patient weighs more than 310 lbs use Bolus Mode on Graesby pump

Baseline   H.R. ___ bpm B.P. ___ mmHg

Time (min) from start of infusion	Heart rate	Blood pressure	Comments/side effects
1			
2			
Isotope inj. 3			
4			
5			
Stop Adenosine 6			
7			

Total mL. Infused over 6 min (#1) _____ × 3mg = _____ mg infused
Side Effects:
  Onset _____ min   Duration _____ min
  Aminophylline amount ____ mg   Time inj. _____ min

CARDIAC EXERCISE LABORATORY DOBUTAMINE PROTOCOL/WORKSHEET

Date: _____

1. Two IV's or Y-connector required
2. Infusion via pump, 3-min stages
3. Radioisotope injected at 40 mcg/kg/min
4. Blood pressure and 12-lead ECG twice per stage and every min at peak infusion

Name: _____   Unit Number: _____

Wt _____ kg

Ht _____ cm

Dobutamine contains 1mg/ml

Use infusion pump

Baseline   H.R. ___ bpm B.P. ___ mmHg

Dose and time from start infusion		Heart rate	Blood pressure	Comments/side effects
10 mcg	1			
	2.5			
20 mcg	4			
	5.5			
30 mcg	7			
	8.5			
40 mcg	10			
	10			

IV atropine given at _____ min; mg given _____ Total dose given _____ mg

Isotope injection time; _____ min

Infusion terminated at; _____ min; Maximal infusion rate: _____ mcg/kg/min

Post Infusion:

1 min			
2 min			
3 min			

Symptons _____

IV Metoprolol* admistered? _____ mg at _____ min

(*May cause bronchconstriction in astmatic patients)

Total Dobutamine infused: _____ ml

infusion cross [conc.]1.0 mg/ml= _____ mg

INTERPRETATION OF STRESS TESTS

Exercise ECG

When interpreting an exercise treadmill test, the following should be considered:

- Exercise duration in minutes
- Exercise stage completed
- Total workload performed in METs
- Peak exercise heart rate achieved
- Blood pressure response
- Symptoms
- ECG changes

First, one should assess whether exercise performance was adequate. The most important variable is the workload achieved. If workload does not exceed 7 METs, the patient either is at high risk or was de-conditioned, unmotivated, or a combination. If there were no objective signs of ischemia or cardiac symptoms during the low level of exercise, the latter were likely the case. Exercise performance should also be viewed in relation to age and gender as shown in **Fig. 5-6** *(13)*.

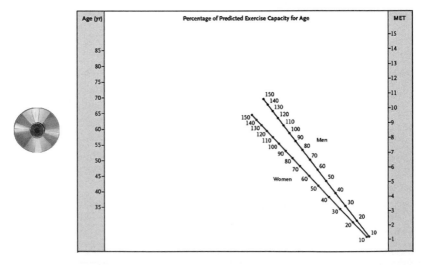

Fig. 5-6. Nomogram showing the percentage of predicted exercise capacity for age in asymptomatic men and women. A line drawn from the patient's age on the lefthand scale to the MET value achieved on the righthand scale will cross the percentage line at the point corresponding to the patient's percentage of predicted exercise capacity for age. (reproduced with permission from ref 13).

Next, one should consider the exercise ECG. For the exercise ECG to be interpretable, the baseline ECG should be normal, without major ST–T changes. Patients on digoxin, or with Wolff–Parkinson–White (WPW) syndrome, are known to have a high percent of false-positive ST-segment responses to exercise. An ischemic ECG response is defined as ≥1 mm horizontal or downsloping ST-segment depression at 0.08 s after the J-point in at least three successive beats.

The results of exercise performance, symptoms, and ECG changes contain important prognostic information. The Duke treadmill score (DTS) incorporates these three variables and is often used as a simple way to categorize patients in low-, intermediate- and high-risk groups after exercise *(14)*. The DTS can be calculated by the following equation or perhaps simpler by the nomogram shown in **Fig. 5-7**.

$$DTS = Exercise\ time(min) - (5 \times maximal\ ST - segment\ depression) - (4 \times angina\ index)$$

(Angina index is derived as follows: 0 = no angina; 1 = non-limiting angina; 2 = exercise-limiting angina).

The DTS typically ranges from –25 to +15. A high-risk score (≤–11) is associated with an average annual mortality of >5%, an intermediate

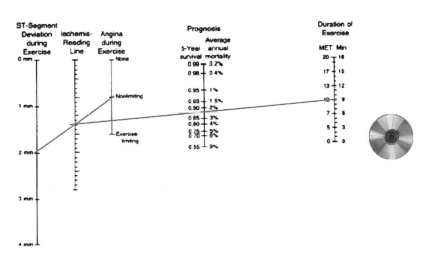

Fig. 5-7. Duke Treadmill score nomogram. Prognosis is determined in five steps: 1. amount of ST segment depression, 2. degree of angina during exercise, 3. connect 1 and 2, find point on ischemia reading line, 4. exercise duration or METs achieved. 5. connect points 4 and 3 and read prognosis on the line in the middle. An example is illustrated by the red lines. (Reproduced with permission from ref 14.)

risk (+45 to −10) is associated with an average annual mortality of 2–3%, and low-risk score (≥ +5) has an average annual mortality of <1%.

Pharmacological Stress

The degree of changes in heart rate and blood pressure during infusion of adenosine or dipyridamole is not a good measure for the degree of hyperemic response achieved and is therefore not of diagnostic significance. Neither are symptoms, in particular chest discomfort, diagnostic of coronary artery disease.

By contrast, ischemic ECG changes, i.e., 1–2 mm of horizontal or downsloping ST-segment depression, during adenosine, dipyridamole, or dobutamine infusion have diagnostic and prognostic significance, even in the absence of myocardial perfusion abnormalities *(15)*.

REFERENCES

1. DePuey GE (ed.) (2006). *Updated Imaging Guidelines for Nuclear Cardiology Procedures 2006*, available at http://www.asnc.org—Menu: "Manage Your Practice": "Guidelines & Standards" (accessed Dec 24, 2006).
2. Ellestad MH (ed.) (1995). *Stress Testing, Principles and Practice*, 4th Edition, FA Davis Co. Philadelphia, PA.
3. Froelicher VF (2000). *Exercise and the Heart*, 4th Edition, WB Saunders Co. Philadelphia, PA.
4. Wackers FJTh (2003). Myocardial perfusion imaging. In Sandler MP, Coleman RE, Patton JA, Wackers FJTh, Gottschalk A (eds), *Diagnostic Nuclear Medicine*, 4th Edition, Lippincott Williams & Wilkins, Philadelphia, PA.
5. Zoghbi GJ, Htay T, Aqel R, Blackmon L, Heo J, Iskandrian AE (2006). Effect of caffeine on ischemia detection by adenosine single-photon emission computed tomography perfusion imaging. *J Am Coll Cardiol* 47:2296–2302.
6. Penell DJ, Maurogeni S, Forbat SM, Karwatowski SO, Underwood SR (1995). Adenosine combined with dynamic exercise for myocardial perfusion imaging. *J Am Coll Cardiol* 25:1300–1309.
7. Samady H, Wackers FJTh, Joska TM, Zaret BL, Jain D (2002). Pharmacologic stress perfusion imaging with adenosine: role of simultaneous low-level treadmill exercise. *J Nucl Cardiol* 9:188–196.
8. Treuth MG, Reyes GA, He ZX, Cwajg E, Mahmarian JJ, Verani MS (2001). Tolerance and diagnostic accuracy of an abbreviated adenosine infusion for myocardial scintigraphy: a randomized, prospective study. *J Nucl Cardiol* 8: 548–554.
9. O'Keefe JH, Bateman TM, Handlin LR, Barnhart CS (1995). Four- versus 6-minute protocol for adenosine thallium-201 single photon emission computed tomography imaging. *Am Heart J* 129:482–487.
10. Ranhosky A, Rawson J (1990). The safety of intravenous dipyridamole thallium myocardial perfusion imaging. *Circulation* 81:1205–1209.
11. Verani MS, Mahmarian JJ, Hixson JB, Boyce TM, Staudacher RA (1990). Diagnosis of coronary artery disease by controlled coronary vasodilation with adenosine and thallium-201 scintigraphy in patients unable to exercise. *Circulation* 82:80–87.

12. Hays JT, Mahmarian JJ, Cochran AJ, Verani MS (1993). Dobutamine thallium-201 tomography for evaluating patients with suspected coronary artery disease unable to undergo exercise or vasodilator pharmacologic stress testing. *J Am Coll Cardiol* 21:1583–1590.
13. Gulati M, Black HR, Shaw LJ, Arnsdorf MF, Bairey Merz CN, Lauer MS, Marwick TH, Pandey DK, Wicklund RH, Thisted RA (2005). The prognostic value of a nomogram for exercise capacity in women. *New Engl J Med* 353:468–475.
14. Mark DB, Hlatky MA, Harrell FE, Lee KL, Califf RM, Pryor DB (1987). Exercise treadmill score for predicting prognosis in coronary artery disease. *Ann Intern Med* 106:793–800.
15. Abbot BG, Afshar M, Berger AK, Wackers FJTh (2003). Prognostic significance of ischemic electrocardiographic changes during adenosine infusion in patients with normal myocardial perfusion imaging. *J Nucl Cardiol* 10:9–16.

6 SPECT Myocardial Perfusion Imaging
Acquisition and Processing Protocols

In view of the diversity of commercially available gamma camera systems, it is difficult to incorporate every acquisition/processing parameter adequately in a few simple charts. Single-headed systems have different acquisition parameters than triple-headed systems, and both are different from dual-headed systems. One must also consider the radiopharmaceutical(s) and imaging protocols one intends to use. Acquisition parameters will vary depending on these variables. This chapter highlights the following:

- Acquisition parameters
- Processing parameters

Key Words: Acquisition SPECT myocardial perfusion images (details), Processing SPECT myocardial perfusion images (details), Radiation Units and conversion, Imaging agents, Imaging protocols, Adjusting dose for weight, Attenuation correction, Quantification myocardial perfusion, Quantification ventricular function, Imaging worksheet.

Once the purchase of a gamma camera has been made, it is advisable that a professional application specialist visits the laboratory to train the technical staff in applying the vendor-recommended acquisition and processing protocols. This is crucial for optimal results.

It has become convention in clinical nuclear cardiology practice to refer to the amount of injected radioactivity as "dose." This is not correct. In radiation physics, "dose" refers to the absorbed radiation by the body and is measured as Rad or Gray (Gy), or as "dose equivalent" and expressed as Rem or Sievert (Sv). Activity is measured as Curie (Ci) or Becquerel (Bq).

From: *Contemporary Cardiology: Nuclear Cardiology, The Basics*
By: F. J. Th. Wackers, W. Bruni, and B. L. Zaret © Humana Press Inc., Totowa, NJ

Table 6-1
Radiation Units and Conversions

Quantity	Unit	New unit (Système International)
Radiation exposure	Roentgen (R)	Coulomb/kg
Absorbed dose	Rad	Gray (Gy)
Dose equivalent	Rem[a]	Sievert (Sv)
Radioactivity	Curie (Ci)	Becquerel (Bq)
Effective dose equivalent = sum of external doses and weighted internal organ doses		

Conversions

$1\,R = 1000\,mR$
$1\,Rad = 1000\,mRad$
$1\,Rad = 0.01\,Gy$
$1\,Rem = 1000\,mRem$
$1\,Rem = 10\,mSv$
$1\,mRem = 0.1\,mSv$
$1\,Gy = 100\,Rad$
$1\,Sv = 100\,Rem$
$1\,Sv = 1\,Gy \times$ Quality Factor

$1\,Ci = 37,000,000,000\,Bq$
$1\,mCi = 37\,MBq$
$1\,Bq = 1$ disintegrations/s (60 disintegrations/m)
$1\,Bq = 2.7 \times 10^{-11}$ disintegrations/s
$1\,Ci = 3.7 \times 10^{10}$ disintegrations/s
$1\,mCi = 3.7 \times 10^{7}$ disintegrations/s $(2.22 \times 10^{9}\,dpm)$
$1\,\mu Ci = 3.7 \times 10^{4}$ disintegrations/s

[a]Rem = roentgen equivalent man.

For clarity, we will continue to use the word "dose" interchangeable with injected activity. Table 6-1 lists radiation units and their conversions.

STRESS–REST MYOCARDIAL PERFUSION IMAGING AGENTS

The radiotracers most commonly used for stress–rest myocardial perfusion imaging are listed in Table 6-2. The basic SPECT imaging protocols are illustrated in **Figs. 6-1** and **6-2**.

Table 6-2
Radiotracers for Stress Myocardial Perfusion Imaging

Radiotracer	Energy	Half-life	Redistribution
Tl-201	80 keV	74 h	Yes
Tc-99m sestamibi	140 keV	6 h	No
Tc-99m tetrofosmin	140 keV	6 h	No
Rb-82	511 keV	72 s	n.a.

Tl-201 is a monovalent potassium analogue that crosses the cell myocytes' cell membrane using the sodium/potassium pump. Tl-201 enters and washes out continuously from the myocytes, which is responsible for the redistribution phenomenon. The initial myocardial uptake of Tl-201 is in proportion to regional myocardial blood flow, whereas late Tl-201 distribution reflects the intracellular potassium pool. The first-pass myocardial extraction fraction of Tl-201 is relatively high at 85%.

Tc-99m-labeled agents such as sestamibi and tetrofosmin are relatively similar. They are lipid-soluble cationic compounds. The first-pass extraction of sestamibi is less than that of Tl-201, whereas the extraction fraction of tetrofosmin is less than that of sestamibi.

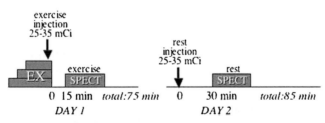

Two-Day Tc-99m-Agent Protocol

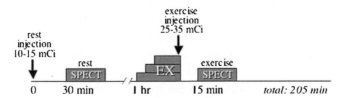

One-Day Tc-99m-Agent Protocol

Fig. 6-1. Schematic representation of the sequence and timing a two-day and one-day Tc-99m-agent imaging protocol.

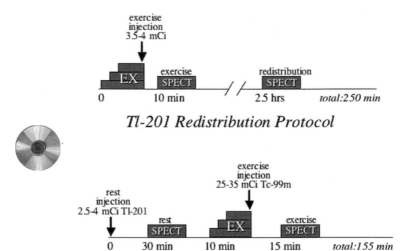

Tl-201 Redistribution Protocol

Dual Isotope (Tl-201/Tc-99m) Protocol

Fig. 6-2. Schematic representation of the sequence and timing of a Thallium-201 (Tl-201) exercise-redistribution and a dual isotope imaging protocol.

The initial myocardial uptake of both compounds is in proportion to regional myocardial blood flow, and intracellular retention depends on mitochondrial transmembrane energy potential. Myocardial washout and redistribution of sestamibi and tetrofosmin are negligible.

Rubidium-82 (Rb-82) is a positron emitter and used for PET myocardial perfusion imaging. Similar to Tl-201, Rb-82 is a potassium analogue with high first-pass extraction fraction. Redistribution of Rb-82 is negligible because of the short half-life of the tracer.

ACQUISITION PARAMETERS

Nuclear cardiology tests are to be performed under general physician supervision. That is, the medical director is responsible on a ongoing basis for the training of non-physician personnel who actually perform the diagnostic procedures, for protocols and policies, and for the appropriate maintenance of necessary equipment and supplies (see pg 22).

All SPECT acquisition parameters listed in Table 6-3 and following tables are based on *Imaging Guidelines for Nuclear Cardiology Procedures (1)*. Additional information on accepted standards for performing myocardial perfusion imaging can be found in the SNM Procedure Guidelines for Myocardial Perfusion Imaging *(2)*. A review of clinical indications for radionuclide myocardial perfusion imaging can be found in the 2003 ACC/AHA/ASNC *Guidelines for Clinical Use of Cardiac Radionuclide Imaging (3)*.

Table 6-3
Acquisition Parameters

	Tc-99m	Tl-201
Activity (dose)	10–30 mCi	3.5–4.5 mCi
Collimator	High-resolution parallel-hole	Low-energy all-purpose parallel-hole
Matrix	64 × 64	64 × 64
Peak	140 keV 20% centered	78 keV 30% centered
Gating	16 or 8 frames/cycle	8 frames/cycle
Number of projections	60–64	32
Orbit	180°	180°
Orbit type	Circular	Circular
Acquisition type	Step and shoot or continuous	Step and shoot or continuous
Pixel size	6.4 ± 0.2 mm	6.4 ± 0.2 mm
Time/projection	25 s for low doses and 20 s for high doses	40 s (at least)
Attenuation correction	Sealed sources or CT	Sealed sources or CT

Two-day or One-day Protocols

Tl-201 stress–redistribution imaging is always 1-day protocol. Post-stress imaging is performed following one single injection of radiopharmaceutical during stress and after several hours of delay: redistribution imaging (**Fig. 6-2**). The dual-isotope imaging protocol is also a 1-day protocol (**Fig. 6-2**).

For imaging with Tc-99m-labeled myocardial perfusion imaging agents, two separate injections are required. One injection during stress and one at rest. Ideally, stress and rest imaging with Tc-99m-labeled agents are performed on two different days, the 2-day protocol (**Fig. 6-1**). One can then administer for each imaging session the maximally allowed amount of radioactivity (30–40 mCi/day). Thus, images be expected to be of optimal quality, i.e., good count density and not contaminated with "shine-through" previously administered radioactivity. For the 1-day imaging protocol, the total dose must be divided over two injections: a low dose first and a high dose later. A minimally contaminated second image is obtained by acquiring the first image after injection of about 1/4 of the total dose, i.e., 10–15 mCi, the second image after injection of 3/4 of the total dose, i.e., 30–35 mCi (**Fig. 6-1**).

Time Interval Between First and Second Injection

For the 1-day imaging protocol, either stress or rest injection/ imaging may be performed first. As indicated in Table 2-3, the conventional time interval between the first injection and second injection is 1h to allow for decay of activity of the first injection. The 2006 updated ASNC imaging guidelines suggest that with the distribution of the total amount of activity as 1/4 for first injection and 3/4 for second injection, this time interval is not critical and that the second injection may be administered without delay after the first imaging session is finished.

Injected Activity (Dose)

With the increasing prevalence of obesity among patients referred to the nuclear cardiology laboratories, it has become more and more difficult to acquire optimal quality SPECT images. It is prudent to institute weight limits for the choice of imaging agents, Tl-201 or Tc-99m agents, and imaging protocols, 1-day or 2-day protocols (Table 6-4). In obese patients, imaging with Tc-99m agents is preferred over imaging with Tl-201, and in the very obese patients, a 2-day protocol is preferred over the 1-day protocol.

When a patient is markedly obese, even the standard dose of 25 mCi per day of a Tc-99m agent may not be adequate. In these obese patients, the dose can be adjusted according to the patient's weight. It is advisable to check with the RSO about such upward dose adjustments. Table 6-5 summarizes examples of dose adjustments on the basis of weight used in our laboratory. The weight limits are based on practical experience. Because in females more of the increased weight is generally in the upper body, the adjusted doses are higher in females than in males.

Table 6-4
Suggested Weight Limits for Selecting Appropriate Imaging Agents and Protocols

Male	*Female*	*Agent/Protocol*
≤225 lb (102 kg)	≤150 lb(68 kg)	Tl-201 or Tc-99m agent 1-day or 2-day protocol
226–275 lb (103–124 kg)	151–175 lb (69–79 kg)	Only Tc-99m agent 1-day or 2-day protocol
>276 lb(125 kg)	>176 lb(80 kg)	Only Tc-99m agent Only 2-day protocol

Table 6-5
Suggested Dose Adjustment of Tl-201 and Tc-99m-Labeled Agents on
the Basis of Body Weight or Chest Circumference

	Male mCi	Female mCi
Tl-201		
Weight (lbs)		
125–150 lb (56–68 kg)	3.0	4.0
151–175 lb (69–79 kg)	3.5	4.5[a]
176–200 lb (80–90 kg)	4.0	4.5[a]
201–225 lb (91–102 kg)	4.5	4.5[a]
> 226 lb(103 kg)	4.5[a]	4.5[a]
Chest circumference		
≤ 44 in(112 cm)	3.5	3.5
45–48 in (113–122 cm)	4.0	4.0
> 48 cm(123 cm)	4.5[a]	4.5[a]
Tc-99m-labeled agents (2-day protocol, daily dose)		
Weight		
< 175 – 200 lb(79–90 kg)	25	30
201–250 lb (91–113 kg)	25	30
251–275 lb (114–124 kg)	25	35[a]
276–300 lb (125–136 kg)	30	40[a]
301–325 lb (137–147 kg)	35[a]	40[a]
326–350 lb (148–159 kg)	40[a]	40[a]

[a] It may be advisable to increase acquisition time per stop as well.

In addition to adjusting the injected activity, one may also increase acquisition time per stop to improve image quality.

Nevertheless, in some obese patients, it is very difficult to acquire diagnostic quality images with single-photon agents and PET imaging may be the only solution.

Deviation from Standard Radiopharmaceutical Dosing

It is recommended that all deviations from the standard dosing are discussed with the RSO and/or medical director. If it appears to be desirable to inject a greater than standard amount of activity due to obesity, the deviation should be approved by the RSO as appropriate. Document this decision also on the patient's imaging worksheet. This may be useful when the patient comes back in the future for repeat imaging procedures.

Doses for pediatric patients should also be discussed with the RSO. A patient under 18 years of age would have a dose adjusted with the following formula:

$$\frac{\text{Patient weight in lb} \times \text{standard dose (mCi)}}{150\,\text{lb}} = \text{pediatric dose (mCi)}$$

Collimator

Low-energy high-resolution (LEHR) collimators provide better resolution but have reduced sensitivity. Therefore, they are usually used with the Tc-99m-labeled agents, which yield higher count rates. Low-energy-all-purpose (LEAP) collimators provide more sensitivity and are routinely used to imaging with Tl-201.

When performing dual-isotope studies, one should use the same collimator for both the rest Tl-201 and the stress Tc-99m study. The high-resolution collimator is preferred in this circumstance.

Note: Collimator sensitivity = counts/min/μCi. For Tc-99m, the sensitivity of a LEHR collimator is 220–280 cpm/μCi and of a LEAP collimator 280–350 cpm/μCi.

Matrix

A 64×64 matrix is standard for SPECT imaging. A 128×128 matrix also can be used; however, this substantially increases the required computer disk storage space. In addition, processing time will increase significantly.

ECG Gating

CHEST ELECTRODES

For ECG gating, the computer should receive a clear R-wave signal. Usually, three electrodes are used: right and left subclavicular and one on the lateral lower chest, either right or left. If this conventional electrode placement does not work, the electrodes should be moved around to a position that results in a more distinct R-wave. (Make sure that in patients with abnormal ECG or peaked T-waves no double signal is detected.)

NUMBER OF FRAMES PER R-R CYCLE

In many laboratories, the acquisition of 16 frames/cycle is presently the standard acquisition mode. The lower limit of normal left ventricular ejection fraction (LVEF) is 0.50. Acquisition of 8 frames/cycle is an acceptable option for gated SPECT and requires less hard drive and archiving space and can be processed on older computers. However, it should be realized that LVEF is systematically underestimated by about 0.05 because of suboptimal temporal resolution.

NUMBER OF PROJECTIONS

When performing high-resolution studies with Tc-99m perfusion agents, it is recommended acquiring 60–64 projections over a 180° arc. Lower resolution studies acquired with Tl-201 need only 32 projections.

It should be noted that the number of recommended projections might vary from this, depending on the manufacturer and the number of camera heads on the system. Adherence to the standardized number of projections is an important element for a successful application for ICANL accreditation.

ORBIT

A circular orbit is the most commonly used orbit. This orbit maintains the camera head at a fixed distance from the patient. Noncircular or elliptical orbits should be used with caution, because they may create artifacts due to varying depth resolution resulting from varying detector–heart distance.

In the ASNC Guidelines for cardiac SPECT image acquisition, acquisition with 180° orbits is recommended (45° RAO to 45° LPO), and a 360° orbit is optional. The reason for this is that acquisition with a 180° orbit avoids the degrading effects of scatter and attenuation from the posterior projections. This is especially relevant when low-energy Tl-201 imaging is performed.

However, using Tc-99m agents, a 180° acquisition orbit may create in some patients image distortion and inhomogeneity in the most apical short axis slices. In our experience, these artifacts can be avoided by acquiring SPECT images with a 360° orbit.

ACQUISITION MODE

The step-and-shoot acquisition mode is most commonly used and is standard because it allows for ECG-gated acquisition. During the step-and-shoot mode, the camera moves to a position, stops and acquires an image for a set time, and then moves on to the next angle. No image acquisition occurs during the motion of the camera. In continuous acquisition mode, the camera acquires image data constantly while moving slowly along the orbit. This acquisition mode at the present time on some systems generally does not allow for ECG-gated acquisition. Some systems now have a continuous step-and-shoot mode that provides the benefits of both acquisition types.

Pixel Size

A 6.4 ± 0.2-mm pixel size for a 64×64 matrix provides adequate image resolution and is considered standard.

Time Intervals

The time intervals from radiopharmaceutical injection to start of imaging for different imaging agents, after exercise and pharmacological stress, and at rest are summarized in Table 6-6.

Time per Projection

The time per projection must be long enough to obtain sufficient counts for producing images of optimal quality. Reducing the time per projection too much will result in low-count density and suboptimal image quality. The time per projection depends on the number of projections acquired over the orbit. For Tc-99m-labeled agents, the standard time per stop is 25 s for low dose and 20 s for high dose. For Tl-201 SPECT, the time per stop should be at least 40 s. However, depending on count density and the patient's weight, it may have to be as long as 60 s. The limiting factor is the amount of time that one can expect a patient to lie immobile on the imaging table. Generally, total imaging time should not exceed 20 min. The significant advantage of multi-headed camera systems is that image data are acquired simultaneously at different angles, thus maximizing image quality (= counts) within less time. Adherence to above standardized times per projection is an important element for a successful application for ICANL accreditation.

Attenuation Correction Map

Attenuation correction (AC) technology is very different from standard emission myocardial perfusion imaging. Because different camera systems use different techniques to perform SPECT AC, it is important to refer and adhere to optimized acquisition parameters as

Table 6-6
Time Intervals from Injection of Radiopharmaceutical to the Start of Imaging

	Exercise	Pharmacological stress	Rest
Tl-201	<10 min	<10 min	30 min
Tc-99m agent	15 min	45 min	45 min

defined by the manufacturer. An applications specialist should visit the imaging facility and train the technical staff on-site on proper use of AC.

It is well recognized that SPECT images should not only be corrected for non-uniform tissue attenuation but also for scatter- and depth-dependent resolution.

Not all vendors apply all three corrections.

AC of SPECT myocardial perfusion images has presently matured and is now routinely used in many laboratories.

The basic concept of AC involves the following:

1. Acquisition of transmission images of the thorax using external photon source(s).
2. Generation of non-uniform tissue attenuation maps.
3. Mathematical correction on a pixel-by-pixel basis of cardiac emission images on the basis of the non-uniform attenuation maps.

Currently two general methodologies are available for the acquisition of non-uniform tissue attenuation maps.

External Sealed Sources. This methodology makes use of fixed or moving external radioactive sources in shielded rod-shaped containers that can be opened and closed. These rods are mounted on standard collimated SPECT imaging equipment in different configurations (**Fig. 6-3**). The most commonly used external source is Gadolinium-153 (Gd-153), but other radioisotopes may be used as well (see Table 6-7). This methodology is often referred to as sealed-source or scanning line sources.

X-ray Computerized Tomography (CT). The second methodology uses an X-ray tube in conjunction with a one- or four-slice CT scanner. This CT device is usually incorporated in the gantry of a conventional multiple detector head SPECT camera (**Fig. 6-4**).

Advantages and disadvantages of the two methodologies are listed in Table 6-8. An important advantage of external sealed radioisotope transmission sources is that acquisition of transmission and emission images is performed *simultaneously* and that misregistration is not an issue. By contrast, because X-ray CT is acquired after SPECT emission imaging is completed, misalignment, or registration of emission and transmission images, may occur because a patient may be more inclined to move during the prolonged imaging time. Using CT imaging with SPECT, there is a discrepancy in technical image quality. The CT images are of higher spatial resolution than the blurred low-resolution SPECT emission images and may therefore not align or register perfectly well. When CT transmission maps and SPECT images are

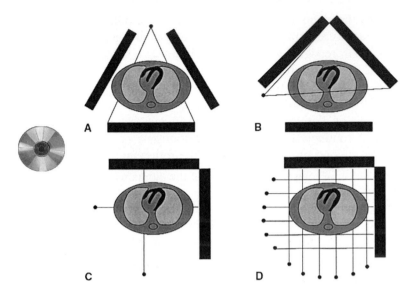

Fig. 6-3. Various configurations for SPECT attenuation correction devices using sealed isotopic transmission sources. The radioactive transmission source(s) are indicated by the black dots. (A) Fixed transmission source opposite a fan-beam collimator, (B) Off-axis fixed source, (C) Two scanning (moving) line sources with windowed opposite parallel collimators, (D) Array of multiple fixed line sources. (Reproduced with permission from ref. 8).

misregistered, special software is needed to move images relative to each other to optimize alignment. Misregistration of attenuation maps and emission images may create artifactual defects depending on the degree and direction of misregistration (see also Chapter 16 p. 255).

An important drawback of external radioisotope sources is the decrease of the strength of the transmission source over time due to radioactive decay. The cost of renewal of the sealed source is not negligible.

Table 6-7
External Radioactive Sources Used for Attenuation Correction

Source	keV	Half-life
Gd-153	99, 103	242 days
Co-57	122	270 days
Am-241	59	458 years
Ba-133	356, 382	10.7 years
Tc-99m	140	6 h

Am, americium; Ba, barium; Co, cobalt; Gd, gadolinium; Tc, technetium.

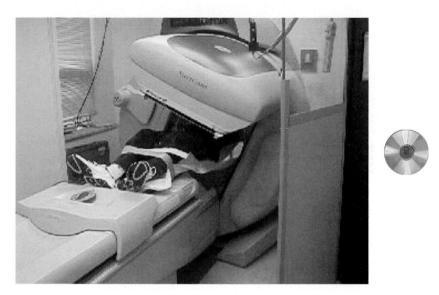

Fig. 6-4. Hybrid SPECT-CT camera (*movie*). After emission SPECT imaging is completed a 1- or 4-slice CT scan is acquired to generate transmission data.

Table 6-8
Advantage and Disadvantages of Radioactive Sealed Sources Versus X-ray CT for Acquisition of Attenuation Maps

	Sealed source	*X-ray CT*
Acquisition transmission/ emission	Simultaneous	Sequential
Misregistration attenuation map	No	Relatively frequent
Photon flux	Marginal	High
Scatter/crosstalk	High	Low
Source renewed regularly	Yes	No
Acquisition time	Duration of SPECT	3–5 min extra
Truncation	Possible	No
Erroneous values due GI activity	Possible	No

GI, gastrointestinal.

Table 6-9
Acquisition and Processing QC for Attenuation Correction with Sealed Sources

Count density, quality attenuation map
Truncation
Appropriate ECG gating
Appropriate photopeak, windows (primary, scatter, and crosstalk)
Patient motion
Transmission scan uniformity

Acquisition Protocols with AC

SEALED SOURCES

Acquisition of transmission and emission data is started simultaneously. A fixed line source is usually used in conjunction with a triple-head camera system. One of the three detector heads, equipped with a converging collimator, opposite the fixed source exclusively acquires transmission image data. Because of the limited FOV, truncation may occur. The other two detector heads, equipped with parallel-hole collimators, acquire emission data as usual.

For the moving or scanning line source(s), parallel-hole collimators are used. The detector head opposite the line source, or rod, is used for the acquisition of both transmission and emission image data. As the rod moves along, a row of pixels directly opposite the line source is electronically windowed for the transmission peak and acquires transmission data, and then, as the rod moves on, the pixels are re-windowed to acquire emission-imaging data. No additional imaging time is required using sealed sources. Table 6-9 lists acquisition and processing QC issues for AC with sealed sources.

X-RAY CT

SPECT emission images are acquired in the usual manner, using standard setup and acquisition times. Immediately after the SPECT emission imaging is completed, acquisition with X-ray CT is started. Depending on the number of slices acquired, i.e., one or four, CT imaging may require 5 to 2 additional minutes. QC using CT AC should focus mainly on correct alignment of emission and CT images (see also Chapter 16 under "attenuation correction errors").

PROCESSING PARAMETERS

Processing parameters are listed in Table 6-10. The following subsections are comments on the individual parameters listed.

Table 6-10
Processing Parameters

Filtering	Filtered back projection is standard; cutoffs and frequencies arc vendor dependent
Motion correction	After applying motion-correction program, slices must be evaluated for motion artifacts. Many motion-correction programs are not adequate
Reconstruction	Filtered back projection is standard; iterative reconstruction is an option. Iterative reconstruction is standard for attenuation-correction devices. After reconstruction tomographic slices are reoriented into vertical and horizontal long axis and short axis planes
Slice alignment	Aligning stress slices to the corresponding rest slices
Normalizing slices	Scaling of images so the heart is visualized optimally
Attenuation correction	Acquisition of transmission map for correction of non-uniform tissue attenuation using sealed sources or X-ray CT. Different approaches by different vendors
Quantification	Based on measuring count density of each tomographic slice
Normal database	Allows extent and severity of defect to be calculated
Left ventricular ejection fraction	Automated estimate of myocardial systolic function
Left ventricular volume	The software that computes ejection fraction also estimates left ventricular end diastolic and end systolic volumes
Archiving	Raw and processed data

Filtering

The purpose of image filters is to remove noise and blur before and after back projection of raw SPECT data. The standard filter for SPECT imaging is the Butterworth filter. The optimal order and cutoff of this filter are different for each vendor (**Fig. 6-5**). Excellent reviews about filters are available in the works of Zubal *(4)* and Hanson *(5–7)*.

Motion Correction

Motion on SPECT studies can be detected in a number of ways. Some systems provide the option of displaying a "sinogram." Breaks or irregularities in the sinogram indicate motion. This display method

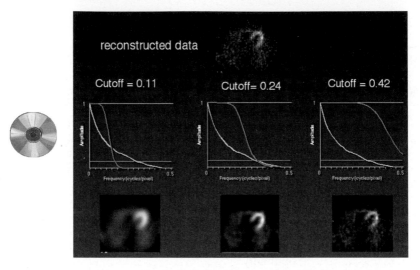

Fig. 6-5. The effect of different cut-offs for a low-pass Butterworth filter is well illustrated in this figure. The preferred cutoff for this particular image is 0.24. A lower low cut-off, e.g. 0.11, results in a markedly blurred image with loss of detail. A higher cut-off value, e.g. 0.42, results in a noisy image. It is recommended to experiment with various filter cutoff values using equipment in the laboratory to appreciate the differential effect of filters on image quality.

is not always easy to interpret. Sinograms do not show horizontal motion but only vertical or Y-axis motion.

A simple, and more commonly used method for detecting patient motion, involves inspection of the cine display of all planar projection images, also known as rotating images. This simple method allows for the detection of both X-axis and Y-axis motion.

If motion is detected, a motion correction program can be applied. Each vendor may have a slightly different approach to motion correction. One should consult with the vendor for instructions on how to run the program. Motion-corrected cine should be viewed to determine if the motion was corrected. Under certain conditions, the correction program may not work, and in some instances, it may create even worse artifacts. If the program does not correct motion adequately, the entire imaging study should be repeated. Even if it appears that the program has corrected the motion on cine display, the reconstructed slices should be inspected for motion artifacts. Typical motion artifacts are gaps at the apex of the long axis slices and breaks in the short axis slices to make them look disjointed. See chapter 16 for examples.

Note that some motion correction programs are very specific and work only on certain types of acquisition data. For instance, not all programs are capable of correcting ECG-gated image data and some correct only 180° acquisition data and not 360° acquisition data.

Reconstruction

The traditional method for reconstruction of SPECT images is (filtered) back projection. A number of the assumptions for back projection are in fact incorrect, such as absence of attenuation, scatter, and infinite number of projections. Nevertheless, an extensive clinical experience is based on this reconstruction method. With the introduction of non-uniform tissue AC, iterative reconstruction has gained greater acceptance. These algorithms are based on more realistic assumptions with regard to radionuclide images and are able to incorporate attenuation, scatter, and varying depth resolution. Initially, there was the practical problem that considerable more computing power was required. However, presently computer speed no longer is an important issue. Nevertheless, no clinical study has as yet proven that iterative reconstruction is superior to filtered back projection in patient imaging. Iterative reconstruction is optional for conventional SPECT imaging but must be used for AC.

For display of tomographic slices of the heart, the reconstructed data are reoriented according to the three anatomical axes of the patient's heart. Horizontal long axis, vertical long axis, and short axis slices are created. It is important that stress and rest slices are reconstructed in identical manner in order to allow for comparison of the same myocardial segments (**Fig. 6-6**).

Slice Alignment

The stress and rest slices must be aligned or matched. The first apical slice of the stress study must match the first apical slice of the rest study and continue on through to the last basal slice. If the slices are misaligned, the study may be misinterpreted.

Normalizing Slices

This step is particularly important when imaging with the Tc-99m-labeled agents. Often, particularly after pharmacological stress, liver or bowel, and not the heart, is the organ with the greatest activity. The heart is then hardly visible unless images are scaled properly to increase the intensity of the heart image.

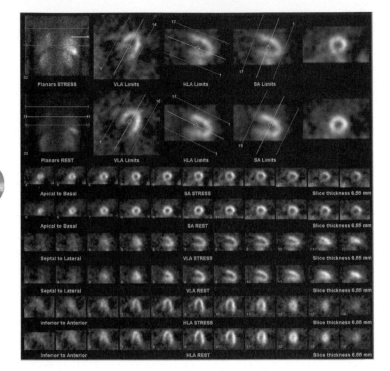

Fig. 6-6. Computer screen capture of the reorientation of reconstructed tomographic slices to the anatomical axis of the heart. The boundaries of the window of reconstruction are indicated by red lines. The green lines indicate the angles of tomographic slicing for the vertical long axis (VLA), horizontal long axis (HLA), and the short axis (SA).

Attenuation Correction, Processing

It is recommended that the myocardial perfusion image data be processed (and displayed) without and with AC. The processing is largely automated. It is very important to refer and adhere to optimized processing parameters defined by the manufacturer. An applications specialist should visit the imaging facility and train the technical staff on-site on proper use of AC. For reconstruction of attenuation corrected image data, iterative reconstruction must be used. While attenuation-corrected images are often very helpful, the technology is demanding *(8)*. Attenuation-corrected images may at times contain artifacts or overcorrections. In particular with X-ray CT AC, an important aspect of QC is the inspection of fused emission and CT images and to identify misregistration or motion (**Figs. 6-7** and **6-8**). Dedicated software exists that allows for realignment of emission and transmission images by moving images in three directions until best alignment is achieved. After accurate co-registration is ensured, the CT image is blurred to generate an attenuation map that matches the resolution of the SPECT emission image (**Fig. 6-9**).

Quantification Relative Radiotracer Uptake

The relative distribution of a radiopharmaceutical in reconstructed myocardial slices can be quantified using a number of commercially available software packages (see Chapter 10). Regional relative radiotracer uptake is compared with regional lower limits of normal uptake. For accurate and reproducible quantitative results, it is important that the apical and basal slices are chosen appropriately in accordance with the vendor's manual.

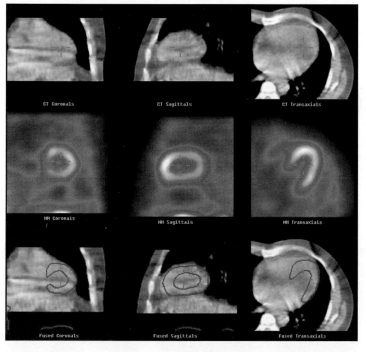

Fig. 6-7. Fusion images for quality control of SPECT-CT. Top: 4-slice CT images for creation of transmission map in (from left to right) coronal, sagittal and transaxial planes. Middle: Tc-99m-tetrofosmin emission images in the same tomographic planes. Bottom: Fusion of transmission and emission images to verify correct coregistration. Quality control is facilitated by automatically generated isocount contours of the emission images. These contours fit well within the boundaries of the heart on the CT scan. In case of misregistration, dedicated software makes it possible to shift the images relative to each other until corrected aligned is achieved.

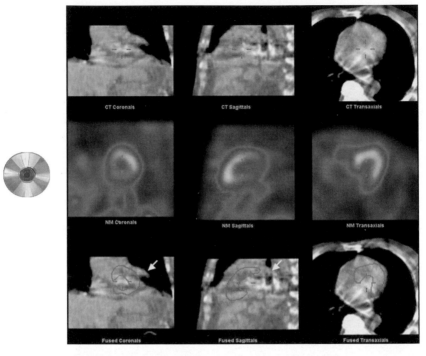

Fig. 6-8. Fusion image of SPECT-CT. The format is the same as in Fig. 6-7. The patient moved during the acquisition of the CT image. A spike-like (arrow) artifact is visible on the coronal and sagittal CT slices .

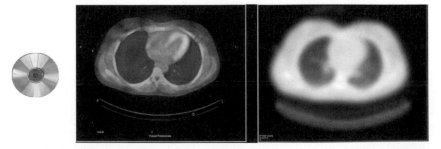

Fig. 6-9. Left: Fusion image of 4-slice CT scan and Tc-99m tetrofosmin SPECT image. Right: blurred CT attenuation map to be used for attenuation correction of SPECT image.

Normal Database

A normal database is generated from images of normal subjects with low (< 3%) likelihood of coronary artery disease, based on age, gender, absence of symptoms and risk factors, and normal exercise ECG. From the relative count distribution on images of these normal subjects, a lower limit of normal count distribution, i.e., mean minus 2 standard deviations, can be derived.

Left Ventricular Ejection Fraction

A number of commercially available software packages exist for calculation of LVEF from ECG-gated SPECT images. Accurate assessment of LVEF depends on stable heart rate, adequate counts, and good image quality. One has the option of acquiring a gated SPECT study with either 16 or 8 frames per R-R cycle. The lower limit of normal LVEF using a 16-frame study is higher (0.50) than for a 8-frame study (0.45) *(9)*. Intense non-cardiac activity and small hearts may render calculation of LVEF inaccurate *(10)*.

Left Ventricular Volumes

Left ventricular volumes are estimated from the endocardial boundaries used for calculation of ejection fraction. End diastolic and end systolic volumes derived from ECG-gated SPECT studies often appear to be relatively small. Nevertheless, several studies have shown good correlations with volumes derived by other modalities *(11)*. Left ventricular volumes can be used to calculate transient post-stress left ventricular dilation (transient ischemic dilation or TID).

Archiving

All raw image data should be archived daily. It is recommended to archive processed and quantified data for comparison with future studies.

TECHNOLOGIST'S WORKSHEETS

Worksheets are useful for documentation of the details of an imaging procedure, such as patient body habitus, dose, time of injection, time of imaging, and other details.

Sample Technologist's Worksheet

Below is a sample of the worksheet for myocardial perfusion imaging used in our laboratory.

SPECT MYOCARDIAL PERFUSION WORKSHEET

Patient Name _____

     Unit # _____   Weight _____   Height _____

     Floor _____   Chest _____   Cup _____

    One Day ☐   Two Day ☐   Camera _____

STRESS IMAGING	REST IMAGING
Date _____	Date _____
☐ Exercise ☐ Adenosine ☐ Aden/Ex Other _____	☐ Rest ☐ Redist
MIBI _____ mCi Initials: _____ TI-201 _____ mCi Other _____ _____ mCi	MIBI _____ mCi Initials: _____ TI-201 _____ mCi Other _____ _____ mCi

Inject Time: _____
      TT: _____
	Inject Time: _____
	      TT: _____

_____ SPECT Time _____ Radius _____ Table Height _____ sec/stop _____ GATED	_____ SPECT Time _____ Radius _____ Table Height _____ sec/stop _____ GATED
PLANARS 5 min TIME Angle _____ LATS (0)_____ _____ LATD (90)_____	PLANARS 5 min TIME Angle _____ LATS (0)_____ _____ LATD (90)_____
DEFECT SCORE	**DEFECT SCORE**
__ __ __ __ __ Api Mid Bas Apx Gbl	__ __ __ __ __ Api Mid Bas Apx Gbl
WLCQ EF: _____ QGS (opt.): _____	WLCQ EF: _____ QGS (opt.): _____
Technologist _____	Technologist _____

COMMENTS:

REFERENCES

1. DePuey GE (2006). *Imaging Guidelines for Nuclear Cardiology Procedures*, available at http://www.asnc.org—Menu: "Manage Your Practice": "Guidelines and Standards" (accessed February 2007).
2. Society of Nuclear Medicine Procedure Guidelines for Myocardial Perfusion Imaging (2002). Available at http://www.snm.org—Menu: "Practice Management": "Procedure Guidelines"; "Myocardial Perfusion Imaging 3.0" (accessed December 2006).
3. *Guidelines for Clinical Use of Cardiac Radionuclide Imaging* (2003). Available at http://www.acc.org—Menu: "Quality and Science": "Clinical Statements/Guidelines"; "Imaging, Cardiac": "Cardiac Radionuclide Imaging." In ACC/AHA/ASNC *Guidelines for Clinical Use of Cardiac Radionuclide Imaging* (accessed December 2006).
4. Zubal IG, Wisniewski G (1997). Understanding Fourier space and filter selection. *J Nucl Cardiol* 4:234–243.
5. Hanson CL (2002). Digital image processing for clinicians, part I. Basics of image formation. *J Nucl Cardiol* 9:343–349.

6. Hanson CL (2002). Digital image processing for clinicians, part II. Filtering. *J Nucl Cardiol* 9:429–437.
7. Hanson CL (2002). Digital image processing for clinicians, part III. SPECT reconstruction. *J Nucl Cardiol* 9:542–549.
8. Hendel RC, Corbett JR, Cullom J, DePucy EG, Garcia EV (2002). The value and practice of attenuation correction for myocardial perfusion imaging: a joint position statement from the American Society of Nuclear Cardiology. *J Nucl Cardiol* 9:135–143.
9. Germano G, Kiat H, Kavanagh PB, Moriel M, Mazzanti M, Su HT, VanTrain KF, Berman DS. Automatic quantification of ejection fraction from gated myocardial perfusion SPECT. *J Nucl Med* 36:2138–2147.
10. Vallejo E, Dione DP, Sinusas AJ, Wackers FJTh (2000). Assessment of left ventricular ejection fraction with quantitative gated SPECT: accuracy and correlation with first-pass radionuclide angiography. *J Nucl Med* 7:461–470.
11. Iskandrian AE, Germano G, VanDecker W, Ogilby JD, Wolf N, Mintz R, Berman DS (1998). Validation of left ventricular volume measurements by gated SPECT 99m Tc-labeled sestamibi imaging. *J Nucl Cardiol* 5:574–578.

7 Planar Myocardial Perfusion Imaging
Acquisition and Processing Protocols

Although the use of planar myocardial perfusion imaging has decreased drastically in the last 10 years, it is not obsolete and some patients can be imaged only using the planar imaging technique. These are patients with claustrophobia, patients who are too heavy for the SPECT imaging table, and patients who cannot remain immobile on the imaging table for an extended period of time. For extremely obese patients, the regular imaging table can be removed and the patients can be imaged lying on a stretcher or even in their hospital bed. When needed, planar imaging can be performed also with the patient sitting in upright position.

Key Words: Acquisition planar myocardial perfusion images (details), Processing planar myocardial perfusion images (details), Patient positioning.

When performed with optimal technique and attention to details, planar imaging can result in good-quality myocardial perfusion images and diagnostic information that approaches that of SPECT imaging. A substantial portion of the literature on radionuclide myocardial perfusion imaging until the early 1990s is based on with planar imaging.

All acquisition parameters listed in the following tables are based on the *Imaging Guidelines for Nuclear Cardiology Procedures (1)*.

PLANAR MYOCARDIAL PERFUSION IMAGING

Table 7-1 lists the acquisition parameters for planar imaging.

From: *Contemporary Cardiology: Nuclear Cardiology, The Basics*
By: F. J. Th. Wackers, W. Bruni, and B. L. Zaret © Humana Press Inc., Totowa, NJ

Table 7-1
Acquisition Parameters for Planar Imaging

	Tc-99m	Tl-201
Activity	10–30 mCi	3.5–4.5 mCi
Collimator	High resolution	Low energy, medium resolution
Zoom	No zoom 10 inch FOV or 1.2–1.5 zoom LFOV	No zoom 10 inch FOV or 1.2–1.5 zoom LFOV
Matrix	128 × 128	128 × 128
Peak	140 keV 20% centered	78 keV 30% centered
Gating	8 or 16 frames/cardiac cycle	8 frames/ cardiac cycle
Imaging time	5 min (10 min ECG-gated)	8–10 (10 min ECG-gated)
Imaging counts	At least 1 million	At least 600,000–800,000

Positioning

View	Detector Position	Patient Position
LAO	Best septal	Supine
Anterior	Best septal minus 45°	Supine
Left lateral	0°	Right decubitus

Key factors to ensure optimal quality planar myocardial perfusion imaging:

1. Adhere to the above-listed acquisition parameters
2. Bring the camera head as close to the patient's chest as possible
3. Acquire adequate counts
4. Reproduce exactly stress and rest patient positioning

Soft Tissue Attenuation in Planar Imaging

BREAST

Soft tissue attenuation, in particular by breasts, is an important problem with planar imaging. In order to recognize breast attenuation, one can acquire in addition to the conventional three-view planar image low-count images—without moving the patient—with a line source in the FOV that outlines the outer contour of the breast (see **Fig. 7-1**).

DIAPHRAGM

Soft tissue attenuation by the left diaphragm is also an important problem with planar images. However, this problem can be entirely

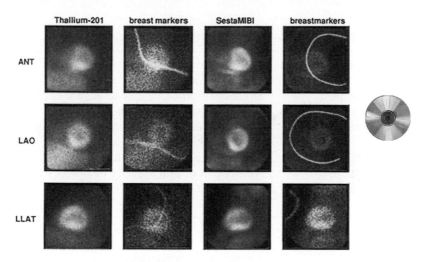

Fig. 7-1. Breast markers (i.e. radioactive line sources) applied to planar Tl-201 (thallium-201) and Tc-99m Sestamibi images. The breast markers are taped to a patient's chest should indicate the outer contour of the breast. If an anterior defect (e.g. on the anterior view of the Tl-201 image) matches with position of the breast marker, the defect is very likely due to breast attenuation.

avoided by acquiring left lateral images with the patient in right side decubitus position (see **Fig. 7-2**).

Table 7-2 lists the processing steps for quantification of planar images.

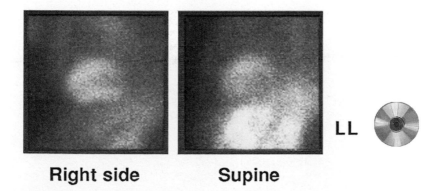

Fig. 7-2. Diaphragmatic attenuation is demonstrated in this patient by acquiring two planar left lateral (LL) images in supine and right-side decubitus position. The supine LL image (right) shows an apparent inferobasal perfusion defect. This defect is not present on a second LL image (left) taken a few minutes later with the patient in right side decubitus position. The latter image is normal. Therefore, in supine position inferior attenuation is present.

Table 7-2
Processing Steps for Quantification of Planar Images

Background subtraction	ROI 4 pixels from heart, interpolative background algorithm applied
Image alignment	Slight rotation of images to ensure stress and rest segments correspond accurately
Normalizing images	Scaling of images so the heart is visualized optimally
Quantification	Plot of image count density
Normal database	Allows extent and severity of defect to be calculated
Archiving	Raw and processed data

Background Subtraction

On planar myocardial projection images, there is substantial foreground and background activity projected over the images of the heart. Quantification of regional myocardial uptake cannot be performed without removal of the extra-cardiac activity. For this

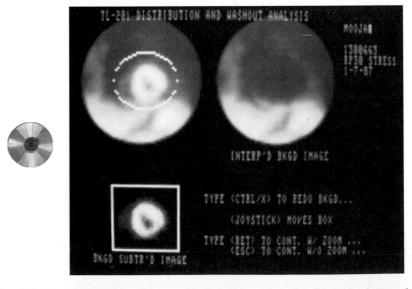

Fig. 7-3. Computer screen capture of the process of interpolative background subtraction. The top left image shows an elliptical region of interest placed around the heart for sampling of background counts. The top right image shows the created background image, which is to be subtracted from the original image. The bottom image shows the resulting background-subtracted image of the heart.

purpose, "interpolative background correction" was developed *(2)*. A background image is created on the basis of the sampling in multiple areas immediately adjacent to the heart and interpolating this information into a new background image. This background image is subsequently subtracted from the raw projection images. The final result of interpolative background correction is a planar image without substantial background that allows for quantitative comparison with normal image files and radiotracer washout (see **Figs. 7-3** and **7-4**).

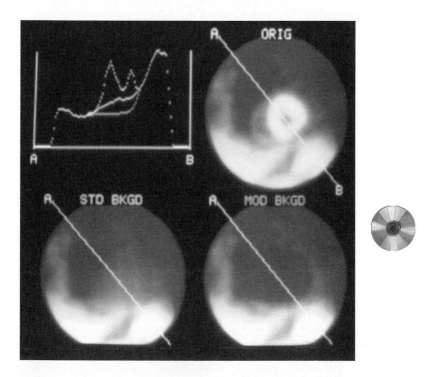

Fig. 7-4. Creation of interpolated background images. The top right image shows the original LAO Tc-99m Sestamibi planar myocardial perfusion image. The top left graph shows count profiles through the images from A to B: white=count profile of the original image.. The bottom images show background images created by interpolative substraction. Bottom left: result of standard interpolative background (STD BKGD) as used for Tl-201 (yellow curve in graph) Bottom right: result of modified interpolative background (MOD BKGD) as developed for Tc-99m agents (orange curve in graph). Standard interpolative background subtraction consists of gradually increasing subtraction from low extra-cardiac counts (lung) to high extra-cardiac counts (gastro-intestinal), thereby leaving a substantial amount of background in the cardiac region. The modified interpolative background substraction subtracts initially a smaller amount of counts from the cardiac region only to increase when high extra-cardiac count area is immediately adjacent *(3)*.

Image Alignment

For paired quantification of images, it may be necessary to rotate the rest or redistribution image slightly in order to match appropriately with the stress image. Rotation should generally not exceed 20° (see **Fig. 7-5**).

Normalizing Images

Rescaling of the images may be necessary when non-cardiac activity is more intense than in the LV (see **Fig. 7-6**).

Normal Database

A normal database is generated from images of normal subjects with low (<3%) likelihood of coronary artery disease, based on age, gender, absence of symptoms and risk factors, and normal exercise

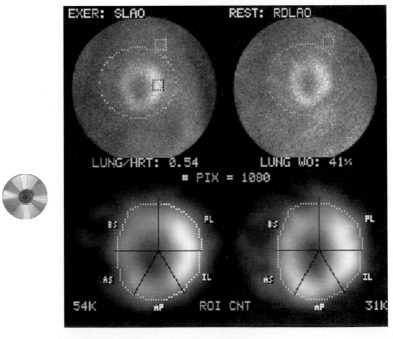

Fig. 7-5. First steps in quantification of planar Tl-201 images. Top images: "raw" left anterior oblique (LAO) planar exercise (EXER) and delayed (REST) Tl-201 images. An elliptical region of interest (ROI) is placed around the heart for interpolative background subtraction. The small square ROIs are for calculation of lung/heart (HRT) ratio and lung washout (WO). Bottom images: interpolative background subtracted images of the heart. The exercise and rest images are aligned and 5 segments are superimposed on the images.

NORMALIZATION TC-99M SESTAMIBI IMAGE

Exercise   Rest

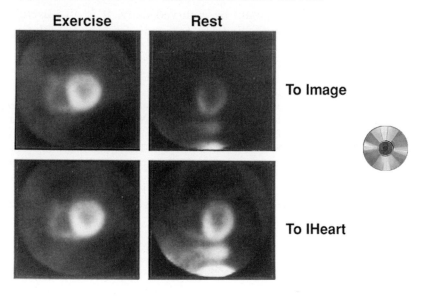

To Image

To IHeart

Fig. 7-6. Normalization of exercise and rest Tc-99m Sestamibi images. Top: images are normalized to highest counts anywhere within the images. In the exercise image maximal counts are located within the left ventricle. Consequently the heart is visualized using the full range of the gray scale. In the rest image maximal counts are located outside the left ventride in the gastrointestinal organs in the bottom of the image. Consequently the heart is poorly visualized using only the lowcr end of the gray scale. Bottom: Both exercise and rest images are normalized to maximal counts within the left ventricle. Exercise and rest images can now be compared and interpreted.

ECG. From the relative count distribution on images of these normal subjects, a lower limit of normal count distribution, i.e., mean minus 2 standard deviations, can be derived.

Quantification

After interpolative background subtraction, regional distribution of radiotracer uptake is quantified relative to the myocardial area with maximal uptake. For this purpose, the circumference of the LV is divided in a number of segments. The average counts in each segment (from center to periphery) may be displayed as circumferential or transverse profiles that are normalized to local maximal counts. The patient's count distribution profiles can be displayed with a lower limit of normal profile. Defect size can then be calculated relative to the normal data files.

Archiving

All raw image data should be archived daily. It is also useful to archive processed and quantified data for ready comparison with future studies.

REFERENCES

1. DePuey GE (2006). *Imaging Guidelines for Nuclear Cardiology Procedures*, Available at http://www.asnc.org—Menu: "Manage Your Practice": Guidelines and Standards" (accessed February 2007).
2. Watson DD, Campbell NP, Read EK, Gibson RS, Teates CD, Beller GA (1981). Spatial and temporal quantitation of plane thallium myocardial images. *J Nucl Med* 22:577–584.
3. Koster K, Wackers FJTh, Mattera J, Fetterman R (1990). Quantitative analysis of planar Tc-99m-Sestamibi myocardial perfusion images using modified background subtraction. *J Nucl Med* 31:1400–1408.

8 Planar Equilibrium Radionuclide Angiocardiography

Acquisition and Processing Protocols

Planar equilibrium radionuclide angiocardiography (ERNA), also known as radionuclide ventriculography (RVG), gated blood pool imaging (GBPI), or multigated acquisition (MUGA), is performed less frequently than radionuclide myocardial perfusion imaging in most laboratories. Nevertheless, ERNA is the most reproducible, accurate, and simplest method for noninvasively assessing LVEF *(1,2)*.

Key Words: Acquisition planar equilibrium radionuclide angiocardiography (details), Processing planar equilibrium radionuclide angiocardiography (details), Blood pool labeling, ECG gating, Ventricularvolume curve, Calculation right and left ventricular ejection fraction.

ERNAs are clinically used for serial assessment of LVEF in patients who undergo chemotherapy and assessment of global function and regional wall motion in patients with recent or old myocardial infarction, in patients with congestive heart failure, and in patients who are potential candidates for implantation of an internal cardiac defibrillator (ICD).

Right ventricular function can be evaluated only by visual inspection on ERNA. Because of overlap by other cardiac structures, right ventricular ejection fraction (RVEF) cannot be calculated reliably. The ECG-gated first-pass method is an alternative means of calculating RVEF *(3)*. Recently, SPECT ERNA has been validated as a methodology to measure RVEF (see Chapter 9).

From: *Contemporary Cardiology: Nuclear Cardiology, The Basics*
By: F. J. Th. Wackers, W. Bruni, and B. L. Zaret © Humana Press Inc., Totowa, NJ

All acquisition parameters listed in the following tables are based on the ASNC *Imaging Guidelines for Nuclear Cardiology Procedures (4)* and guidelines published by the SNM *Gated equilibrium radionuclide ventriculography 3.0 (5)*.

Clinical indications for equilibrium radionuclide angiography can be found in the 2003 ACC/AHA/ASNC *Guidelines for Clinical Use of Cardiac Radionuclide Imaging (6)*.

ACQUISITION

ERNAs are acquired either by planar technique in multiple views or by tomographic SPECT technique (see Chapter 9). Acquisition parameters for planar imaging are listed in Table 8-1. Detector positions and angulations during acquisition are detailed in Table 8-2.

Injected Activity and Labeling

Red blood cells can be labeled using three techniques:

1. In vivo
2. Modified in vivo
3. In vitro

Table 8-1
Acquisition Parameters

	Rest	*Stress*[a]
Activity	25–30 mCi	
Collimator	LEHR parallel hole	LEHS parallel hole
Matrix	64 × 64	64 × 64
Zoom	No zoom 10-inch FOV or 1.5–2.2 zoom LFOV	No zoom 10-inch FOV or 1.5–2.2 zoom LFOV
Peak	140 keV 20% centered	140 keV 20% centered
Frame rate	16 frames/cycle	16 frames/cycle
R–R window	10–15%	20–25%
Beat rejection	Buffered beat or on the fly	Buffered beat or on the fly
Acquisition mode	Frame mode	Frame mode
Acquisition length	>4 million counts standard FOV	2–2.5 min/stage
Pixel size	<4 mm/pixel	<4 mm/pixel

LEHR, low-energy high resolution; LEHS, low-energy high sensitivity; FOV, field of view.

[a]Acquisition parameters for stress ERNA are shown for completeness. In actual clinical practice, exercise ERNAs are infrequently performed in most laboratories.

Table 8-2
Positioning and Angulation

View	Detector position	Patient position
First pass	5–10° RAO	Supine
LAO	Best RV/LV separation (also known as "best septal")	Supine
Anterior	Best RV/LV separation minus 45°	Supine
Left lateral	Best RV/LV separation plus 45°	Right decubitus

LAO, left anterior oblique; RAO, right anterior oblique; RV, right ventricle; LV, left ventricle.

For each of these methods, stannous ion (in the form of stannous pyrophosphate) is used as a reducing agent to facilitate the binding of pertechnetate to hemoglobin.

IN VIVO LABELING

- Inject 2–3 mg of cold stannous pyrophosphate IV.
- After 15–30 min, inject 20–30 mCi of Tc-99m pertechnetate directly intravenously.

(The labeling efficiency for this method is 60–70%.)

MODIFIED IN VIVO LABELING

- Inject 2–3 mg of cold stannous pyrophosphate IV.
- After 15–30 min, draw 3 mL of venous blood into a shielded syringe containing the anticoagulant acid-citrate-dextrose and 20–30 mCi of Tc-99m pertechnetate.
- Incubate at room temperature for at least 10 min.
- Re-inject radiolabeled blood into patient.

(The labeling efficiency for this method approaches 90%.)

IN VITRO LABELING

(The labeling efficiency for this method is >97%.)

Presently, commercial kits (e.g., Ultratag®) are available that have simplified this method. *We believe that this technique is the method of choice.*

Three components are required: (i) a vial with stannouschloride dihydrate, sodium dihydrate, and sodium citrate dihydrate, (ii) a syringe I with sodium hypochlorite, and (iii) a syringe II with citric acid monohydrate and sodium citrate dihydrate.

- Draw 1–3 mL of venous blood into syringe with heparin or anticoagulant citrate dextrose (ACD).
- Add blood to vial and wait 5 min.
- Add content of syringe I to vial and gently mix and invert.
- Add content of syringe II to vial and gently mix and invert.
- Add dose of Tc-99m pertechnetate to vial (in lead shield container) and gently mix and invert.
- Wait 20 min.
- Re-inject blood into patient.

The following subsections are comments on the individual acquisition parameters listed in Table 8-1.

Collimator

The parallel-hole LEHR collimator is used for a rest ERNA. However, when performing exercise ERNAs, the short acquisition time (2 min) of stress images requires the use of a low-energy high-sensitivity (LEHS) collimator in order to assure adequate count statistics. When performing rest and stress ERNAs, one should use the same collimator for both parts. A LEAP collimator can be used to increase the sensitivity while still providing adequate image resolution.

Matrix

A matrix of 64×64 16-bit (word) pixels is standard.

ECG Gating

CHEST ELECTRODES

For ECG-gating, the computer should receive a clear R-wave signal. Usual three electrodes are used: right and left subclavicular and one on the lateral lower chest (either right or left). If this conventional electrode placement does not work, one should move the electrodes around to a position that results in one more distinct R-wave. (Make sure that in patients with abnormal ECG or peaked T waves no double signal is detected).

NUMBER OF FRAMES

Not less than 16 frames/cardiac cycle should be acquired for accurate assessment of LVEF. Although 24 or more frames per cardiac cycle have better temporal resolution and result in better time-activity curves, the acquisition files are too large for most present-day nuclear medicine computers.

R-R WINDOW

The R-R intervals can be displayed on the computer screen as a histogram. With normal heart rate variability, this will be a relatively narrow peak displaying Gaussian distribution. A 10–15% window around the R-R peak is standard and accommodates physiologic heart rate variability. Increasing the window beyond this may cause the ejection fraction (EF) to be less accurate. Nevertheless, during exercise acquisition, the window is expanded to 25% in order to accommodate the quickly changing heart rate. The R-R peak also needs to be adjusted at the beginning of each stage in response to the increasing heart rate.

Beat Rejection

Buffered beat rejection means that each beat is temporarily stored in computer memory to determine whether the beat falls within the acceptable R-R window. If the beat is not within the window, it is rejected without contaminating the acquisition. This is the preferred method of beat rejection. Some systems reject beats "on the fly," which means the beat is determined to be bad and rejected as it is seen but not before a small portion of it is added to the acquisition.

Acquisition Mode

Forward or forward/backward framing is standard on most systems. An alternative acquisition method is list mode. List mode allows all beats to be accepted and then the operator selects the beat length to use. This offers more flexibility in window selection but usually requires extra processing time to convert the list mode to frame mode for LVEF calculation. List mode studies also take up much more disk space than frame mode studies. List mode should be used for ECG-gated first-pass studies, which is commonly used for assessment of RVEF.

Atrial Fibrillation

Meaningful ERNA data can be acquired in patients with atrial fibrillation using standard ECG-gated acquisition. The calculated LVEF then represents the average LVEF during the time of acquisition. Due to the varying R-R interval in atrial fibrillation, there is considerable beat-to-beat variation in LVEF values. List mode acquisition can be used to select beats within a specific range of R-R interval.

ECG-Gated First Pass for RVEF

The injection of the Tc-99m-labeled blood cells is used for this purpose. The gamma camera and computer are set up as for acquisition of ERNA *(3)*. Acquisition is started and the radiolabeled blood is injected rapidly in an anticubital vein. One can either stop acquisition when the radioactive bolus passes through the pulmonary artery as can be assessed on the persistence scope or acquire the entire study in list mode and reformat the data later.

Acquisition Time

Rest ERNAs are usually acquired for counts, not time. For instance, when the spleen is enlarged, most counts/time emanate from the spleen and not from the heart. It is of crucial importance to have adequate count statistics within the LV to ensure reliable and reproducible assessment of LVEF. Using 25–30 mCi, it takes about 5 min to acquire a total of approximately 3–4 million counts with a small FOV camera equipped with a high-resolution collimator. When assessing the final quality of an ERNA, background corrected LV counts in the end diastole are important. The statistical error is affected by the value of LVEF. Studies with normal LVEF should have approximately 3000–4000 counts in the LV end-diastolic region of interest (ROI), whereas studies with abnormal LVEF require at least 20,000 counts for similar reliable LVEF.

For stress ERNAs, the acquisition time necessarily is shortened and fixed. Stress ERNAs are acquired during the last 2 min of each 3 min stage of stress (Table 8-1). Consequently, exercise ERNAs are often relatively low in counts.

Pixel Size

Pixel size should be kept under 4 mm/pixel. Depending on the size of the FOV of the camera, one may have to use a zoom factor to reduce pixel size to <4 mm. Typically, a small FOV of 10 inches does not require any zoom. A large FOV can require a zoom from 1.5 to 2.2 depending on the size of the FOV.

PROCESSING

Similar to acquisition parameters, processing parameters may vary slightly from vendor to vendor. While the processing steps may be different on each computer system, the overall methodology should be similar. The following tables outline the options computer systems

Table 8-3
Processing Parameters

Smoothing	9-point spatial and temporal
Background subtraction	ROI 5–10 pixels from diastolic ROI
ED and ES ROIs	Manual or automated
Volume curve generation	Over ROIs, background subtracted
RVEF/LVEF calculation	Global or regional
LV diastolic function	Peak filling rate and time to peak filling rate
LV volumes	End-diastolic and end-systolic volumes
Cine or movie generated	Assessment of wall motion
Archiving	Raw and processed data

ED, end diastolic; ES, end systolic.

should provide. These processing parameters are also based on the ASNC *Imaging Guidelines for Nuclear Cardiology Procedures (4)*.

Table 8-3 lists the processing parameters. The following subsections are comments on the individual items.

Background Subtraction

There exists variation among vendors with respect to placement of left ventricular background ROI. In some programs, the ROI is placed automatically four pixels outside the lateral border of the end-diastolic ROI; in others, the operator is asked to place the background ROI manually. Regardless of the method, the operator must make sure that the background ROI is not placed over an exceedingly hot area, e.g., spleen or descending aorta. Misplaced background region significantly affects the calculation of LVEF. When the background is too high, LVEF will be erroneously high; conversely when background is lower, LVEF will be lower.

For this reason, it is important to archive data that document the selection of background. Background selection should be checked for reproducibility when comparing LVEF on serial studies.

LV End-Diastolic and End-Systolic ROI

Many systems have semi or fully automatic programs that will draw end-diastolic and end-systolic ROI. All ROIs must be checked for accuracy and redrawn manually as necessary (see **Fig. 8-1**).

LV VOLUME CURVE GENERATION

The appearance of the left ventricular volume curve must be the first item to be checked as part of routine quality control. The

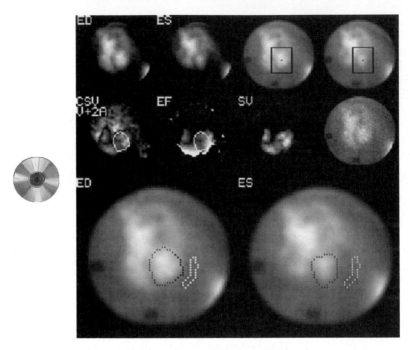

Fig. 8-1. Computer screen capture of processing parameters of a normal ERNA. On the top right are raw end diastolic (ED) and end systolic (ES) frames. The rectangle over the left ventricle is used for automatic search of ED and ES edges. The ED and ES edges are displayed in two larger images on the bottom of the figure for quality control. The automatically placed background region (white dots) is also shown. The images on the top left are functional images that may be helpful for assessing whether the edges were assigned correctly.

curve should start at end-diastole (highest counts), then descend to a well-defined and narrow end-systolic through (lowest counts), and then demonstrate a smooth diastolic upslope and finally an "atrial kick" that merges with end-diastole (**Fig. 8-2**). It is acceptable that one last frame contains less counts due to respiratory variation in heart rate.

However, if a larger number of frames at the end of the cardiac cycle contain low counts due to arrhythmia during acquisition, the diastolic portion of the volume curve is significantly distorted. The volume curve is then unreliable for calculation of diastolic filling parameters. The LVEF is calculated as follows:

$$\frac{\text{End-diastolic counts (bc)} - \text{End-systolic counts (bc)}}{\text{End-diastolic counts (bc)}}$$

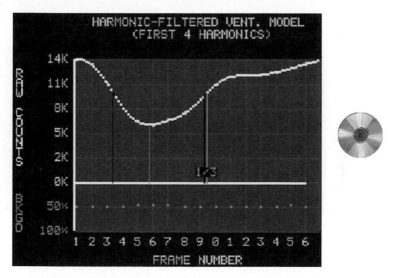

Fig. 8-2. Computer screen capture of normal left ventricular volume curve. The curve should be inspected whether it displays an appropriate "physiologic" shape.

where bc is background corrected. The lower limit of normal for LVEF derived from planar ERNA is 0.50. Background counts have the greatest effect on the denominator. Thus, the higher the background counts the higher the calculated LVEF.

PEAK FILLING RATE

If ERNAs are acquired with sufficient temporal resolution (24 frames per R-R cycle) or if Fourier curve fitting is performed to 16-frame ERNAs, diastolic filling parameters can be calculated. The lower limit of normal peak filling rate is 2.5 end-diastolic volumes/s.

VOLUMES

Left ventricular volumes can be derived from ERNAs using a number of methods. This may involve either the acquisition and counting of a reference blood sample, or measuring pixel size for calibration. The upper limit of normal of end-diastolic left ventricular volume is generally between 100 and 140 mL. Discussion of the details of determining volumes is beyond the scope of this book and can be found in the literature *(7)*.

RVEF

For determination of RVEF, the gated first-pass data are displayed. A large initial ROI is drawn over the RV for identifying the end-systolic

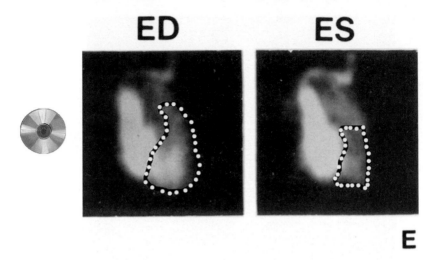

Fig. 8-3. Gated first pass study for determining RVEF. Manually drawn regions of interest outlining the end diastolic (ED) and end systolic (ES) borders of a normal right ventricle are shown. One should be careful to include the right ventricular outflow tract in the regions of interest.

frame. Separate ROIs are drawn outlining the end-diastolic and end-systolic contours (**Fig. 8-3**). RVEF is calculated in the usual manner from end-diastolic and end-systolic counts. No background subtraction is necessary. Note that count density may be suboptimal in about 10% of patients. If counts in the end-diastolic ROI are < 1000, RVEF should not be calculated.

The lower limit of normal RVEF is 0.42 *(3)*.

ARCHIVING

All raw data should be archived daily. Storage of documentation of processing and quantified data for comparison with future studies is recommended.

REFERENCES

1. Wackers FJTh, Berger HJ, Johnstone DE, Goldman L, Reduto LA, Langou RE, Gottschalk A, Zaret BL (1979). Multiple gated cardiac blood pool imaging for left ventricular ejection fraction: validation of the technique and assessment of variability. *Am J Cardiol* 43:1159–1166.
2. Van Royen N, Jaffe CC, Krumholz HK, Johnson KM, Lynch PJ, Natale D, Atkinson P, Deman P, Wackers FJTh (1996). Comparison and reproducibility of visual echocardiographic and quantitative radionuclide left ventricular ejection fraction. *Am J Cardiol* 77: 843–850.
3. Winzelberg GG, Boucher CA, Pohost GM, McKusick KA, Bingham JB, Okada RD, Strauss HW (1981). Right ventricular function in aortic and mitral

valve disease: relation of gated first pass radionuclide angiography to clinical and hemodynamic findings. *Chest* 79:520–528.

4. DePuey GE (2006). *Imaging Guidelines for Nuclear Cardiology Procedures*, available at http://www.asnc.org—Menu: "Manage Your Practice": "Guidelines & Standards" (accessed February 2007).

5. Scheiner J, Sinusas A, Wittry MD, Royal HD, Machac J, Balon HR, Lang O (2007). Gated equilibrium radionuclide ventriculography 3.0. Available at http://www.snm.org—Menu: "Practice Management": "Procedure Guidelines" (accessed May 2007).

6. *Guidelines for Clinical Use of cardiac Radionuclide Imaging* (2003). Available at http://www.acc.org—Menu: "Quality and Science": "Clinical Statements/Guidelines"; "Imaging, Cardiac":"Cardiac Radionuclide Imaging": ACC/AHA/ASNC Guidelines for clinical use of cardiac radionuclide imaging (accessed June 2007).

7. Levy WC, Cerqueira MD, Matsuoka DT, Harp GD, Sheehan FH, Stratton JR (1992). Four radionuclide methods for left ventricular volume determinations: comparison of a manual and automated technique. *J Nucl Med* 33:763–770.

9 SPECT Equilibrium Radionuclide Angiocardiography
Acquisition and Processing Protocols

SPECT ERNA is presently performed in many nuclear cardiology laboratories in addition to planar ERNAs. The equipment used for the acquisition of ECG-gated SPECT myocardial perfusion images can also be used for acquisition of ECG-gated SPECT ERNA. No modifications of hardware are needed. Several reconstruction and processing software packages for SPECT ERNA are now commercially available. The greatest attraction of SPECT ERNA is in the ability to evaluate cardiac chambers and regional wall motion without overlap of other structures. This is very useful in patients with extensive LV wall motion abnormalities and in patients with abnormal RV function and morphology. In pediatric patients with surgically corrected congenital heart disease, we have found SPECT ERNA to be useful for more accurate assessment of contractile function of both ventricles.

Key Words: Acquisition SPECT equilibrium radionuclide angiocardiography (details), Processing SPECT equilibrium radionuclide angiocardiography (details).

All acquisition parameters listed in the following tables are based on the ASNC *Imaging Guidelines for Nuclear Cardiology Procedures (1).* Additional information about accepted standards for performing ERNAs can be found in the SNM guidelines for *Gated Equilibrium Radionuclide Ventriculography 3.0 (2).*

Clinical indications for nuclear cardiology imaging can be found in the ACC/AHA/ASNC *Guidelines for Clinical Use of Cardiac Radionuclide Imaging (3).*

From: *Contemporary Cardiology: Nuclear Cardiology, The Basics*
By: F. J. Th. Wackers, W. Bruni, and B. L. Zaret © Humana Press Inc., Totowa, NJ

ACQUISITION PARAMETERS

Table 9-1 lists the acquisition parameters for ECG-gated SPECT ERNA. The following subsections comment on the individual parameters. Imaging can be performed with either a single-head or dual-head camera.

Collimator

Because of the abundance of counts, a parallel-hole LEHR collimator with resolution of 8–10 mm full-width half-maximum (FWHM) is preferred. With the use of single detector, a parallel-hole LEAP collimator is recommended.

Pixel Size

Usually a 64 × 64 matrix with the appropriate zoom will produce a better than 4 mm/pixel. Depending on the size of the FOV of the camera, one may have to adjust the zoom to obtain the correct pixel size. Typically, a small FOV of 10 inches does not require any zoom. A large FOV can require a zoom from 1.5 to 1.75 depending on the exact size of the FOV.

Table 9-1
Acquisition Parameters

Activity (dose)	30 mCi
Collimator	Parallel-hole LEHR (dual head)
	Parallel-hole LEAP (single head)
Matrix	64 × 64
Zoom	No zoom 10-inch FOV or 1.5-2.2 zoom LFOV
Peak	140 keV 20% centered
Frame rate	16 frames/cycle
R-R window	15–35%
Beat rejection	On the fly
Acquisition mode	Frame mode
Number of stops	60–64 (30–32 per detector head)
Time/stop	30 s (dual head), 40 s (single head)
Pixel size	4.8–6.6 mm
Orbit	Circular 180°
Planar LAO	5 min acquisition (for calculation of LVEF)

ECG Gating

CHEST ELECTRODES

For ECG gating, the computer should receive a clear R-wave signal. Usual three electrodes are used: right and left subclavicular and one on the lateral lower chest (either right or left). If this conventional electrode placement does not work, one may move the electrodes around to a position that results in one more distinct R-wave. (Make sure that in patients with abnormal ECG or peaked T-waves, no double signal is detected.)

NUMBER OF FRAMES

Sixteen frames per cardiac cycle are preferred over 8 frames/cycle. As is the case for SPECT myocardial perfusion-derived LVEF (see pg 85), image data acquired with 8 frames/cycle underestimates the value of LVEF by about 0.05.

R-R WINDOW

The window width is larger for SPECT ERNA than for planar ERNA in order to increase the count statistics. A 15–35% window is standard; however, it may vary with different camera systems and with the patient's rhythm.

Beat Rejection

This parameter may also differ from system to system. An "on the fly" beat rejection where the abnormal beat and the subsequent beat are rejected is preferred.

Acquisition Mode

Frame mode is standard on most systems.

Number of Projections

Thirty to thirty-two projections per head over 180° are adequate. For dual headed systems with the camera heads at 90°, a total of 60–64 stops are acquired.

Time per Stop

For a dual-headed system acquiring 64 projections, each stop should be 30 s. Total acquisition time of an ERNA SPECT study is approximately 20 min.

PROCESSING PARAMETERS

Table 9-2 lists the processing parameters. The following subsections comment on the individual parameters.

Filtering

The purpose of image filters is to remove noise and blur before and after back projection of raw SPECT ERNA data. The standard filter for SPECT ERNA imaging is the Butterworth filter. The optimal order and cutoff of this filter is different for each vendor.

Motion Correction

Not all programs are capable to correct ECG-gated data for motion. Check with vendor. After applying the program to the data, always check the reconstructed slices for motion artifacts. The programs are not fool proof and are not always successful.

Reconstruction

Image data are reconstructed using filtered back projection or, optional, iterative reconstruction. Subsequently, tomographic slices are reoriented according to the three anatomical axes of the heart. Horizontal long axis, vertical long axis, and short axis slices are created.

Table 9-2
Processing Parameters

Filtering	Filtered back projection is standard; cutoffs and frequencies are vendor dependent
Motion correction	Some programs are not able to correct motion of ECG-gated data
Reconstruction	Reorientation of tomographic data into vertical and horizontal long axis and short axis planes of the heart
Normalizing cine	The gray scale setting normalized to heart activity
Ejection fraction	Derived from count-based volume changes within the 3-D ventricular region of interest
Volumes	Simpson's rule: sum of pixels within each slice, summed for all slices
Archiving	Raw and processed data

Normalizing Slices

This step may be necessary if the patient has intense radiotracer uptake in the spleen. When images are normalized to the spleen, the heart may not be visible. The gray scale setting must be normalized to the maximal pixel value within the heart for optimal visualization of cardiac structures.

Left Ventricular Volume Curve Generation

A left ventricular volume curve for determination of LVEF can be derived by adaptation of the processing methodology used for planar ERNA, by generating multiple ROIs over the summed short axis slices, including the entire LV and excluding the left atrium. However, this approach is considered outdated. Newer automated or semi-automated software packages consider the LV a count-based 3-D volume object that can be traced throughout the cardiac cycle. Various algorithms have been used to determine the border of the ventricular cavity throughout the cardiac cycle. Some are based on count and temporal gradients and others on count density level thresholds *(4–9)*.

The change in ventricular volume is used to calculate ejection fractions.

LVEF

LVEF can be determined from the 3-D volume-based method using the conventional equation:

$$\frac{\text{End-diastolic volume} - \text{end-systolic volume}}{\text{End-diastolic volume}}$$

Because the background in reconstructed SPECT ERNA images is extremely low, no background subtraction is necessary. Because of lack of atrial overlap, LVEF by SPECT ERNA is slightly higher than that derived from planar ERNA, *(4,5)*. The lower limit of normal SPECT ERNA LVEF is about 0.55. The reproducibility of SPECT ERNA-derived LVEF is excellent. Interobserver variability is about 2–3% (EF units) *(8,9)*.

Because SPECT ERNA-derived LVEF currently has not been not fully validated in larger clinical studies, one has the option to acquire a conventional planar LAO ERNA image for assessment of LVEF using the traditional well-validated software (Chapter 8). The tomographic slices may then be used for visual assessment of chamber sizes and regional wall motion.

RVEF

Calculation of RVEF, which is not reliable by planar ERNA technique, is feasible with SPECT ERNA because the RV is spatially separated from other cardiac structures. Recently, semi-automatic, operator-interactive methods have been described and validated in comparison with EBCT and MRI ventricular volumes *(10,11)*. Quantification of right ventricular function and volume is probably most useful application of SPECT ERNA.

Ventricular Volumes

Right and left ventricular volumes can been determined from SPECT ERNA by summing the calibrated voxels within the LV volume of interest. Further clinical validation is still required.

Archiving

All raw data should be archived daily. It is also recommended that processed and quantified data are stored for comparison with future studies.

REFERENCES

1. DePuey GE (2006). *Imaging Guidelines for Nuclear Cardiology Procedures*, available at http://www.asnc.org—Menu: "Manage Your Practice": "Guidelines & Standards" (accessed June 2007).
2. Scheiner J, Sinusas A, Wittry MD, Royal HD, Machac J, Balon HR, Lang O (2002). *Gated Equilibrium Radionuclide Ventriculography 3.0*. Available at http://www.snm.org—Menu: "Practice Management": "Procedure Guidelines": "Gated equilibrium radionuclide ventriculography 3.0" (accessed June 2007).
3. ACC/AHA/ASNC *Guidelines for Clinical Use of Cardiac Radionuclide Imaging* (2003). Available at http://www.acc.org—Menu: "Quality and Science": "Clinical Statements/Guidelines"; "Imaging, Cardiac": "Cardiac Radionuclide Imaging" (accessed June 2007).
4. Bartlett ML, Srinivasan G, Barker WC, Kitsiou AN, Dilsizian V, Bacharach SL (1996). Left ventricular ejection fraction: comparison of results from planar and SPECT gated blood-pool studies. *J Nucl Med* 37:1795–1799.
5. Groch MW, DePuey EG, Belzberg AC, Erwin WD, Kamran M, Barnett CA, Hendel RC, Spies SM, Ali A, Marshall RC (2001). Planar imaging versus gated blood-pool SPECT for assessment of ventricular performance: a multicenter study. *J Nucl Med* 42:1773–1779.
6. Van Kriekinge SD, Berman DS, Germano G (1996). Automatic quantification of left ventricular ejection fraction from gated blood pool SPECT. *J Nucl Cardiol* 6:498–506.
7. Daou D, Van Kriekinge SD, Coagulla C, Lebtahi R, Fourme T, Sitbon O, Parent F, Slama M, Le Guludec D (2004). Automatic quantification of right ventricular function with gated blood pool SPECT. *J Nucl Cardiol* 11:293–304.

8. Vanhove C, Franken PR, Defrise M, Momen A, Everaert H, Bossuyt A (2001). Automatic determination of left ventricular ejection fraction from gated blood-pool tomography. *J Nucl Med* 42:401–407.
9. Daou D, Harel F, Helal BO, Fourme T, Colin P, Lebtahi R, Mariano-Goulart D, Faraggi M, Slama M, Le Guludec D (2001). Electrocardiographically gated blood pool SPECT and left ventricular function: comparative value of 3 methods for ejection fraction and volume estimation. *J Nucl Med* 42:1043–1049.
10. Nichols K, Saouaf R, Ababneh AA, Barts RJ, Rosenbaum MS, Groch MW, Shoyeb AH, Bergmann SR (2002). Validation of SPECT equilibrium radionuclide angiographic right ventricular parameters by cardiac magnetic resonance imaging. *J Nucl Cardiol* 9:153–160.
11. Clements IP, Brinkmann B, Mullan BP, O'Connor MK, Breen JF, MCGregor CGA (2006). Operator-interactive method for simultaneous measurement of left and right ventricular volumes and ejection fraction by tomographic electrocardiograph-gated blood pool radionuclide ventriculography. *J Nucl Cardiol* 13:50–63.

10 Display and Analysis of SPECT Myocardial Perfusion Images

The display and nomenclature of nuclear cardiology images have been standardized. The analysis of nuclear cardiology images should follow a systematic approach and sequence as outlined in the ASNC *Imaging Guidelines for Nuclear Cardiology Procedures, 2006 (1)*.

Display of SPECT myocardial perfusion images should include the following at a minimum:

- Rotating planar projection images
- Reconstructed slices
- Movie display of selected ECG-gated slices
- 3-D condensation of image data

Key Words: Display and analysis SPECT images, Rotating planar projection images, Reconstructed slices, ECG-gated movies, Nomenclature, Semi-quantitative analysis, Quantitative analysis, Attenuation correction, Co-registration.

Interpretation of SPECT myocardial perfusion images should follow a systematic approach.

1. Inspection of rotating planar projection images.
2. Analysis of reconstructed tomographic short-axis, vertical, and long-axis slices.
3. Analysis of co-registration of emission and transmission images (if applicable).
4. Comparison of non-corrected and attenuation-corrected images (if applicable).
5. Analysis of regional and global left ventricular function.
6. Incorporation of quantitative myocardial perfusion and functional data.
7. Incorporation of clinical and stress data.
8. Final interpretation and report.

From: *Contemporary Cardiology: Nuclear Cardiology, The Basics*
By: F. J. Th. Wackers, W. Bruni, and B. L. Zaret © Humana Press Inc., Totowa, NJ

The following subsections are comments on the parameters listed above.

ROTATING PROJECTION IMAGES

The raw unprocessed planar projection images (**Fig. 10-1**) should be viewed on computer screen in a rotating endless loop cine format and inspected for the following:

1. Overall quality of images
2. Motion and effectiveness of motion correction
3. Gastrointestinal uptake
4. Breast attenuation
5. Diaphragmatic attenuation
6. Count density within the heart
7. Presence of non-cardiac radiotracer uptake in:
   a. Lungs,
   b. Thyroid gland,
   c. Salivary glands,
   d. Kidneys,
   e. Tumors and lymph nodes, etc.

The overall quality of SPECT images is determined by a number of interrelated variables, such as presence of patient motion and adequacy of

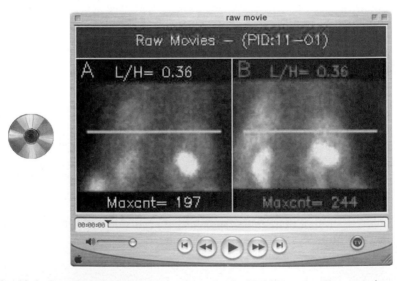

Fig. 10-1. Rotating planar projection images of a SPECT study. The stress images are on the left, the rest images are on the right. The maximal counts per pixel (Maxcnt) within the heart are displayed. The lung-to-heart count ratio (L/H) is also displayed. (**movie**)

motion correction, the intensity and location of gastrointestinal uptake, breast or diaphragmatic attenuation, and very importantly count density in the heart.

Evaluation of Rotating Planar Projection Images

COUNT DENSITY AND IMAGE INSPECTION

There are several ways to assess count density, e.g., total counts in entire SPECT study or per planar projection image. We have found empirically that the maximal counts per pixel within the LV is a useful measure of quality. When maximal counts in the heart are < 100/pixel, reconstructed slices are frequently noisy and of suboptimal quality. Count density can be enhanced either by administering a higher dose of radiopharmaceutical or by prolonging acquisition time. However, in obese patients, even if measured counts are adequate, scattered photons may degrade image quality substantially.

PATIENT MOTION

Patient motion can best be recognized on the rotating planar projection images. This is done by visual inspection. A horizontal line that is aligned with the left ventricular apex is very helpful (see also Chapter 16, p. 237).

GASTROINTESTINAL UPTAKE

Images acquired with Tc-99m-labeled agents, in particular those acquired at rest and after pharmacological stress, at times display substantial subdiaphragmatic gastrointestinal uptake. The most disturbing image pattern is that of a bowel loop with intense radiotracer uptake immediately adjacent to the left ventricular inferior wall. This may obscure visualization of the inferior wall. The intense uptake may also create artifactual inferior defects due to errors in filtered back projection. On the contrary, fixed inferior defects may appear reversible due to scattered photons from adjacent intense non-cardiac uptake. No good remedies exist to avoid these problems. In our experience, the best solution is either to wait and repeat imaging later or to have the patient drink large amounts of fluid in order to move radioactivity further down the gastrointestinal tract.

BREAST SHADOW

When viewing the cine display of the rotating planar projection images, one may see the shadow of the left breast moving over the heart from the LAO to left lateral projections. On planar images, breast attenuation is a serious problem that may make images not interpretable. However, on SPECT imaging, because of the limited number of projections affected, breast attenuation artifacts are not a serious problem most of the time.

INFERIOR ATTENUATION

On cine display of the rotating planar projection images, one may see sudden disappearance of the inferior wall in the left lateral projections. Such a sudden disappearance favors diaphragmatic attenuation, whereas a gradual appearance of an inferior wall defect makes it more likely that a true myocardial perfusion defect is present.

ECG-GATING PROBLEMS

ECG-gating problems may be suspected by reviewing the cine display of the planar projection images. Sometimes, a "flashing" effect occurs, caused by brighter and darker projection images. If the heart rate during SPECT image acquisition was irregular, not all 8 or 16 bins of an ECG-gated SPECT study accumulated the same number of counts per stop, resulting in darker and lighter images. However, one should be aware that ECG-gating irregularities are often subtle and may not be spotted directly from planar projection images.

LOCALIZED NON-CARDIAC RADIOTRACER UPTAKE

Depending on the size of the FOV, rotating projection images also display part of the chest and upper abdomen. When inspecting rotating images, one should pay attention to normal and abnormal extra-cardiac radiotracer accumulation. One may see varying degrees of uptake in the salivary glands, thyroid gland, and stomach mucosa. This is not abnormal and is due to the presence of free unlabeled Tc-99m pertechnetate. At times, the skeleton may be faintly visualized; the significance of the latter is unclear. However, localized radiotracer accumulation in the mediastinum, breast(s), and axilla should be considered abnormal and may indicate malignancy. Such abnormal extra-cardiac uptake should be mentioned in the final report to the referring physician, and further clinical work-up should be suggested.

INCREASED LUNG UPTAKE

Increased radiotracer lung uptake, in particular when present on stress images and not on rest images, is a sign of transient left ventricular dysfunction during stress. Lung uptake is quantified as lung/heart ratio. The lower limit if normal lung/heart ratio is 0.50 for Tl-201 and 0.42 for Tc-99m sestamibi.

INCREASED SPLEEN UPTAKE

In patients with malignancies, the spleen is frequently enlarged and may have increased radiopharmaceutical uptake.

DECREASED LIVER UPTAKE

In patients with cirrhosis of the liver, one may observe complete lack of uptake of radiopharmaceutical. Regional lack of uptake may be seen in patients with liver cysts.

RECONSTRUCTED SLICES

The display of reconstructed SPECT slices has been standardized *(1–3)* (**Fig. 10-2**). Three sets of tomographic slices are reconstructed: short-axis slices, horizontal long-axis slices, and vertical long-axis slices. The stress (A) and rest or delayed (B) images are displayed in two rows of images (stress on top and rest below) to facilitate comparison (**Fig. 10-3**). The short-axis images are displayed from apex (left) to base (right), the vertical long-axis slices are displayed from

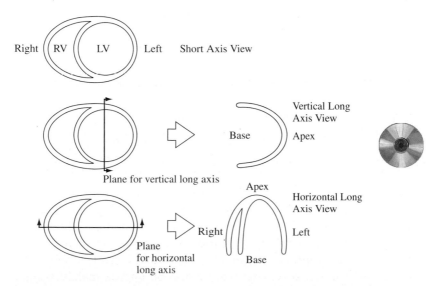

Fig. 10-2. Standardized planes of cut for reconstructed SPECT slices (Reproduced with permission from ref. 2).

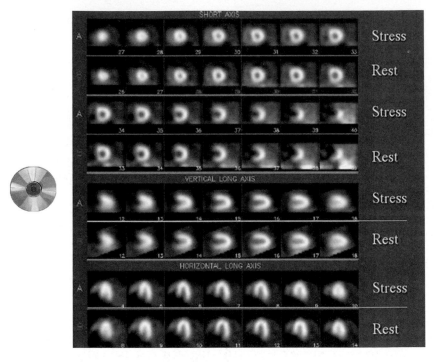

Fig. 10-3. Reconstructed SPECT slices.

septum (left) to lateral wall (right), and the horizontal long-axis are displayed from inferior wall (left) to anterior wall (right).

Images are preferably displayed on computer screen in color or "white on black" using a linear gray scale. It is important that the display of images is standardized and not changed randomly. Certain color scales have a tendency to exaggerate subtle differences in myocardial radiotracer uptake; other color scales may have the opposite effect.

If AC has been applied, both uncorrected and corrected reconstructed tomographic slices must be viewed for interpretation.

DISPLAY OF SPECT MYOCARDIAL PERFUSION IMAGES

Reconstructed slices (**Fig. 10-3**) should be checked as to whether tomographic cuts were performed along appropriately selected left ventricular anatomical axes. Inappropriate orientation should be suspected when the morphology of the LV is apparently distorted.

In addition, appropriate alignment of stress and rest slices should be verified: left ventricular cavity size should be approximately similar on companion of stress–rest short-axis slices. Also paired stress–rest long-axis slices should have similar morphology. Obviously, when

TID is present, stress and rest images are different and this should be distinguished from misalignment.

ECG-gated SPECT slices are displayed in color and played as an endless loop movie (**Fig. 10-4** and on CD-ROM). Gradual change in color intensity during the cardiac cycle correlates with left ventricular regional myocardial thickening. Display in black and white is often helpful to analyze motion of regional myocardial borders. Problems with ECG-gating should be suspected when the transition from one frame to another shows an abrupt change in intensity ("flashing").

3-D rendering of myocardial perfusion is shown in **Fig. 10-5**. A composite 3-D rendering of myocardial perfusion information from all reconstructed slices is often helpful when myocardial perfusion abnormalities are large. Visualization of abnormal areas in three dimensions makes it easier to understand the full anatomic involvement of the LV.

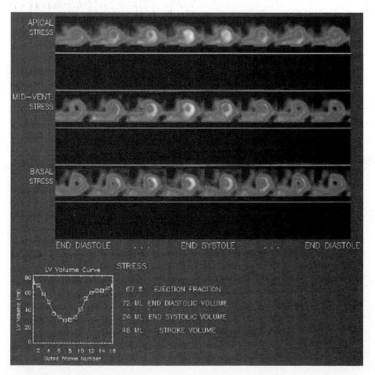

Fig. 10-4. Display of wall motion and LVEF of ECG-gated SPECT.

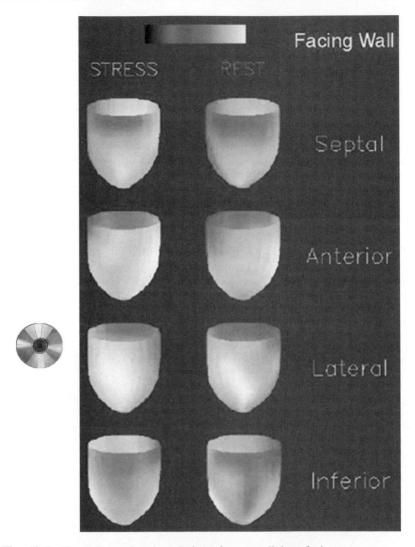

Fig. 10-5. Three dimensional rendering of myocardial perfusion.

ANALYSIS OF SPECT IMAGES

After QA of the rotating planar projection images and of reconstructed slices as outlined above, we recommend that the SPECT slices are first analyzed visually and then, when available, by quantitative analysis.

Stress and rest reconstructed slices are often divided in 17 segments according to standards developed by the AHA, ACC, and ASNC *(3)*.

Specific segments can be assigned to various coronary artery perfusion territories as shown in **Fig. 10-6**.

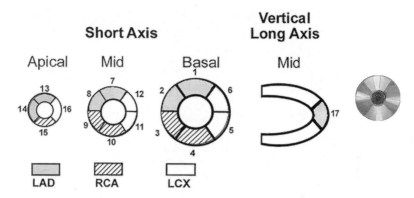

Fig. 10-6. Assignment of myocardial segments to the territories of the left anterior descending (LAD), right coronary artery (RCA), and the left circumflex coronary artery (LCX). (Reproduced with permission from ref 1.).

Because of the many reconstructed SPECT images available for analysis, it is useful to compress all information into *one* image. This can be done either by displaying a 3-D rendering of myocardial perfusion of the LV (**Fig. 10-5**) or by generating color-coded polar maps or "bull's-eye" images (**Fig. 10-7**).

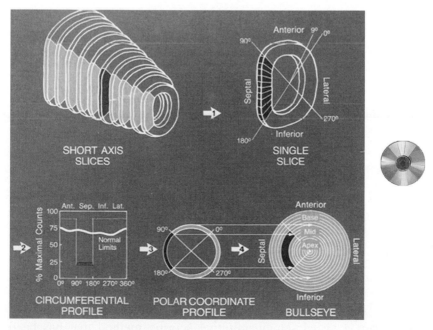

Fig. 10-7. Steps involved in generating a "bull's eye" map (reproduction by permission of General Electric, Milwaukee, WI).

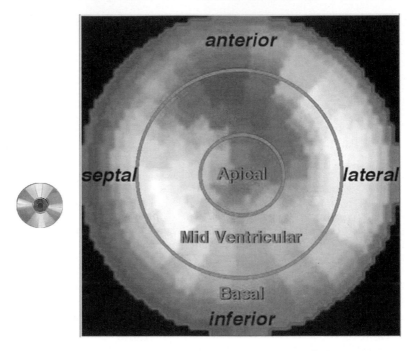

Fig. 10-8. Bull's eye display of tomographic myocardial perfusion images.

A bull's eye display of tomographic myocardial perfusion images is shown in **Fig. 10-8**. Myocardial perfusion image data are projected onto one plane. Image data of the apex are projected in the center of the bull's eye. Image data of the base of the LV are projected on the periphery of the bull's eye, whereas mid-ventricular image data are projected between these two areas. The location of the anterior, lateral, inferior, and septal walls are indicated.

A standardized segmentation and nomenclature for bull's eye display or circumferential polar plot of tomographic myocardial perfusion images *(2,3)* is shown in **Fig. 10-9**.

Figure 10-10 shows a bull's eye display and assignment of coronary artery territories.

Semiquantitative Analysis

Myocardial perfusion images should not be interpreted simply in a binary fashion as either "normal" or "abnormal" but should be characterized by the degree of decreased radiotracer uptake. Table 10-1 summarizes a visual semiquantitative scoring method that has been widely used.

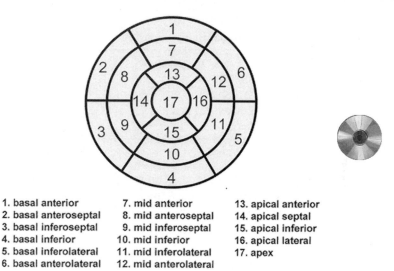

1. basal anterior
2. basal anteroseptal
3. basal inferoseptal
4. basal inferior
5. basal inferolateral
6. basal anterolateral

7. mid anterior
8. mid anteroseptal
9. mid inferoseptal
10. mid inferior
11. mid inferolateral
12. mid anterolateral

13. apical anterior
14. apical septal
15. apical inferior
16. apical lateral
17. apex

Fig. 10-9. Standardized segmentation and nomenclature. (Reproduced with permission from ref 1).

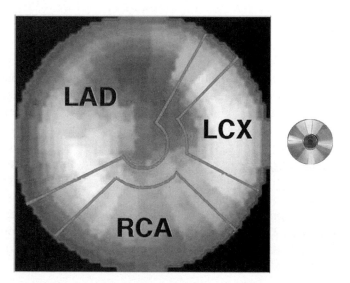

Fig. 10-10. Bull's eye display and assignment of coronary artery territories.

Applying the scoring system for each segment of the 17-segment model to both rest and stress images, one can derive a summed stress score (SSS), a summed rest score (SRS), and a summed difference score (SDS).

Table 10-1
Semiquantitative Scoring

Normal	0
Mildly reduced	1
Moderately reduced	2
Severely reduced	3
Absent uptake	4

These semiquantitative scores have been shown to provide important prognostic information. A normal image thus has a score of "0," whereas the maximal abnormal score is "68" (no heart visualized). A summed score of < 8 is considered small, 9–13 moderate, and > 13 large.

Quantitative Analysis

Radionuclide imaging is an intrinsically digital imaging technique that is ideally suited for quantification. A number of validated software packages are commercially available for quantification of SPECT myocardial perfusion and function (QPS-QGS™ , Emory Toolbox™, 4D-MSPECT™, and Wackers-Liu CQ™) and are distributed by the major vendors of nuclear medicine imaging equipment *(4–7)*.

The basic principles of SPECT quantification are similar for each of these software packages. Normalized relative radiotracer uptake in reconstructed slices is quantitatively compared against normal data files. Relative radiotracer uptake on SPECT images is displayed either as polar plots or bull's eye plots, as was shown above, or as circumferential count distribution profiles. The size of myocardial perfusion defects can be expressed either as percent of LV or as computer-generated summed defect scores.

Each commercially available software package also includes software for computation of LVEF and left ventricular volumes from ECG-gated SPECT images. EF calculations are based on applying Simpson' rule to computer-derived endocardial edges and volumes throughout the cardiac cycle.

EXAMPLES OF COMMERCIAL QUANTITATIVE SOFTWARE

Figures 10-11 to **10-37** show representative screen captures of display of four commercially available software packages. Although all examples show anterior wall perfusion abnormalities, the image data are from different patients.

CEDARS SINAI QPS AND QGS® (COURTESY GUIDO GERMANO, PhD)

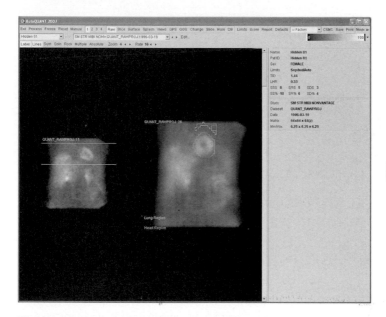

Fig. 10-11. Cedars-Sinai QPS and QGS. Rotating projection images of separate acquisition dual isotope SPECT. Regions of interest for calculating lung/heart ratio are shown.

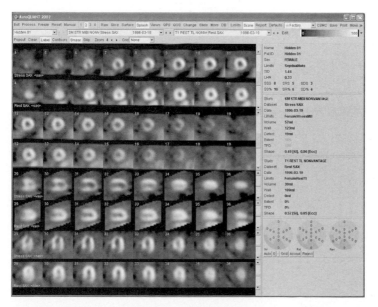

Fig. 10-12. Cedars-Sinai QPS and QGS. Standard display of reconstructed tomographic slices. A reversible anteroapical defect is present. On the right quantitative parameters are displayed.

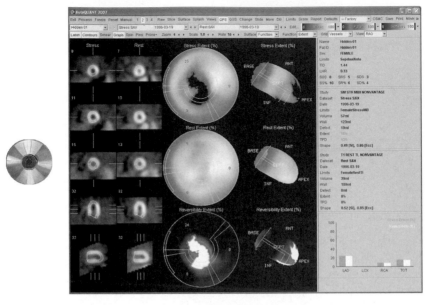

Fig. 10-13. Cedars-Sinai QPS and QGS. Quantification of myocardial perfusion. Computer-generated left ventricular contours are displayed on the left. Two-dimensional polar plots (bull's eyes) and three-dimensional rendering of myocardial perfusion are shown in the middle and on the right. On the far right are quantitative results. Summed stress score is 8, or 10 % of LV, predominantly in the LAD territory.

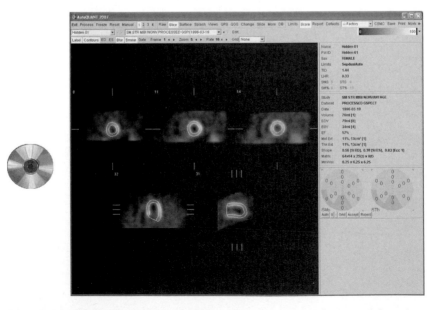

Fig. 10-14. Cedars-Sinai QPS and QGS. Left ventricular contours used for calculation of LVEF are displayed. LVEF is 57%.

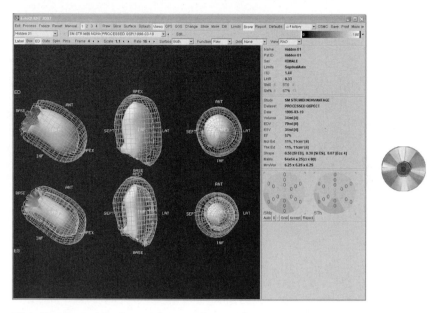

Fig. 10-15. Cedars-Sinai QPS and QGS. Three dimensional rendering of left ventricular function. The end diastolic volume is shown as a bird cage.

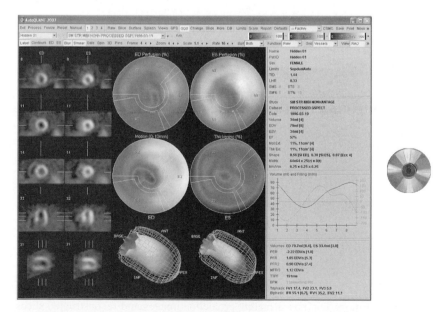

Fig. 10-16. Cedars-Sinai QPS and QGS. Summary of quantification of left ventricular perfusion and function. LVEF = 57%.

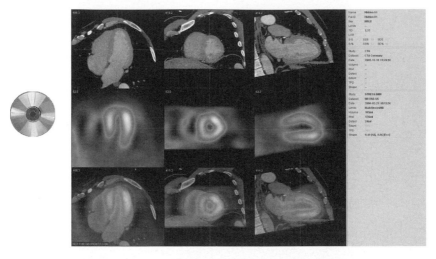

Fig. 10-17. Hybrid imaging using the Cedars-Sinai software package of a different patient than in figs. 10-10 to 10-16. Contrast CT left ventriculography is displayed at the top; Tc-99m-sestamibi SPECT images in the middle and fusion images at the bottom.

EMORY TOOLBOX® (COURTESY ERNEST V. GARCIA, PhD)

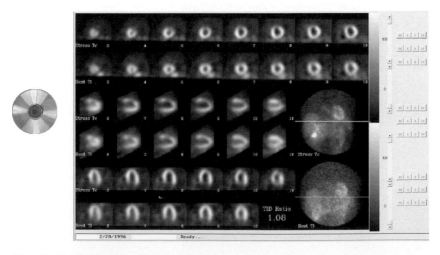

Fig. 10-18. Emory Toolbox. Rotating projection images and reconstructed slices of separate acquisition dual isotope SPECT are displayed. A largely reversible anteroapical myocardial perfusion defect is present.

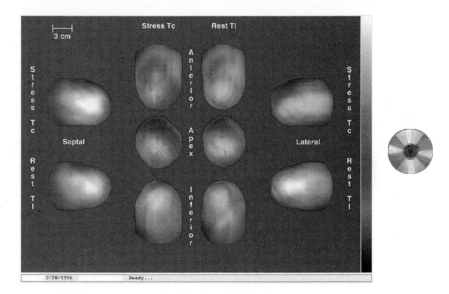

Fig. 10-19. Emory Toolbox. Three dimensional display of myocardial perfusion. The darkened area represents the anteroapical perfusion defect.

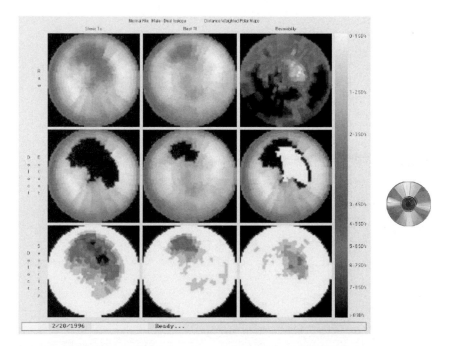

Fig. 10-20. Emory Toolbox. Bull's eye display of results of quantification of myocardial perfusion. The anteroapical defect is mostly reversible with small residual rest defect.

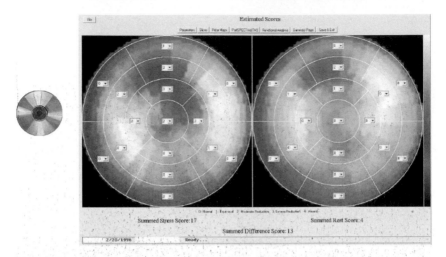

Fig. 10-21. Emory Toolbox. Results of quantification. Stress and rest score are computed for each of 17 segments. The summed stress score is 17; summed rest score is 4 and the summed difference score is 13.

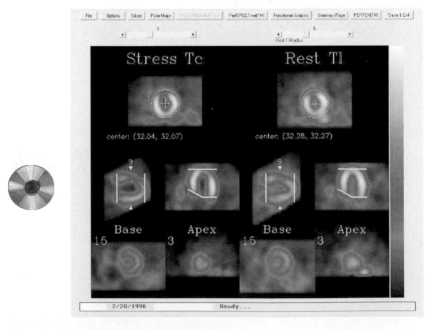

Fig. 10-22. Emory Toolbox. Parameters used for computing LVEF from ECG-gated SPECT.

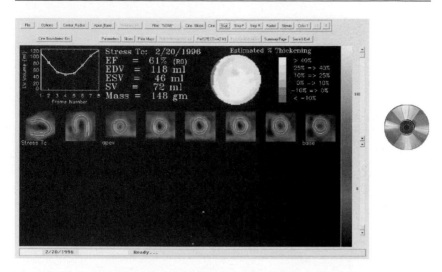

Fig. 10-23. Emory Toolbox. Calculated LVEF and percent wall thickening. LVEF is 61% with normal (>40%) wall thickening. End diastole volume is calculated as 118 ml.

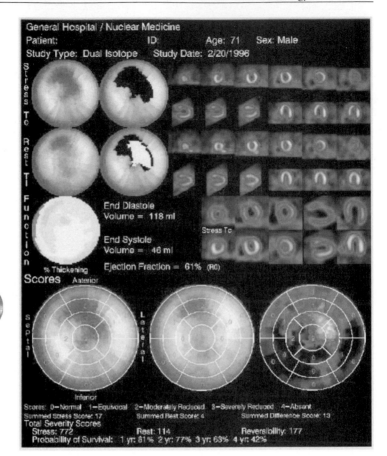

Fig. 10-24. Emory Toolbox. Summary screen displaying quantitative myocardial perfusion and function. There is a large, almost completely reversible, anteroseptal myocardial perfusion defect with preserved global and regional left ventricular function.

4DM-SPECT® (Courtesy Edward Ficaro, PhD)

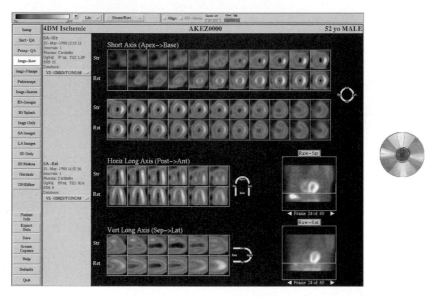

Fig. 10-25. 4DM-SPECT. Rotating planar projection images and selected reconstructed slices.

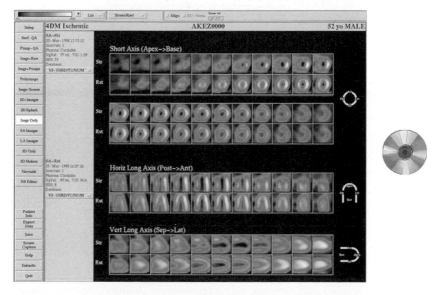

Fig. 10-26. 4DM-SPECT. Standard display of reconstructed slices. A reversible antero-apical and septal myocardial perfusion defect is present.

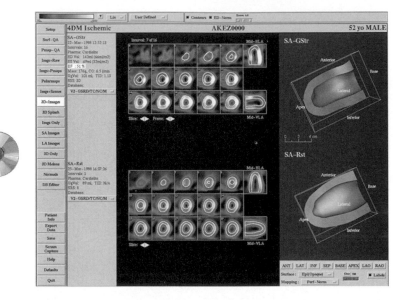

Fig. 10-27. 4DM-SPECT. Left ventricular contours for quantifying myocardial perfusion (left) and three-dimensional rendering (right).

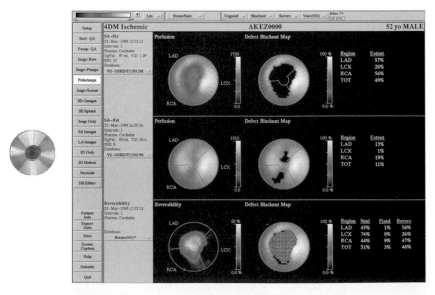

Fig. 10-28. 4DM-SPECT. Left column: polar maps of stress (top) and rest (middle) myocardial perfusion and defect reversibility (bottom). Middle column: blackout maps for stress and rest myocardial perfusion in comparison to normal database. Defect sizes in various coronary artery territories are shown on the right.

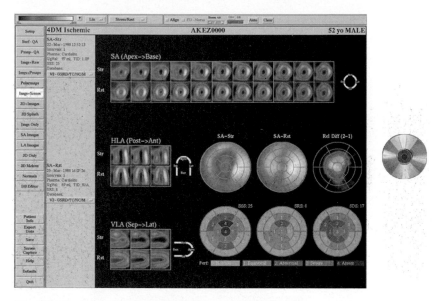

Fig. 10-29. 4DM-SPECT. Summary screen of quantitative myocardial perfusion. Summed stress defect size is 25.

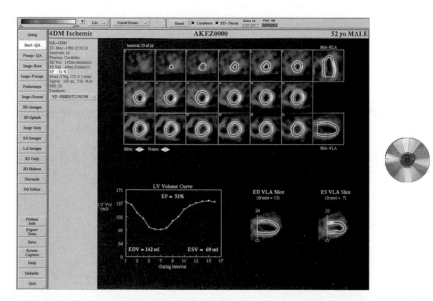

Fig. 10-30. 4DM-SPECT. Quantification of left ventricular function. Endocardial and epicardial edges are displayed. Left ventricular volume curve, calculated LVEF and end diastolic and end systolic volumes are shown.

WACKERS–LIU CIRCUMFERENTIAL PROFILES QUANTIFICATION (WLCQ®)

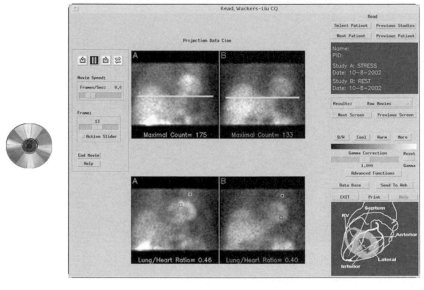

Fig. 10-31. WLCQ. Rotating planar projection images and regions of interest for calculating lung/heart ratio.

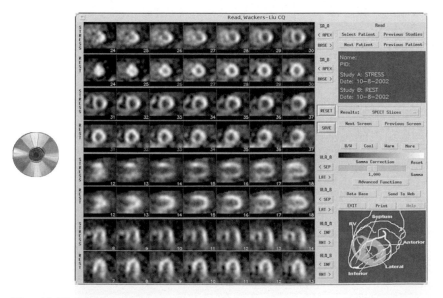

Fig. 10-32. WLCQ. Standard display of reconstructed slices of same-day rest-stress Tc-99m-Sestamibi SPECT images. A large reversible anteroseptal and lateral and inferoseptal myocardial perfusion defect is present.

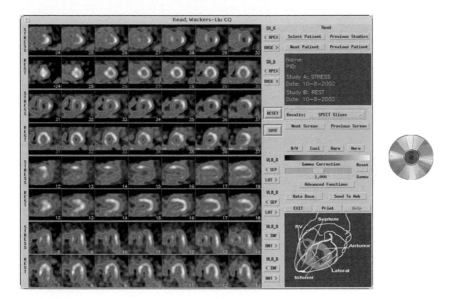

Fig. 10-33. WLCQ. Color display of the reconstructed slices displayed in Fig. 11-31.

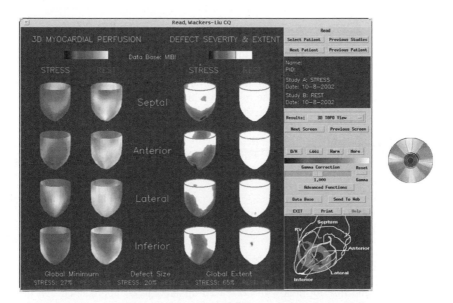

Fig. 10-34. WLCQ. Three dimensional rendering of stress and rest myocardial perfusion. From the top to bottom the septal, anterior, lateral and inferior walls are facing the observer. On the left, regional radiotracer uptake is normalized to maximal count density within the left verticle. The darkened areas represent decreased myocardial perfusion. On the stress images a large anteroseptal, lateral.

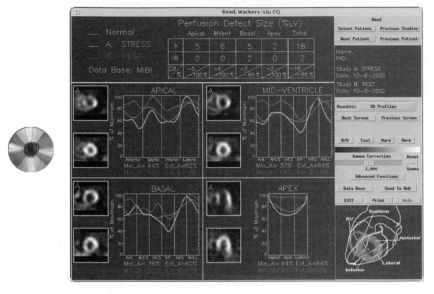

Fig. 10-35. WLCQ. Quantification of myocardial perfusion using circumferential count distribution profiles. The yellow curves represent regional count distribution on the stress images. The red curves represent rest images. The white curve depicts the lower limit of normal Tc-99m-labeled radiotracer distribution. The stress curve is below the lower limit of normal in the apical slices in the anterior, and lateral regions. The rest curve in the apical slices is within normal range. In the mid ventricular short axis slices, the stress curve is below to the lower limit of normal in the anterior, inferior, and lateral regions. The mid ventricular rest curve is within normal range. In the basal slices the stress curve is below normal in the inferior and lateral region. The rest curve in the basal slices is largely within normal range. At the apex a reversible defect is present. Stress and rest defect size are quantified in the table at the top. The stress defect is large and involves 18% of the left ventricle,, the rest defect is very small at 2%. This is an example of a large reversible anteroapical, anteroseptal, lateral, and inferior defect.

Fig. 10-34. and inferior area with decreased uptake can be appreciated. On the rest images mildly decreased uptake in the inferior wall consistent with attenuation is present. On the right, regional myocardial perfusion is compared to a normal database. Areas with less than normal myocardial uptake are displayed in color. On the stress images a large anteroseptal, lateral and inferior myocardial perfusion defect can be appreciated. The stress images are normal.

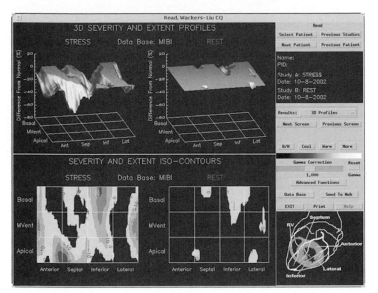

Fig. 10-36. WLCQ. Three dimensional display of circumferential count distribution profiles. The images on top display 36 circumferential count profiles from apex (front) to base (back). The limit of normal myocardial perfusion is displayed as a flat plane. Where the circumferential profile breaks through the normal limits, i.e. abnormal perfusion, valleys are shown. On the stress profiles (left), abnormal perfusion ("valleys") is present in the anterior, septal and lateral regions. On the rest images (right) only mild impressions are present at the base in the inferolateral walls. The bottom images show color-coded projections of the image on top. Dark-blue is normal. Abnormal perfusion is indicated by shades of color. This rectangular display is similar to the concentric bull's eye display. However, the apical myocardial perfusion data are displayed at the bottom of the rectangle and the basal perfusion data are displayed at the top of the rectangle. This leads to less distortion of the extent of myocardial perfusion abnormalities than with the concentric bulls eye display. The marked reversibility of stress-induced myocardial perfusion abnormality can be appreciated.

COMPARATIVE QUANTIFICATION OF SPECT IMAGES

Stress and rest myocardial perfusion abnormalities may be expressed as percent of left ventricular volume or as SSSs and SRSs. One should be aware that defect size calculated using one method differs from that calculated by other methods (see Table 10-2, p. 156).

IMPORTANCE OF QUANTITATIVE IMAGE ANALYSIS

Reliable quantification of myocardial perfusion images, by any method, is extremely important and should be used for the following reasons:

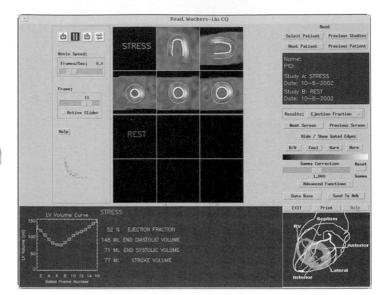

Fig. 10-37. WLCQ. Display of stress ECG-gated SPECT and computed endocardial edges for regional wall motion analysis and calculation of LVEF. In this patient LVEF is preserved at 52%, with anteroapical dyskinesis and anteroseptal hypokinesis. In addition the motion of the septum is paradoxical due to prior cardiac surgery. The end diastolic volume of 146 ml is relatively large.

- Quantification provides *greater confidence* in interpretation. Graphic display of relative count distribution, compared with a normal database, serves as an objective and consistent "second observer." The normal database serves as a consistent "benchmark" against which images are compared.
- Quantification provides enhanced intraobserver and interobserver interpretive reproducibility.
- Quantification provides a reproducible means of measuring the *degree of abnormality*. This is important because it is well established that the more abnormal a myocardial perfusion image, the poorer is patient outcome.
- Quantification of rest LVEF from myocardial perfusion images provides additional important prognostic information *(9,10)*.

In our view, quantitative analysis is complementary to visual analysis.

Interpretation should start with visual inspection of images using the following systematic approach:

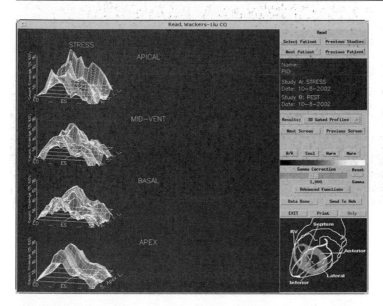

Fig. 10-38. WLCQ. Three dimensional thickening profiles. In order to judge the quality of an ECG-gated SPECT study, in particular to recognize technical gating problems, inspection of the count recovery or thickening curves is useful. The figure shows families of thickening curves for apical, mid-ventricular and basal short axis slices, and the apex (derived form horizontal log axis slice). The y-axis shows counts normalized to end diastolic (ED) counts. The three-dimensional display shows the increase in count in end systole (ES) and decrease in ED as circumferential profiles from anterior (A), septum (S), inferior (I) and lateral (L) wall. In a gated SPECT study with good ECG-synchronization, the thickening profiles start and end at the same count level. Thickening curves can thus be used as a method to recognize technical ECG-gating problems.

Table 10-2

Comparative Characterization of Abnormal SPECT Results (Modified from Ref. 8

	Defect size		
	Small	*Moderate*	*Large*
Vascular territories	≤ 1	1–2	2 or 3
SSS	4–8	9–13	> 13
Polar maps (% of LV)[a]	< 10%	10–20%	> 20%
Circumferential profile (% of LV)[b]	< 5%	5–10%	> 10%

SSS, summed stress score.

[a]Compared with gender-matched normal file and reflects extent only.

[b]Based on Yale-CQ: Sum of defects in 36 interpolated slices. Compared with normal data files and incorporates both extent and severity.

1. Visual inspection of the unprocessed rotating planar images.
2. Visual analysis of reconstructed SPECT slices in three orthogonal cuts. Images should be inspected for overall quality and the presence of possible artifacts.
3. Quantitative display then serves to confirm and enhance the visual impression.

Quantitative analysis generally should not necessarily be expected to provide entirely new information. However, quantitative analysis may frequently be helpful clinically in adding a level of certainty in differentiating equivocal image features from abnormal or normal studies. We refer to this process as "quantitative analysis with visual overread."

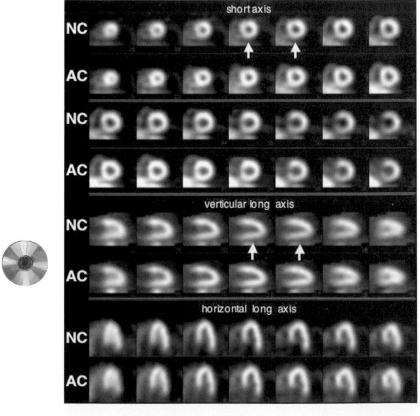

Fig. 10-39. Non corrected (NC) and X-ray CT attenuation-corrected (AC) stress SPECT images. The NC images show mild inferior attenuation (arrows), which is appropriately corrected on the AC images.

Analysis of Attenuation-Corrected SPECT Images

AC devices have become more robust over the last couple of years *(11)*. AC is used routinely in many laboratories. Clinical studies have shown that AC improved diagnostic accuracy by enhanced artifact recognition. Sensitivity usually was only slightly higher by AC, but specificity and normalcy rates were substantially better *(12)*. Attenuation-corrected images are often of better quality, in part due to the use of iterative reconstruction.

When interpreting attenuation-corrected images, it is strongly recommended to review also the uncorrected images. It may be helpful when one suspects an attenuation artifact on the non-corrected images, to see this confirmed by correction on the attenuation-corrected images (**Figs. 10-39** to **10-47**). On the contrary, QA of the attenuation map and correct co-registration are important. As can be expected, attenuation-corrected images are more uniform than non-corrected images. Therefore, when quantification is performed, one must use a specifically generated attenuation-corrected normal database.

AC not only corrects for artifacts, it may also bring out abnormalities not apparent on uncorrected images (**Figs. 10-48** to **10-52**). In particular in the latter situation, appropriate quality control is important to enhance reader confidence.

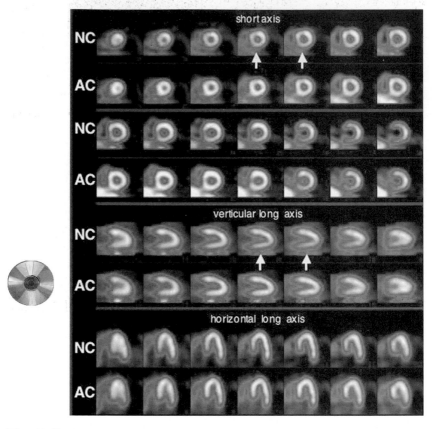

Fig. 10-40. Same images as in Fig 10-39 in color.

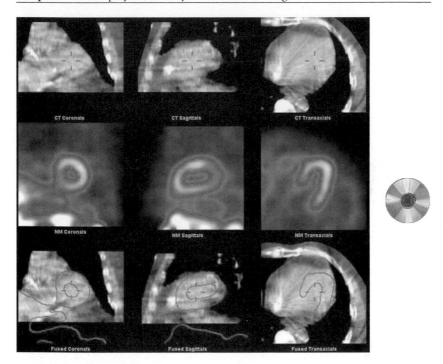

Fig. 10-41. Fusion of CT and SPECT images of the patient shown in Figs 10-39 and 10-40. Single-slice x-ray CT transmission images are shown on top in coronal, sagittal and transverse slices. The middle row shows Tc-99m-tetrofosmin SPECT emission images in the same orientations. The bottom row shows the fusion of emission (contours) and transmission images. Alignment of the two images is acceptable for attenuation correction.

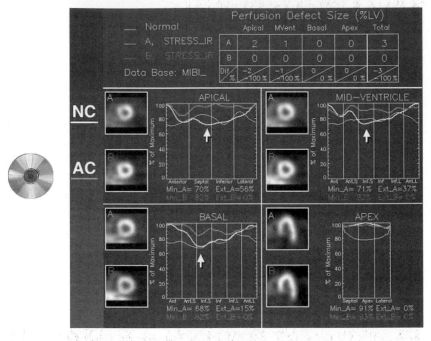

Fig. 10-42. Circumferential count profiles of the images shown in Fig. 10-39 and 10-40. The profiles of the non-corrected (NC) images are shown in yellow; the profiles of the attenuation-correction (AC) images are shown in red. The white curve indicates the lower-limit-of–normal of AC SPECT images. The arrows mark the mild (3%) inferior defect on the NC images. The AC profile is well within the normal range.

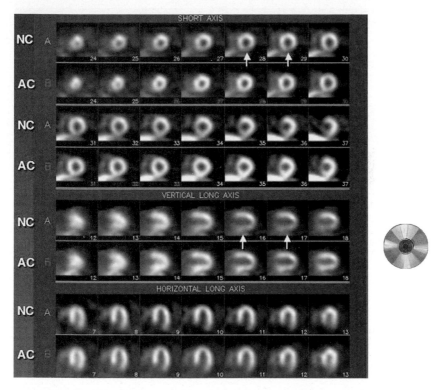

Fig. 10-43. Non corrected (NC) and X-ray CT attenuation-corrected (AC) stress SPECT Images. The NC images show a moderate inferior defect (arrows). On the AC images no defect is present.

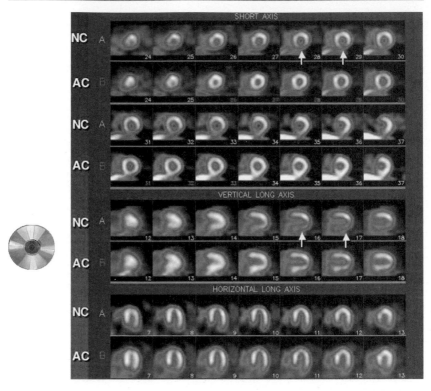

Fig. 10-44. Same images as in Fig 10-43 in color.

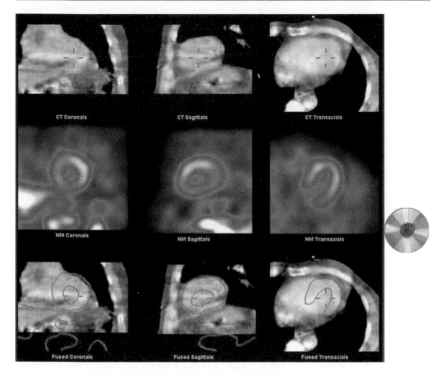

Fig. 10-45. Fusion images of the same patient as in Figs. 10-43 and 10-44. The format is the same as in Fig 10-41.

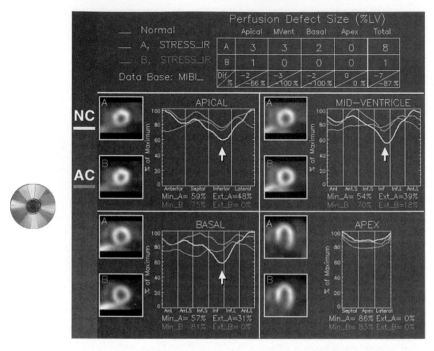

Fig. 10-46. Circumferential count profiles of the images shown in Fig. 10-43 and 10-44. The format is the same as in Fig. 10-42. The arrows mark a moderate (8%) inferior defect on the NC images. The circumferential profile of the AC images is largely within the normal range.

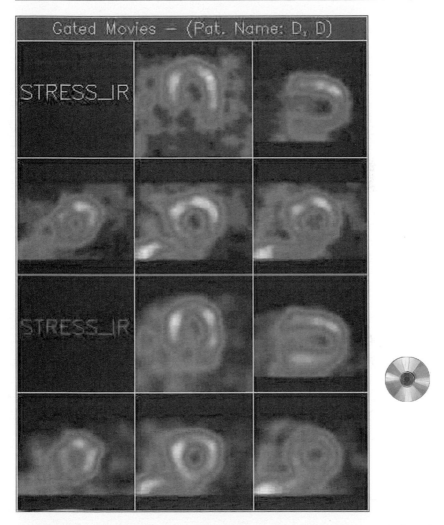

Fig. 10-47. ECG-gated SPECT movie of the images shown in Figs. 10-43 and 10-44. Overall, global left ventricular function is normal (LVEF %). Regional wall motion, particularly of the inferior wall (with defect on NC images) is normal.

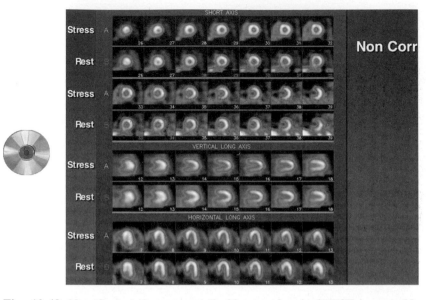

Fig. 10-48. Non Corrected stress-rest Tc-99m-tetrofosmin SPECT images. No defect is present.

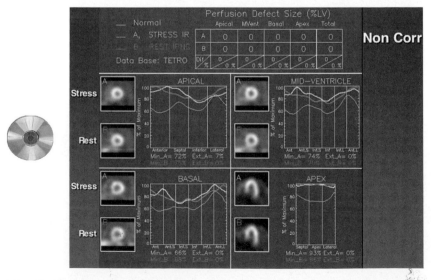

Fig. 10-49. Circumferential count profiles of the images shown in Fig. 10-48. The stress (yellow) and rest (rest) profiles are above the lower limit of normal curve (white), confirming the absence of a perfusion abnormality.

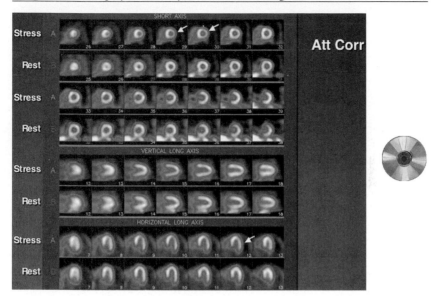

Fig. 10-50. Attenuation-corrected stress-rest Tc-99m-tetrofosmin images of the same patient shown in Fig. 10-48. A mild reversible lateral wall defect (arrows) is present.

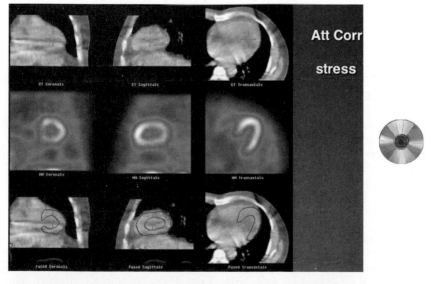

Fig. 10-51. Fusion images of the same patient as in Figs. 10-48 and 10-49. Alignment is correct.

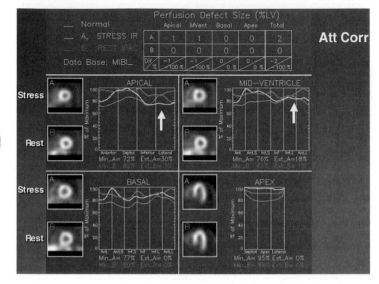

Fig. 10-52. Circumferential count profiles of the images shown in Fig. 10-50. The format is the same as in Fig. 10-42. The arrows mark a mild (2%) lateral wall defect on the attenuation corrected images. On cardiac catheterization the patient had 3-v CAD with the most severe obstruction in the left circumflex coronary artery.

REFERENCES

1. DePuey EG (2006). *Imaging Guidelines for Nuclear Cardiology Procedures 2006*, available at http://www.asnc.org Menu: "Manage Your Practice": "Guidelines & Standards".
2. American Heart Association, American College of Cardiology, and Society of Nuclear Medicine (1992). Standardization of cardiac tomographic imaging. *Circulation* 86:338–339.
3. Cerqueira MD, Weissman NJ, Dilsizian V, Jacobs AK, Kaul S, Laskey WK, Pennell DJ, Rumberger JA, Ryan T, Verani MS; American Heart Association Writing Group on Myocardial Segmentation and Registration for Cardiac Imaging (2002). Standardized myocardial segmentation and nomenclature for tomographic imaging of the heart. *Circulation* 105:539–542 and *J Nucl Cardiol* 9:240–245.
4. Germano G, Kavanagh PB, Waechter P, Areeda J, Van Kriekinge S, Sharir T, Lewin HC, Berman DS (2000). A new algorithm for the quantification of myocardial perfusion SPECT I: technical principles and reproducibility. *J Nucl Med* 41:712–719.
5. Germano G, Kiat H, Kavanagh PB, Moriel M, Mazzanti M, Su HT, Van Train KF, Berman DS (1995). Automatic quantification of ejection fraction from gated myocardial perfusion SPECT. *J Nucl Med* 36:2138–2147.
6. Faber TL, Cooke CD, Folks RD, Vansant JP, Nichols KJ, DePuey EG, Pettigrew RI, Garcia EV (1999). Left ventricular function and perfusion images: an integrated method. *J Nucl Med* 40:650–659.

7. Liu YH, Sinusas AJ, DeMan P, Zaret BL, Wackers FJ (1999). Quantification of SPECT myocardial perfusion images: methodology and validation of the method. *J Nucl Cardiol* 6:190–204.
8. Iskandrian AE (1999). Risk assessment of stable patients (panel III). In: Wintergreen panel summaries. *J Nucl Cardiol* 6:93–155.
9. Berman DS, Hachamovitch RH, Kiat H, Cohen I, Cabio JA, Wang FP, Friedman JD, Germano G, Van Train K, Diamond GA (1995). Incremental value of prognostic testing in patients with known or suspected ischemic heart disease: a basis for optimal utilization of single-photon emission computed tomography. *J Am Coll Cardiol* 26:639–647.
10. Vanzetto G, Ormezzano O, Fagret D, Comet M, Denis B, Machecourt J (1999). Long term additive prognostic value of thallium-201 myocardial perfusion imaging over clinical and exercise stress test in low-to-intermediate risk patients. Study in 1,137 patients with 6 year-follow-up. *Circulation* 100:1521–1527.
11. Hendel RC, Corbett JR, Cullom J, DePuey EG, Garcia EV, Bateman TM (2002). The value and practice of attenuation correction for myocardial perfusion SPECT imaging: a joint position statement from the American Society of Nuclear Cardiology and the Society of Nuclear Medicine. *J Nucl Cardiol* 9:135–143.
12. Massood Y, Liu YH, Depuey G, Taillefer R, Araujo LI, Allen S, Delbeke D, Anstett F, Peretz A, Zito MJ, Tsatkin V, Wackers FJTh (2005). Clinical validation of SPECT attenuation correction using x-ray computed tomography-derived attenuation maps: multicenter clinical trial with angiographic correlation. *J Nucl Cardiol* 12:676–686.

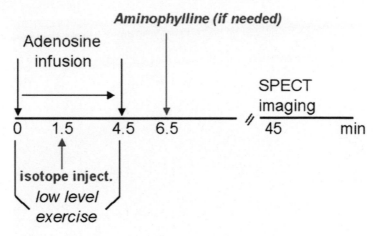

Color Plate 1, Short adenosine infusion protocol. (see Fig. 5-4).

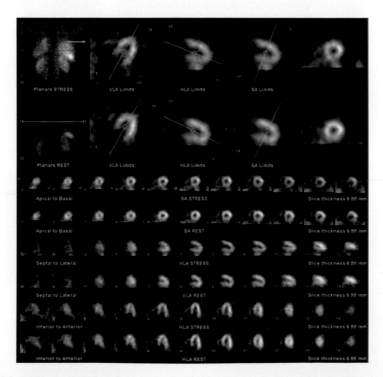

Color Plate 2, Tomographic slicing (see Fig. 6-6).

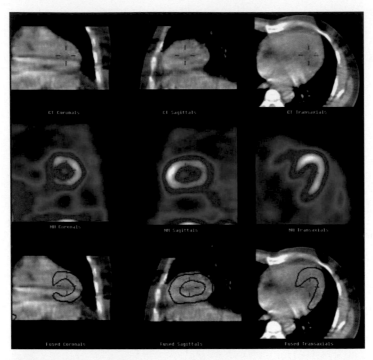

Color Plate 3, Fusion image SPECT CT (see Fig. 6-7).

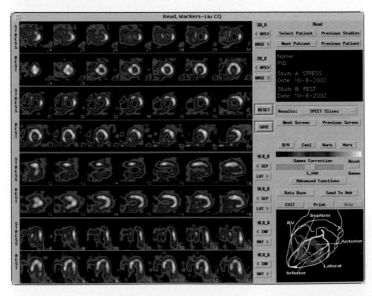

Color Plate 4, WLCQ. Color display of the reconstructed slices displayed in **Fig. 10-31** (see Fig. 10-33).

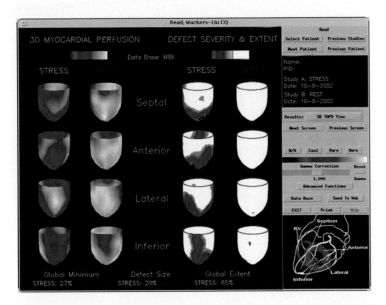

Color Plate 5, WLCQ. 3-D rendering of stress and rest myocardial perfusion (see Fig. 10-34).

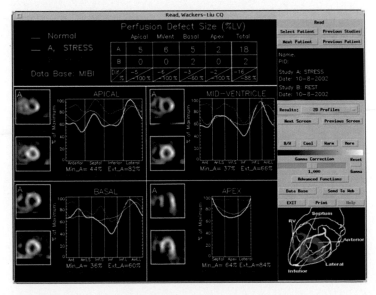

Color Plate 6, WLCQ. Quantification of myocardial perfusion using circumferential count (see Fig. 10-35).

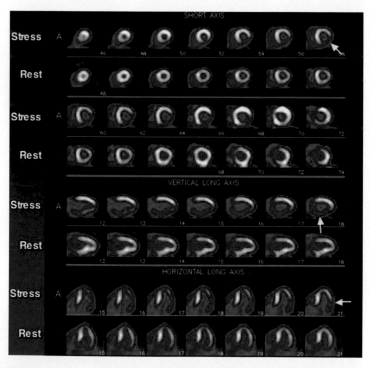

Color Plate 7, Abnormal PET inferolateral ischemia color (see Fig.11-12).

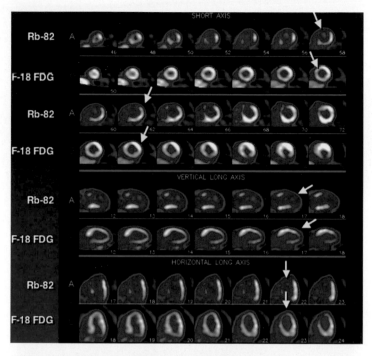

Color Plate 8, Rb/FDG mismatch Berg (see Fig. 11-20).

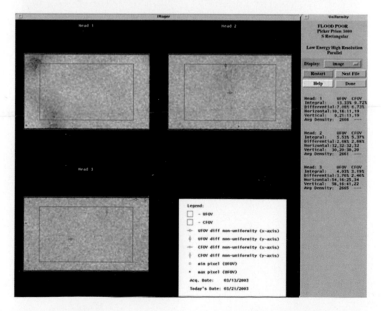

Color Plate 9, Daily flood triple-head camera (see Fig. 19-3).

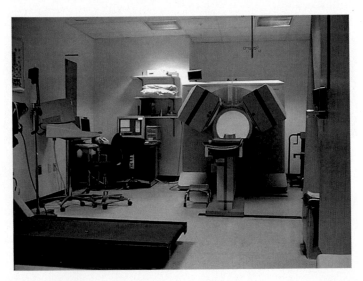

Color Plate 10, Imaging and procedure room in chest pain center (see Fig. 21-2).

11 Acquisition, Processing, Display, and Analysis of PET Images

Although the aim of this book is to provide basic and practical information about the operation of a conventional nuclear cardiology laboratory in which SPECT is operative, it is now also appropriate to address basic operational aspects of PET as well. While PET imaging now plays a major role in oncology, the clinical use of PET myocardial perfusion imaging, particularly of PET/CT, has increased substantially in recent years. The marked proliferation of PET centers, not only in academic centers but also in physicians' offices, is due to the appreciation of PET imaging as a well-validated and a Centers for Medicare & Medicaid Services (CMS)-reimbursable cardiac imaging modality *(1–5)*.

Key Words: Space requirements for PET imaging, PET camera, Acquisition PET images, Rubidium-82 generator, Staff training, Rubidium-82 PET myocardial perfusion imaging, Fluor-18 FDG PET myocardial viability imaging, PET imaging protocol, Glucose loading, Analysis PET images.

ADVANTAGES OF CARDIAC PET IMAGING

State-of-the art PET imaging has several practical advantages over conventional SPECT imaging:

- Improved image quality, especially in obese patients
- Relatively short rest–stress imaging protocol
- Routine attenuation correction
- Higher sensitivity and particularly specificity for detecting coronary artery disease
- Potential to perform additional CT-based diagnostic imaging, that is, coronary artery calcium scoring and noninvasive coronary angiography

From: *Contemporary Cardiology: Nuclear Cardiology, The Basics*
By: F. J. Th. Wackers, W. Bruni, and B. L. Zaret © Humana Press Inc., Totowa, NJ

It is nearly impossible to encompass all specific technical parameters of all available PET systems in this brief summary. PET/CT imaging is relatively new, and the technology continues to evolve rapidly. Nevertheless, many of the requirements for PET imaging are similar to those of SPECT imaging.

This chapter will focus on those aspects of PET that are different or additional.

The following items will be discussed:

- Space requirements
- Specialized training
- Hardware and software options
- Acquisition and processing parameters
- PET radiotracers for myocardial blood flow and viability

SPACE REQUIREMENTS

PET/CT equipment is substantially larger and heavier than SPECT cameras. Furthermore, the total required imaging space is about twice that for a regular SPECT camera. In addition to a large imaging room (20×16 ft, 6.1×4.8 m), a separate adjacent processing/monitoring room (12×4 ft, 3.6×1.2 m) is also needed (**Fig. 11-1**). Because of

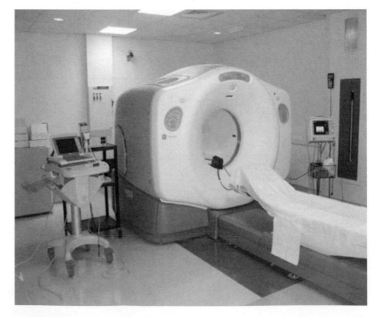

Fig. 11-1. Imaging room with PET-CT camera.

the use of X-ray radiation, walls, floor, and ceiling need appropriate shielding. A small room (8 × 8 ft, 2.5 × 2.5 m) in which patients can be prepared for imaging and in which they can be observed after the test if needed as well.

SPECIALIZED TRAINING

Appropriate training in PET imaging technology is important. PET imaging technology is different from standard nuclear imaging, and it is crucial that technologists have a good understanding of how the equipment works to prevent imaging artifacts.

In some states, only certified X-ray technologists may operate CT scanners. Therefore, it makes sense to have technologists on staff with expertise and certification in both nuclear medicine and X-ray or have individual technologists with dual certification. Dual expertise will allow for the performance of diagnostic CT scans in conjunction with PET imaging.

After the purchase of a PET camera, one should insist that the vendor's PET application specialist spends sufficient time in the imaging facility for adequate teaching of equipment-specific acquisition and processing parameters, as well as trouble-shooting and QA. It may be particularly helpful to perform the first patient studies with the application specialist present in the laboratory and to acquire and process these first "real" patient studies with her/his assistance. Attenuation correction (AC) is an absolute necessity for PET imaging, but it has the potential of creating artifacts. It will be particularly useful to review in detail the process of AC with the application specialist.

HARDWARE

Each vendor has different hardware options for PET imaging. Each option has its advantages and disadvantages, which should be discussed with the vendor.

Dedicated PET cameras are no longer widely used. There is general agreement that hybrid PET/CT scanners for the acquisition of attenuation maps are faster than those acquired with the traditional radioisotope transmission sources, and they are considered to be more accurate. The CT scanner also provides the important additional potential of performing coronary calcium scoring and/or noninvasive CT angiography after the cardiac PET examination is complete.

Detector Crystals

Currently, three types of detector crystals are available for PET imaging:

1. Bismuth germanate (BGO)
2. Lutetium oxyorthosilicate (LSO)
3. Gadolinium oxyorthosilicate (GSO)

The BGO is the conventional type crystal; the LSO and GSO are newer types of crystals. Each type has advantages and disadvantages. One should discuss these with the vendor and ensure that the crystal that is purchased is optimal for the type of imaging that will be performed, that is, 3-D or 2-D imaging. Detailed discussion of these options and pertinent issues can be found in the ASNC guideline "PET emission tomography myocardial perfusion and glucose metabolism imaging" *(5)*.

Number of Crystal Rings and Axial FOV

PET cameras have a number of rings of hundreds of small crystal detectors. The number of rings is different for each vendor and may vary from 24 to 44. For imaging of the heart, the axial FOV is of practical relevance and should be large enough for imaging enlarged hearts without truncation. The axial FOV must be at least 15 cm.

2-D Versus 3-D Imaging

The crystal rings in the PET camera are separated by lead or tungsten septa. Imaging with the septa in place (conventional imaging mode) is now called 2-D imaging. Some newer scanners have retractable septa, which, when retracted, increase count rate substantially. This is now called 3-D imaging. However, this increased sensitivity of 3-D imaging is achieved at the cost of greater amount of scatter and randoms (i.e., false coincidences). The 2-D acquisition mode remains standard for cardiac PET.

Number of CT Slices

The number of CT rings determines whether CT scans are suited only for AC or also are of "diagnostic quality." Diagnostic quality CT scans (16-slices or more) have sufficiently high spatial resolution to allow for diagnostic interpretation of the entire thorax. Six-slice CT is a minimal requirement for performing coronary calcium scoring. A minimum of 64-slice CT is preferred for performing noninvasive CT coronary angiography.

Patient Weight Limit

Verify the maximal patient weight that the table can support. Consider the average weight of the patients in your practice. Maximal acceptable weight limit is generally 350–400 lb (160–180 kg).

Gantry Size and Weight

An engineer must authorize the floor's capacity to support the scanner weight. Reinforcement of the floor may be necessary, which adds to the overall cost of the purchase and extends the installation time. PET/CT scanners weigh considerably more than standard gamma cameras.

Power Requirements

Most scanners have special electrical power needs. Check with the manufacturer.

Universal Power Supply

Even if the electrical power supply is stable, a UPS is a good optional feature.

Air Conditioning

PET/CT scanners have specific air conditioning requirements. The CT portion of the scanner generates a substantial amount of heat that needs to be dissipated adequately.

Hardware Service

Is local service available for the equipment? What is their response time? What is their backup or support? Contact other hospitals/users in your geographic area that have the same PET service and ask about the average downtime of the system, the service response times, and the capabilities of the service technicians. Negotiate for a guaranteed minimal downtime in the service contract.

Computer Speed and Memory

Computer speed should be at least 2 GHz with at least 2 GB of RAM and 500 GB disk memory space.

Networking Capabilities

Can the new imaging computer system be interfaced readily with the existing network system in the laboratory/hospital? It is particularly useful if PET images can be viewed on the same workstations where the other SPECT perfusion studies are interpreted. If the new system can be interfaced seamlessly with laboratory network, there is no need for additional and separate workstations for reviewing both SPECT and PET studies.

Display Computer

Cardiac PET images must be interpreted from a high-resolution (1280 × 1024 pixels) color monitor (24-bit or higher true color). Multiple color scales, including linear gray scale, should be available.

Storage of Digital Data

The PET workstation should have sufficient on-computer memory space (at least 500 GB) for easy access to recent studies. Raw image data may be stored on 2.3–4.2 GB optical disks or large 1.7 TB RAID archiving system. Processed data may be kept on 700 MB CDs.

SOFTWARE CONSIDERATIONS

Software considerations are the same as those for conventional SPECT computer systems, with the following additional issues.

Ease of Changing Pre-Set Acquisition Protocols

Some systems do not allow changing the order of CT transmission scans or eliminating some of the CT transmission scans. For example, the acquisition software may be programmed for the acquisition of transmission scans before *and* after PET imaging. The software may not allow for acquiring a single-transmission scan after PET image acquisition.

Ability to Align Transmission and Emission Data

It is crucial to ensure that the emission and transmission data are aligned properly. Some software algorithms allow for manipulation and realignment of the imaging data. This is important if a patient has moved slightly between emission and transmission images. If the software does not allow for this, one has to consider repeat acquisition of the transmission scan.

Fusion Software

To fuse SPECT, MR, or other CT data with the PET images, additional software may be needed. Ensure that the standard software package has the all capabilities and features needed.

Screen Captures

The capability to obtain screen captures of processed images and of processing results may be a useful feature when communication images with other healthcare providers. It also may be valuable when preparing slides for a presentation.

CT Software

If the CT scanner is used only for AC, additional CT software may not be needed. However, for the performance of coronary calcium scoring or CT coronary angiography, additional CT acquisition and or processing software may be needed.

ECG MONITOR AND STRESS EQUIPMENT

Size and Portability

If the PET camera is shared with other disciplines, for example, oncology, it may be useful to have a small portable ECG machine that is easily stored or moved and out of the way to accommodate oncology patients.

Software Options

The ECG machine should be easily programmed and modified for various stress protocol options. Can laboratory-specific protocols be inserted in the program? For example, printing ECGs at predetermined time intervals or the printing of certain parameters in the final report.

Test Setup

Is the setup of a patient, that is, entering patient information in the computer, placement of electrodes, and arrangement of ECG cables, easily performed?

Stress Protocol Options

Ensure that the standard software has all required features. For some portable ECG machines, it may necessary to purchase additional stress software.

AUTOMATIC BLOOD PRESSURE MACHINE

Using the hybrid PET/CT scanner, CT transmission scans are acquired immediately following the infusion of a pharmacologic stress agent. During the CT acquisition, one cannot take a blood pressure measurement manually. Therefore, an automatic blood pressure machine is required.

Additional Blood Pressure Cuff Sizes

It is necessary to have a variety of cuff sizes to accommodate patients with the various body habitus.

Extra-Length Air Tubing

Depending on the layout of the imaging room and the orientation of the patient on the imaging table (i.e., head-first or feet-first), one may need to order extra long (several feet) air tubing to connect patient to the blood pressure machine. Some vendors now offer blood pressure machines specifically designed with PET imaging in mind, with extra-long tubing.

Infusion Pump

The standard stress protocol with PET imaging requires pharmacological vasodilator stress with dipyridamole or adenosine infusion. A reliable infusion pump is necessary (see Chapter 1 p. 9 for tips in selecting a pump).

Crash Cart

Although the risk of medical emergencies with pharmacological stress is relatively low, the same equipment described for medical emergencies in Chapter 1 (p. 10) must be available in the immediate proximity of the PET imaging facility.

RADIOPHARMACY

The performance of PET imaging requires additional hot-lab equipment for handling high-energy PET isotopes. Below is a listing of the required items (refer also to Chapter 1, p. 11).

Hot-lab equipment is available in two varieties: standard lead for single-photon radioisotopes and alternatively thick lead shielding or tungsten for PET radioisotopes.

Dose Calibrator

The dose calibrator should be able to measure a wide range of energies. Ensure that the specifications of the dose calibrator include the energy of positron emitters in addition to that of single-photon isotopes.

Lead Shield with Glass

Because PET isotopes have high energy, special shielding is required.

Syringe Shields

For F-18 fluorodeoxyglucose (FDG) studies, syringes with high-energy shields are needed. Typically, tungsten shields offer the best shielding and yet are lighter in weight than lead.

Lead Pigs and Carrying Cases

Manufacturers supply thick lead-lined carrying cases to hold F-18 FDG activity. However, these cases are very heavy. It is recommended that the F-18 FDG activity is stored in close proximity to the area where F-18 FDG will be injected, to minimize the amount of time/exposure for the technologist by carrying the case back and forth. Relatively light-weight tungsten pigs with a carrying handle for easy transportation are commercially available.

Lead-Lined Trash Containers

These are necessary for the storage and decaying of the radioactive trash. Trash containers are available with thick lead shielding, specifically designed for F-18 FDG storage.

Rb-82 GENERATOR

Rb-82 is commercially available as CardioGen-82® (**Fig. 11-2**). The CardioGen-82® generator contains the parent isotope strontium-82 (Sr-82) that produces Rb-82 by elution with saline. The half-life of Sr-82 is 25.5 days, whereas the half-life of Rb-82 is 72 s.

The generator must be used with the calibrated CardioGen-82 Infusion System. The infusion system consists of a mobile cart that houses the generator in a shielded compartment that has an automated computerized dosing system, thus reducing the amount of personal interaction needed. It thus reduces exposure of the nuclear technologist. The infusion system automatically detects, calibrates, and controls the activity infused into the patient. An application specialist should train technologists in the laboratory on the operation of the infusion system.

The generator requires replacement each month. A new generator has to be installed into the cart and the tubing of the infusion system be attached to the generator.

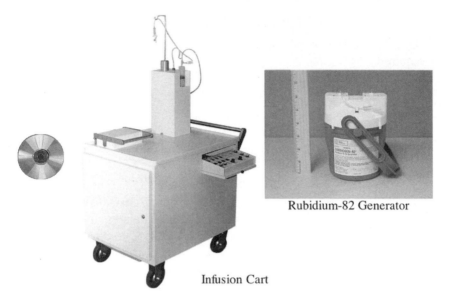

Rubidium-82 Generator

Infusion Cart

Fig. 11-2. Rubidium-82 generator and Rubidium infusion cart.

QC is required *daily* prior to use in patients to ensure that no Sr-82 breakthrough occurs. At the end of the month, the generator is shipped back to the manufacturer with strict adherence to the packing instructions provided by the vendor. In addition to these specific packing instructions, normal radioactive shipping procedures with surveying and wiping of the generator package are to be followed.

ADDITIONAL MISCELLANEOUS SUPPLIES
(IN ADDITION TO THOSE MENTIONED IN CHAPTER 1, P. 18)

Heavy Blankets

Due to the powerful air conditioning of the PET/CT scanner, patients are often cold and require extra blankets to keep warm. If patients are uncomfortable, they may shiver and not be able to hold still during the imaging.

Blood Glucose Testing Supplies

When F-18 FDG studies are performed for assessment of myocardial viability, patient's blood glucose level needs to be monitored and adjusted according to the glucose-loading protocol (see pg. 183 and table 11-3). Portable monitoring machines are available that measure the glucose level quickly and accurately. Syringes, alcohol swabs, test strips, and glucose-control solutions are needed.

Insulin

This is needed to adjust the glucose level of the patient to the desired level according to the glucose-loading protocol.

Glucola or Other Oral Glucose

This may be given orally to the patient at the beginning of an F-18 FDG viability protocol.

IV Tubing

For Rb-82 pharmacological stress testing, special patient tubing for use with the Rb-82 generator is needed. This can be purchased through the generator supplier.

LABORATORY STAFFING

Staff Needed for Rb-82 Stress Testing

The following staff are needed at a minimum:

- One ECG/stress technologist
- Two nuclear technologists
- One registered nurse or physician to monitor the test

The reason that two nuclear technologists are needed for Rb-82 stress imaging is that one technologist operates the Rb-82 generator and another technologist operates the PET/CT camera in the control room. Another option is to have one nuclear technologist and one X-ray technologist

For additional efficiency, some laboratories have found it helpful to have two nurses working in the PET laboratory instead of one nurse and one ECG tech. In this scenario, the first nurse prepares and interviews patient 1 and monitors his/her Rb-82 stress test. In the time that the first patient is being scanned, the second nurse prepares and interviews patient 2. As soon as the first patient is off the table, the second patient is ready to go on the table. Thus, there is no delay in imaging because of the time involved with patient preparation and interviewing prior to the test.

Because a typical rest–stress Rb-82 imaging protocol takes approximately 35 min, the latter scenario with two nurses results in no downtime for the scanner, due to waiting for a patient to be ready. Obviously, two nurses are a more expensive than one nurse and one ECG technician, but the volume of patients that can be imaged is greater.

Staff Needed for Myocardial Viability Imaging

The following staff are needed at a minimum:

- Registered nurse
- Nuclear technologist

A nurse is needed to monitor and adjust a patient's blood glucose, whereas a nuclear technologist is needed to inject the F-18 FDG and to perform imaging. Attending physicians should remain in close proximity to the imaging facility, in case a patient becomes hypoglycemic.

PET LABORATORY LOGISTICS

There are currently two types of clinical studies to perform with cardiac PET imaging:

1. Rest–stress myocardial perfusion imaging for detection of coronary artery disease.
2. Metabolic imaging for myocardial viability.

MYOCARDIAL PERFUSION IMAGING

PET myocardial perfusion studies can be performed with three different isotopes:

1. N-13 ammonia (half-life 10 min)
2. O-15 water (half-life 2 min)
3. Rb-82 (half-life 72 s)

N-13 and O-15 are cyclotron produced and not widely available. Most clinical laboratories use generator-produced Rb-82.

Because of the relative long half-life of F-18 (110 min), F-18 FDG can be purchased from an outside supplier within the geographical area to be delivered on a prespecified day and time. Viability imaging is done with F-18 FDG following a glucose-loading protocol (see pg. 183 and table 11-3).

Time Requirements

One of the attractive aspects of cardiac PET protocols is that they are relatively short compared to standard SPECT imaging (**Fig. 11-3**). Accordingly, the daily schedule for a PET camera is generally simpler than for SPECT cameras. For PET stress imaging, rest imaging is always performed first, followed by stress imaging. All PET studies are 1-day studies. Because of the short half-life of the radiotracer, there is no need

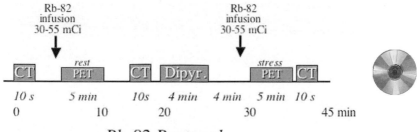

Rb-82 Protocol

Fig. 11-3. Schematic representation of timing and sequence of the Rubidium (Rb)-82 imaging protocol. The amount of Rb-82 infused depends on the age of the generator. CT = X-ray-computerized tomography; PET = positron emission tomography; Dipyr = dipyridamole infusion.

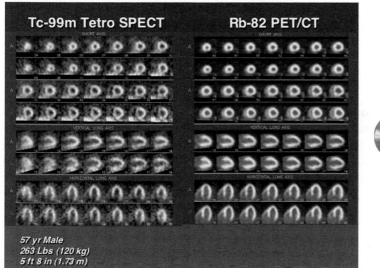

Fig. 11-4. Tc-99m-tetrofosmin stress (A)–rest (B) SPECT imaging in a very obese patient. The quality of the SPECT images (left) is of suboptimal diagnostic quality. The study was repeated one week later with Rb-82 PET (right). The considerable improvement in quality of the PET imaging can be appreciated. The images are unequivocally normal.

for separate stress and rest imaging sessions on two separate days even in obese patients, as is recommended in SPECT imaging. In fact, the high-energy PET tracer is well suited for obese patients and generally provides better image quality than with SPECT imaging (**Fig. 11-4** and **11-5**).

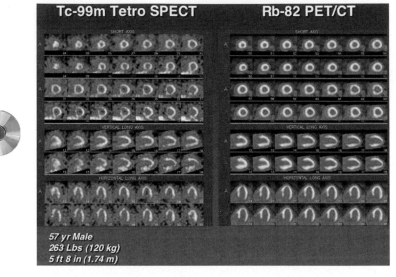

Fig. 11-5. Same images as in Fig. 11-4 in color.

REST–STRESS MYOCARDIAL PERFUSION IMAGING

Rest–stress Rb-82 myocardial perfusion imaging is performed in conjunction with pharmacologic stress. Some investigators have reported N-13 ammonia imaging after treadmill exercise and some others reported on the use of supine bicycle exercise. These methods are not being widely used at this time. Because of the short half-life of Rb-82 (72 s), it is not quite feasible to acquire acceptable quality images after injection at peak treadmill exercise. Count rate decreases rapidly within 5 min to an inadequate count rate for imaging. On the other hand, pharmacological stress (dipyridamole or adenosine) allows for injection during stress with the patient lying under the PET camera allowing for images with optimal count density.

Patient preparation for pharmacologic stress PET studies is the same as the preparation for pharmacologic stress SPECT studies (see Chapter 4).

Dipyridamole, with a half-life of 30–45 min, is currently the vasodilator of choice for Rb-82 stress imaging. Only one IV line is needed. Dipyridamole (0.56 mg/kg) is infused over 4 min. After dipyridamole infusion is completed, there is ample time for positioning of the patient in the camera gantry. At 3–4 min after the completion of dipyridamole infusion, the infusion of Rb-82 infusion is started, and after a short delay of 90 s for blood pool clearance, the acquisition of PET images is started.

Table 11-1
PET Acquisition Sequence

1. Scout X-ray	120 kV, 10 mA	5 s
2. CT	120 kV, 50 mA	10 s
3. Start Rb-82 infusion and delay		90–120 s
4. Rest PET acquisition		300 s
5. Get patient ready		300 s
6. Dipyridamole infusion	0.58 mg/kg	240 s
7. Wait		180 s
8. Scout X-ray	120 kV, 10 mA	5 s
9. CT[a]	120 kV, 50 mA	10 s
10. Start Rb-82 infusion and delay		90–120 s
11. Stress PET acquisition		300 s
12. CT optional if misregistration occurred		

[a]Optional: stress CT transmission scan may be acquired either before or after completion of stress PET imaging.

An alternative vasodilator stressor is adenosine. Adenosine has a very short half-life of 30 s. Rb-82 imaging with adenosine is more complicated than with dipyridamole because the Rb-82 infusion/acquisition has to be started while adenosine is still infused at 1.5 min after the start of adenosine infusion. Adenosine infusion has to continue for the duration of the Rb-82 PET image acquisition. The patient also needs two IV lines when adenosine is used. Refer to Chapter 5 for details about pharmacological stress.

The sequence of a typical dipyridamole Rb-82 PET/CT protocol is shown in Table 11-1.

Short 5-s scout X-ray images are acquired for a quick orientation regarding the position of the heart. The actual transmission CT is acquired for 10 s. It should be noted that the second stress CT transmission scan may be obtained either before or after stress Rb-21 PET imaging. We believe, however, that a CT scan after PET imaging is preferred because patients have tendency to move because of dipyridamole side effects.

ACQUISITION/PROCESSING PARAMETERS

The technology of PET imaging equipment is continually changing. New crystals, electronics, and photo-multiplier tubes are being introduced each year. Each vendor has different approaches for dealing with randoms, dead time, and scatter. Table 11-2 shows acquisition parameters for BGO and LSO PET systems (6).

Table 11-2
Rest–stress Rb-82 PET Acquisition Parameters

Activity (dose)	40–60 mCi
Patient position	Supine, arms over head
Injection rate	Bolus < 30 s
Imaging time	3–6 min
Imaging delay after start Rb-82	• LVEF > 50% = 70 − 90 s
	• LVEF < 50% = 90 − 130 s
	• 130–150 s if LVEF is unknown
Matrix	128 × 128
Imaging mode	Gated static
AC	CT or Ge-68
Reconstruction method	Filtered back projection or iterative expectation maximization
Reconstruction filter	Laboratory specific
Pixel size	2–3 mm

2-D imaging with a BGO crystal is the standard acquisition mode for cardiac PET. 3-D imaging is an alternative acquisition mode with potential of substantially increased count sensitivity. However, this is offset by increased dead time and increased acquisition of scatter and randoms (i.e., false coincident counts).

Injection Rate

The entire amount of activity should be administered as an infusion of less than 30 s.

Imaging Time

Imaging time is relatively short (3–6 min) because of the rapid decay of Rb-82. Imaging must be completed before count rate has become too low.

Imaging Delay

The start of cardiac image acquisition should be delayed for 90 s to ensure clearance of Rb-82 from the blood pool. Patients with lower EFs should be given longer delay (120 s) for adequate clearance. Excessive blood pool activity may cause scatter into myocardial perfusion defects, thus making defects appear smaller.

Imaging Mode

In addition to the conventional standard static acquisition mode, newer generation PET systems allow for dynamic or serial imaging.

Dynamic PET image acquisition is begun immediately after Rb-82 is infused and continues for a set period of time. The acquired imaging serial data may then be reviewed, allowing one to select the time frames to be included or excluded for processing. This provides the option to eliminate or ignore the early phase of blood pool activity and to include only images with adequate blood pool clearance. If dynamic imaging is not feasible, one should use an appropriate imaging delay as mentioned above.

Attenuation Correction

AC of PET images may be performed using either radioactive line sources [Germanium-68 (Ge-68) or Gallium-68 (Ga-68)] on dedicated PET scanners or x-ray CT transmission on hybrid PET/CT scanners. Either method is acceptable as long as a good quality transmission map is acquired, and emission and transmission images are well coregistered.

Matrix

A matrix of 128 × 128 is standard for PET imaging.

Reconstruction Method

Filtered back projection or an iterative expectation maximization reconstruction algorithm can be used.

Reconstruction Filter

Filtering is used to achieve a desired smoothing. This will vary from laboratory to laboratory.

Pixel Size

2–3 mm is standard.

MYOCARDIAL VIABILITY IMAGING

Patient Preparation and Glucose Loading

For F-18 FDG myocardial viability studies, patient preparation prior to actual imaging may be time consuming, especially in patients with diabetes mellitus. However, the actual PET imaging protocol is relatively short: only 15–30 min. Because of the potentially long time involved with glucose loading, it is recommended that a different room be used for patient preparation and injection of F-18 FDG.

To perform optimal F-18 FDG myocardial viability imaging, it is important the patient is prepared appropriately. The myocardium prefers to use free fatty acids as an energy substrate. Thus, a patient must be prepared such that the myocardium will use glucose instead of the free fatty acids. For patients without diabetes mellitus, the most common method to achieve this is through oral glucose loading. As an option, glucose loading may also be done intravenously. The latter is sometimes preferred for patients with diabetes, since the oral method is often not sufficient to adjust their blood glucose levels. We refer for more details to the ASNC guidelines online for IV glucose-loading protocols *(6)*. Table 11-3 shows the glucose-loading protocol followed in our laboratory for myocardial viability assessment.

Myocardial Ischemia

When the purpose of F-18 FDG imaging is to assess the presence of resting myocardial *ischemia*, glucose loading is not recommended. The patient is injected with F-18 FDG during fasting state. If a patient has ongoing regional myocardial ischemia, subsequent F-18 FDG PET imaging may demonstrate "hot spot" uptake in myocardium with enhanced glucose metabolism due to ongoing ischemia.

Table 4 lists the acquisition and procession parameters for F-18 FDG imaging. The following subsections are comments on the individual parameters listed.

Image Acquisition

F-18 FDG imaging is started not earlier than 45 min after injection. At this time, there may still be some blood pool activity, but clearance will continue to improve through 90 min. Too long a delay after injection may result in low-count-density images due to the relative short half-life of F-18 (110 min). To optimize image quality, it is recommended that diabetic patients be imaged after a slightly longer delay, but not later than 60 min. If repeat F-18 FDG studies are performed, imaging parameters should be reproduced at each imaging session. It is recommended to monitor blood glucose levels at 20-min intervals until end of study.

2-D static acquisition for approximately 30 min is standard for F-18 FDG imaging. Assessment of F-18 FDG uptake can be combined with rest–stress Rb-82 myocardial perfusion imaging.

Dynamic image acquisition is an alternative acquisition mode. At least three data sets are acquired and summed to create one static image. If one of the three data sets is of suboptimal quality, for example, due to motion, the data can be excluded and only two summed sets be used for processing.

Table 11-3
Glucose Loading Protocol for Myocardial Viability Imaging

Fasting period	6–12 h	
Oral glucose loading	If fasting blood glucose < 150 mg/dL and no known diabetes, then oral glucose load: 50 g glucose orally and monitor blood glucose	
	If fasting blood glucose > 150 − 200 mg/dL or known diabetic, then oral glucose load: 25 g glucose orally and 2 U regular insulin and monitor blood glucose:	
Check blood glucose	30 min after glucose or insulin, then:	
Monitor blood glucose (check every 15 min)	130–140 mg/dL	No insulin
	150–200 mg/dL	2 U regular insulin
	200–250 mg/dL	2–3 U regular insulin
	250–300 mg/dL	3–4 U regular insulin
	300–350 mg/dL	4–5 U regular insulin (notify attending physician)
F-18 FDG injection	At the time blood glucose level is 100–140 mg/dL (continue to monitor blood glucose level at 20-30 min intervals)	

Pixel Size

2–3 mm per pixel is considered standard.

Attenuation Correction

AC can be performed by radioactive line sources (Ge-68 or Ga-68) on dedicated PET scanners or with a CT transmission scan on PET/CT scanners. Either method is acceptable as long as good quality transmission maps are acquired.

Table 11-4
F-18 FDG Acquisition/Processing Parameters

Activity (dose)	5–15 mCi (185–555 MBq)
Image start time	45–60 min post injection
Patient position	Supine, arms over head
Acquisition duration	30 min
Acquisition mode	2-D static
Total counts	Dependent on machine performance characteristics
Pixel size	2–3 mm
Matrix	128 × 128
Gating	ECG gating recommended
AC	Transmission scan (CT or Ge-68)
Reconstruction method	Filtered back projection or Iterative reconstruction method

Gating

ECG gating of FDG images is feasible and one can assess EF and regional wall motion from these images. A regular heart rate is required for ECG gating.

Patient Position

The patient should be imaged in supine position with the arms placed over the head. Great care should be taken to make sure that the patient is comfortable and is able to remain still for the duration of imaging. If the patient cannot bring the arms over the head, imaging can be performed with the arms down. In the latter situation, the time of transmission scan may have to be extended to ensure good quality. If the patient is on a PET/CT scanner, the arms down position may create beam-hardening artifacts on the transmission scan, which can create artifacts on the attenuation-corrected images.

Reconstruction

Filtered back projection or an iterative expectation maximization reconstruction algorithm can be used.

DISPLAY AND ANALYSIS OF PET IMAGES

The display and analysis of Rb-82 PET rest–stress myocardial perfusion images should include at a minimum

1. Sinogram of Rb-82 images
2. Fusion image of CT and Rb-82 images

3. Reconstructed tomographic slices
4. Display of ECG-gated cine of reconstructed slices

As with SPECT, interpretation of PET myocardial perfusion images should follow a systematic approach.

1. Inspection of the sinogram is important to identify patient motion during Rb-82 (see p. **16–5** and **Fig. 16–12**).
2. Inspection of fusion images for coregistration of Rb-12 emission image and CT heart image.
3. Rotating whole-heart PET images are usually available for inspection, but one should realize that they are in fact 3-D reconstructions and therefore are post-processing and not comparable to SPECT-rotating planar images.
4. Analysis of reconstructed tomographic short axis, vertical, and long axis slices.
5. Analysis of regional and global left ventricular function.
6. Incorporation of quantitative myocardial perfusion and functional data.
7. Incorporation of clinical and stress data.
8. Final interpretation and report.

The following subsections are comments on the parameters listed above. See also Chapter 10 for comments on systematic SPECT interpretation.

Sinogram

The sinogram (**Fig. 16–5** and **16–12**) is a composite image in which each horizontal row of pixels represents the summed counts of an entire projection image on the x-axis. Motion can be recognized by "breaks" in the smooth sinusoid pattern of inhomogeneous activity. Although the acquisition time for Rb-82 perfusion images is substantially shorter than for SPECT imaging, patient motion is still a possibility and may create artifacts.

Fusion Image of Rb-82 Emission and CT Chest Images

Transverse CT images are reviewed in stacked multiple slices scrolling mode for the following (**Fig. 11-6**).

COREGISTRATION RB-82 EMISSION IMAGES AND CT IMAGE OF THE HEART

The emission Rb-82-reconstructed slices are displayed superimposed on the CT image in the same plane. Misregistration, particularly when the lateral wall is superimposed over lung, may result in artifactual lateral wall defects after AC.

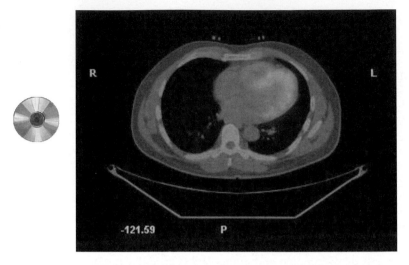

Fig. 11-6. Fusion image of PET Rb-82 myocardial perfusion (red) and chest CT (transverse plane). Inspection of these images are an important part of quality control of PET-CT imaging. Misalignment may result in significant reconstruction artifacts.

Presence of Calcium in Coronary Arteries and Ascending/Descending Aorta

For quantitative calcium scoring, the CT images must be ECG-gated. However, the presence of calcium in the coronary arteries and aorta may be qualitatively assessed on ungated CT images.

Clinically Significant Findings in Lungs, Pleura, Mediastinum, and Pericardium

In order not to miss noncardiac chest pathology, the CT images should be reviewed jointly with a physician well trained in interpreting chest CT.

Reconstructed Slices

Reconstructed PET slices are displayed using identical standardized planes and nomenclature as for SPECT images (see Chapter 10). Because all PET images are attenuation-corrected, normal PET images have greater homogeneity than normal SPECT images.

It is standard to interpret PET images on computer screen in color display (**Figs. 11-7** and **11-8**). Color display tends to exaggerate subtle differences in myocardial radiotracer uptake on SPECT images. However, because of the greater homogeneity of PET images, color display is appropriate for interpretation of PET images.

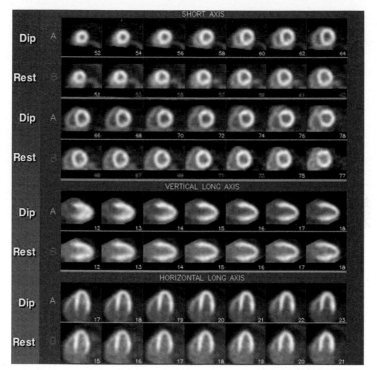

Fig. 11-7. Normal dipyridamole vasodilator stress-rest Rb-82 PET myocardial perfusion images of a 26-yr-old male volunteer. Note the high quality of images of this normal volunteer.

PET-reconstructed slices should be interpreted using the same routine as described for SPECT imaging in Chapter 10. It should be verified whether the tomographic cuts were oriented correctly relative to the anatomical axes of the heart and whether stress and rest slices were appropriately aligned. Cine display of the ECG-gated PET slices should be inspected for potential gating problems as described in Chapter 10.

Analysis of PET Images

Analysis of PET images is not significantly different from analysis of conventional SPECT images. Because PET slices are thinner (3.27 mm) than SPECT slices, more tomographic slices are available for analysis. To make interpretation of PET images similar to that of SPECT images and to avoid extensive back-and-forward scrolling of slices, we sum every two adjacent PET slices for display purpose. In this way, all slices from apex to base can be displayed on one computer screen. The standard 17-segment model may be used for

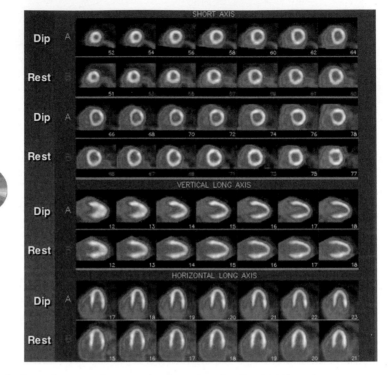

Fig. 11-8. Same images of a normal volunteer as in Fig. 11-7 in color.

semiquantitative analysis. When performing visual analysis of PET slices, one should account for the substantial greater homogeneity in radiotracer uptake of normal Rb-82 images. The description of PET myocardial perfusion defects is similar to that described in Chapter 10 for SPECT.

Quantitative Analysis

Quantitative image analysis may be performed as described for SPECT imaging. Because of the high quality of images (high-count density) and AC, regional differences in normal Rb-82 myocardial uptake are less than for SPECT imaging (**Fig. 11-9**). Accordingly, circumferential count profiles of normal Rb-82 distribution are relatively "flat" compared to those with single-photon agents.

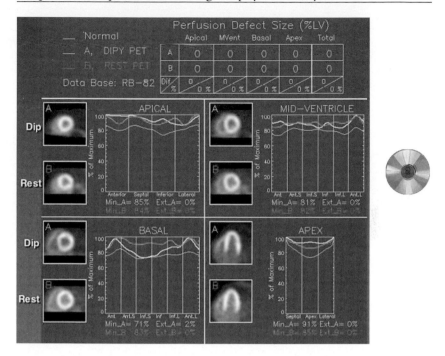

Fig. 11-9. Circumferential count profiles of the images of the normal volunteer shown in Figs. 11-7 and 11-8. The dipyridamole (Dip) stress circumferential profiles are shown in yellow, the rest profiles in red. No perfusion abnormality is quanti- fied (0%). Note that the lower-limit-of–normal curve (white) for Rb-82 is flatter and closer to the 100% line, than for single photon imaging (see e.g. Fig. 10-35).

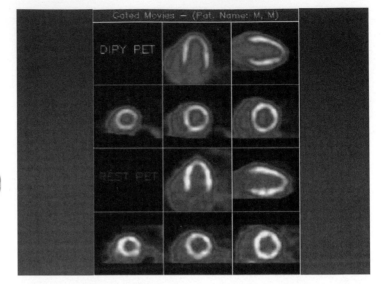

Fig. 11-10. ECG-gated PET movie of the images of the normal volunteer shown in Figs 11-7 and 11-9. Regional wall motion and wall thickening are normal. LVEF is 50%. **(movie)**

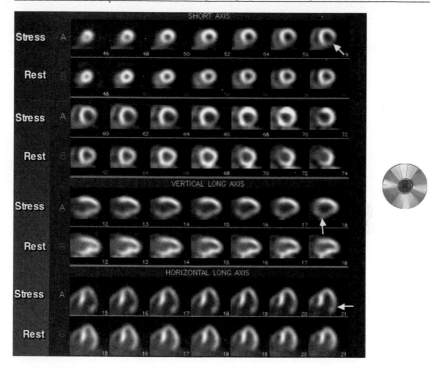

Fig. 11-11. Stress-rest Rb-82 PET images of a 57-yr old male with severe multi-vessel coronary artery disease without previous infarction. The images show a large reversible inferolateral (arrows) myocardial perfusion defect.

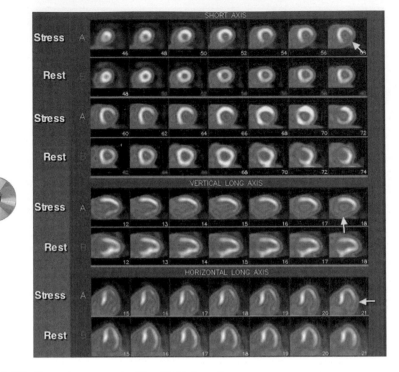

Fig. 11-12. Same images as in Fig. 11-11 in color.

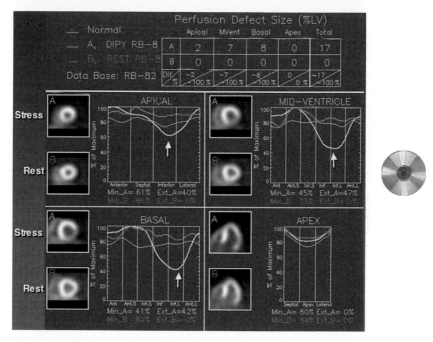

Fig. 11-13. Circumferential count profiles of the images shown in Figs. 11-11 and 11-12. The inferolateral reversible defect (arrows) is quantified as 17% of the left ventricle.

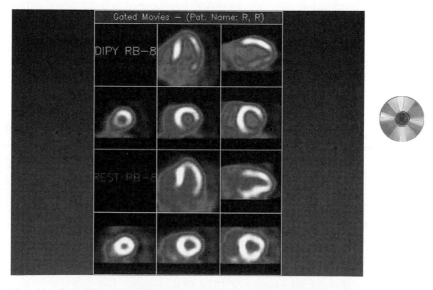

Fig. 11-14. ECG-gated PET movie of the images shown in Figs. 11-11 and 11-12. On the stress images (top) there is hypokinesis of the inferolateral. Regional wall motion reverted to normal at rest (bottom). Global LVEF was 40% after stress and 50% at rest, indicating ischemic dysfunction during dipyridamole vasodilator stress. **(movie)**

Left Ventricular Ejection Fraction

Software used for calculation of LVEF from ECG-gated SPECT images can be used without modification for ECG-gated PET images (**Fig. 11-10**).

Figures 11-11 to **11-15** show abnormal rest–dipyridamole Rb-82 PET myocardial perfusion images in a patient with severe coronary artery disease.

Analysis of F-18 FDG Images

The clinical indication for F-18 FDG imaging is usually the assessment of viable myocardium in an area with left ventricular dysfunction.

FDG imaging is almost always performed in conjunction with rest (sometimes rest–stress) myocardial perfusion imaging with Rb-82.

The analysis may be restricted to the assessment of "match" or "mismatch" between a Rb-82 myocardial perfusion defect and F-18 FDG evidence for myocardial metabolism, that is:

- Match = scar
- Mismatch = viability

However, assessment in conjunction with rest–stress Rb-82 imaging provides more complete information.

It is recommended that one interpret stress–rest Rb-82 myocardial perfusion images first:

- Normal Rb-82 uptake
- Rb-82 reversible defect
- Rb-82 fixed defect
- Regional wall motion and global function

The following preliminary conclusions may be drawn from this assessment:

- Normal Rb-82 uptake with normal regional wall motion implies myocardial viability.
- Normal Rb-82 uptake with abnormal regional wall motion suggest myocardial stunning and myocardial viability.
- Stress-induced (complete or partially) reversible Rb-82 abnormalities (regardless of wall motion) indicate myocardial ischemia and thus imply myocardial viability.
- Fixed rest–stress Rb-82 defects with abnormal regional wall motion do require additional assessment of F-18 FDG uptake, but:
  - If minimal radiotracer uptake within a rest Rb-82 defect is greater than 50% of maximal, it is likely that viable myocardium is present (e.g., within a nontransmural infarct).

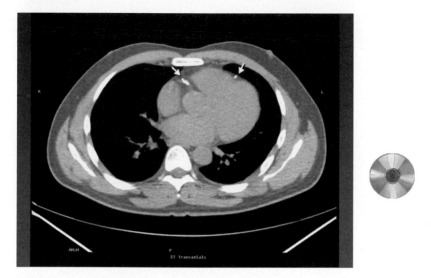

Fig. 11-15. CT image of the same patient as in Figs. 11-11 to 11-15. Moderate coronary calcium is noted in the mid right coronary artery (left arrow) and mid left anterior descending coronary artery (right arrow). Invasive contrast coronary angiography showed severe triple vessel coronary artery disease, most severe in the right coronary artery.

- – If the residual radiotracer is less than 50%, additional F-18 FDG imaging is required.
- F-18 FDG uptake within a fixed Rb-82 defect (pattern of mismatch) indicates metabolic activity and implies myocardial viability.
- Absence of F-18 FDG uptake within a fixed Rb-82 defect (match) generally indicates scar and absence of significant amount of viable myocardium.

Revascularization of areas with mismatch may result in improvement of regional and global left ventricular function. The degree of improvement of ventricular function is related to the extent of ischemic and viable myocardium. When about 25–30% of the LV shows the pattern of Rb-82/F18FDG mismatch one may anticipate a clinically relevant increase of LVEF after revascularization *(7)*. However, this does not mean that with smaller amounts of mismatch, revascularization is not meaningful. Relief of ischemia, even without improved function, may improve outcome in individual patients *(8)*.

Examples of myocardial viability studies with Rb-82 and F-18FDG are shown in **Figs. 11-16** to **11-22**.

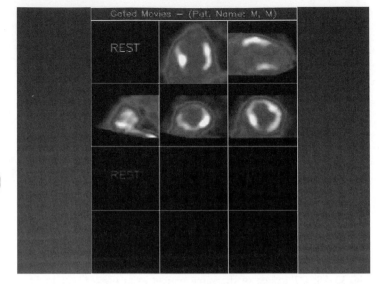

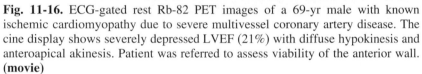

Fig. 11-16. ECG-gated rest Rb-82 PET images of a 69-yr male with known ischemic cardiomyopathy due to severe multivessel coronary artery disease. The cine display shows severely depressed LVEF (21%) with diffuse hypokinesis and anteroapical akinesis. Patient was referred to assess viability of the anterior wall. **(movie)**

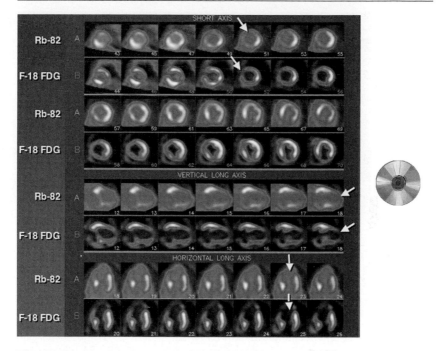

Fig. 11-17. Rest Rb-82 and F-18 FDG imaging of the patient shown in Fig. 11-15. Both the Rb-82 and F-18 FDG images show a similar large defect in the anteroapical and septal walls (arrows): a matched defect of blood flow and cardiac metabolism. There is no evidence of myocardial viability in the akinetic anterior wall.

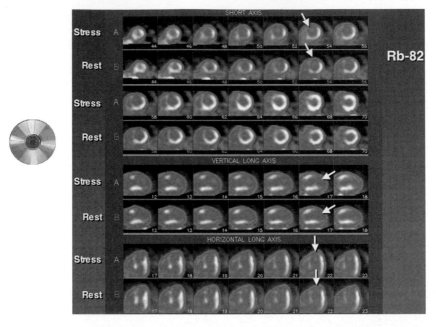

Fig. 11-18. Rest-dipyridamole Rb-82 PET images of a 69-yr-old male with previous anterior infarction and congestive heart failure. The Rb-82 PET images show an enlarged left ventricle with a large fixed anteroseptal and apical defect (arrows).

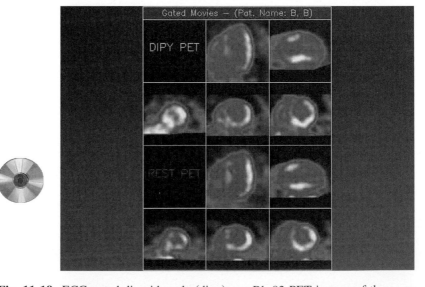

Fig. 11-19. ECG-gated dipyridamole (dipy)-rest Rb-82 PET images of the same patient shown in Fig. 11-18. The left ventricle is enlarged. There is akinesis of the Anteroseptal and apical walls. Wall motion of the remaining segments also is hypokinetic. Global LVEF is depressed at 30%. The patient was referred for assessment of myocardial viability. **(movie)**

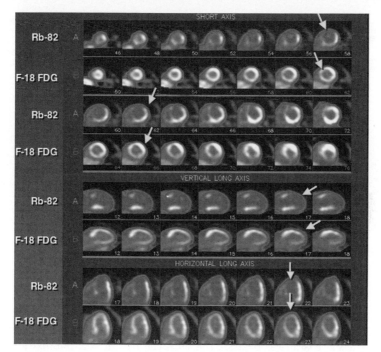

Fig. 11-20. Rest Rb-82 and F-18 FDG imaging of the patient shown in Fig. 11-18. The rest Rb-82 images show the large anteroseptal and apical perfusion defect. The F-18FDG images show FDG uptake in all myocardial segments, particularly in the anterolateral wall: mismatch of perfusion and cardiac metabolism (arrows). This pattern indicates substantial amount of myocardial viability, particularly in the dysfunctional anterolateral-septal and apical walls.

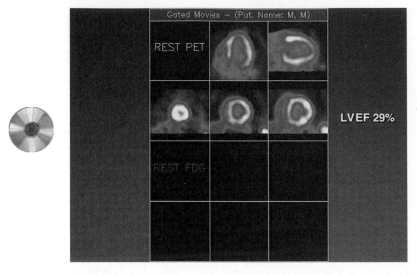

Fig. 11-21. ECG-gated dipyridamole rest Rb-82 PET images of a patient with known multivessel coronary artery disease and recent non ST-segment elevation acute myocardial infarction by elevated MB-CK and troponins. The cine display of the gated PET study shows an enlarged LE with diffuse hypokinesis and anteroapical and septal akinesis. LVEF was depressed at 29%.The patient was referred for assessment of myocardial viability. **(movie)**

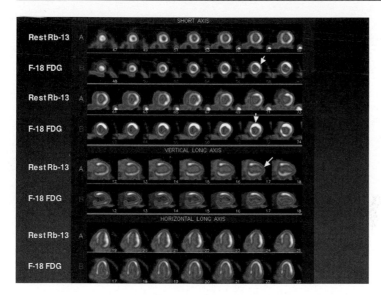

Fig. 11-22. Rest Rb-82 and F-18 FDG imaging of the patient shown in Fig. 11-21. The rest Rb-82 images show no definite myocardial perfusion defect. There is slightly less Rb-82 uptake in the anteroapical and septal walls (arrow). The F-18 FDG PET images show uptake in all myocardial segments, particularly in the mid ventricular and basal anterior wall (arrows). This pattern suggests diffuse hibernating and viable myocardium with severe resting ischemia in the anterior wall.

REFERENCES

1. Schwaiger M, Ziegler SI, Bengel FM (2000). Assessment of myocardial blood flow with positron emission tomography. In Sgaw PM (ed.), *Imaging in Cardiovascular Disease*. Lippincott, Williams & Wilkins, Philadelphia, PA; 195–212.
2. DiCarli M (2004). Advances in positron emission tomography. *J Nucl Cardiol* 11:719–732.
3. Bateman TM, Heller GV, McGhie AI, Friedman JD, Case JA, Bryngelson JR, Hertenstein GK, Moutray KL, Reis K, Cullom SJ (2006). Diagnostic accuracy of rest/stress ECG-gated Rb-82 myocardial perfusion PET: comparison with ECG-gated Tc-99m sestamibi SPECT. *J Nucl Cardiol* 13:24–33.
4. DiCarli MF, Hachamovitch R (2006). Should PET replace SPECT for evaluating CAD? The end of the beginning? *J Nucl Cardiol* 13:2–7.
5. Sampson UK, Dorbala S, Limaye A, Kwong R, Di Carli MF (2007). Diagnostic accuracy of rubidium-82 myocardial perfusion imaging with hybrid positron emission tomography/computed tomography in the detection of coronary artery disease. *J Am Coll Cardiol* 49:1052–1058.
6. DePuey EG (ed.) (2006). *Guidelines for Nuclear Cardiology Procedures. PET Emission Tomography Myocardial Perfusion and Glucose Metabolism Imaging*. Available at http://www.asnc.org– Menu:ManageYour Practice:Guidelines&Standards (accessed May 2007).

7. Bax JJ, Visser FC, Poldermans D, Elhendy A, Cormel JH, Boersma E, Valkema R, van Lingen A, Fioretti PM, Visser CA (2001). Relationship between preoperative viability and postoperative improvement in LVEF and heart failure symptoms. *J Nucl Med* 42:79–86.
8. Samady H, Elefteriades JA, Abbott BG, Mattera JA, McPherson CA, Wackers FJTh (1999). Failure to improve left ventricular function after coronary revascularization for ischemic cardiomyopathy is not associated with worse outcome. *Circulation* 100:1298–1304.

12 Hybrid Imaging

ECG-gated SPECT myocardial perfusion imaging has become the most widely used imaging technique for the noninvasive evaluation of patients with known or suspected coronary artery disease. The clinical use of SPECT myocardial perfusion imaging has continued to grow over the years, because it is valued as a clinically effective and cost-efficient diagnostic method. Hybrid imaging constitutes a new advance in cardiac imaging.

Key Words: Hybrid imaging, SPECT-CT, PET-CT, Attenuation correction, Coronary calcium scoring, Noninvasive multislice CT coronary angiography, Co-registration targeted imaging.

The usefulness of stress SPECT myocardial perfusion imaging for diagnosing coronary artery disease and for predicting cardiovascular events has been documented extensively in the literature.

Nevertheless, SPECT cardiac imaging has important limitations:

- The spatial resolution of conventional imaging equipment is suboptimal (Table 12-1)
- The full range of myocardial blood flow is suboptimally visualized, particularly at higher flow levels
- Nonuniform soft tissue attenuation may mimick regional myocardial perfusion deficits

It is well accepted that stress-induced myocardial perfusion defects indicate hemodynamically and pathophysiologically significant coronary artery disease.

Nevertheless,

- Coronary artery disease develops over the course of many years, and atherosclerotic plaques may be subclinical and asymptomatic until the instance of a major cardiac event.

From: *Contemporary Cardiology: Nuclear Cardiology, The Basics*
By: F. J. Th. Wackers, W. Bruni, and B. L. Zaret © Humana Press Inc., Totowa, NJ

Table 12-1
Spatial Resolution (FWHM) of Various Imaging Modalities

Single-photon planar projection imaging	7 mm
SPECT	10–14 mm
PET	7–10 mm
X-ray CT	0.5–1.0 mm
MRI	0.2–0.5 mm

FWHM, full width half maximum.

- Those (as yet) nonhemodynamically significant manifestations of coronary artery disease cannot be detected by the conventional stress–rest myocardial perfusion imaging.

Consequently, new technology has been developed to address these limitations in cardiovascular imaging.

Recent new directions in nuclear cardiology focus on the following goals:

1. Correction of nonuniform attenuation artifacts.
2. Coronary artery calcium scoring.
3. Noninvasive CT coronary angiography.
4. Imaging atherosclerotic processes on a molecular level in the vessel wall of coronary arteries and other arteries (carotid and aorta) with targeted radionuclide imaging, that is, hot-spot imaging.
5. Anatomic coregistration of hot-spot radiotracer uptake with anatomic imaging techniques that have high spatial resolution.

To achieve these goals, X-ray CT appears a natural match with radionuclide imaging. The imaging approach of combining radiotracer imaging and CT imaging is referred to as hybrid or dual-modality imaging *(1)*.

This new imaging requires specialized and complex equipment that incorporates a X-ray scanner and a gamma camera.

Hybrid imaging equipment

- Is more expensive than conventional nuclear imaging cameras.
- Requires a larger imaging room, as well as a separate monitoring room.
- Is heavier than conventional equipment and requires enforced floor support.
- Requires lead shielding (1/16 inches) of walls, floor, ceiling, and door.
- Is operated by CT-certified X-ray technologists.
- Is interpreted by physicians with specialized training.
- Involves complex imaging QC of CT and nuclear images.

Table 12-2
Present and Future Applications of Hybrid Imaging

- AC
- Coronary artery calcium scoring
- CT angiography
- Anatomic coregistration of CT with hot-spot imaging

Present and future applications of hybrid imaging that may optimize and complement radionuclide imaging are listed in Table 12-2.

ATTENUATION CORRECTION(SPECT/CT AND PET/CT)

The first clinical application of hybrid imaging was its use for SPECT attenuation correction (AC) *(2)*. CT-based AC in conjunction with SPECT and PET myocardial perfusion imaging is discussed in greater detail in Chapters 6 and 10, because it is already routinely used in many laboratories.

SPECT/CT

For AC of SPECT images, 1- or 4-slice CT scanners suffice. Although the CT images provide excellent quality attenuation maps, they have insufficient spatial resolution for diagnostic imaging of the chest. CT-based AC improves overall diagnostic accuracy, largely through improved specificity but also through improved identification of multivessel coronary artery disease *(2)*.

PET/CT

The number of laboratories performing PET/CT imaging is increasing rapidly *(3)*. For PET imaging attenuation, correction is a necessity, and for CT-based attenuation, correction has been adopted readily. Currently available PET cameras are usually paired with high-resolution, high-speed 16- or 64-slice CT scanners. In addition to providing high-quality AC, these scanners also can perform calcium scoring and noninvasive contrast CT coronary angiography. However, the latter two hybrid applications are performed in relatively few centers and are not yet routine procedures. The chest CT images are of high diagnostic quality, and noncardiac abnormalities must not be missed. It is therefore advisable to perform interpretation jointly with individuals well trained in interpreting CT studies, particularly of the thorax *(4)*.

Because the attenuation CT scan is not acquired at the same time as the SPECT or PET images, a very important aspect of QC of this hybrid imaging is verification of accurate coregistration of emission and transmission images.

CORONARY ARTERY CALCIUM SCORING

Although coronary artery calcifications (CACs) are visualized on regular high-resolution CT images, reliable quantification of CAC requires ECG-gated electron beam CT or multislice (at least 16-slice) CT. An important condition for artifact-free images is that the patient has a regular heart rhythm.

The diagnostic information gained from CAC is entirely different from that derived from stress SPECT imaging. CAC provides anatomical information concerning the calcium burden of the coronary artery vessel walls, whereas SPECT imaging assesses the pathophysiologic significance of coronary artery stenoses.

The amount of calcium in the coronary arteries can be quantified based on the attenuation of X-ray and is measured in Hounsfield units. The total coronary artery calcium burden can be expressed either as the widely used Agatston score (Table 12-3) or the calcium volume score.

Patients with CAC score <400 rarely have abnormal stress SPECT myocardial perfusion images. With increasing CAC scores, a greater percentage of patients have abnormal SPECT. However, a substantial number of patients with a CAC score >1000 may still have normal SPECT images.

Thus, CT calcium scoring and stress SPECT imaging are not identical but must be viewed as complementary *(1)*.

An abnormal CAC score provides long-term prognostic information, whereas an abnormal SPECT image provides short-term prognostic information.

Through the detection of subclinical coronary atherosclerosis, one is able to identify patients who may benefit long term from aggressive risk-factor modification.

Table 12-3
Categorization of Agatston Scores

• Insignificant	(≤ 10)
• Mild	(11–100)
• Moderate	(101–400)
• Severe	(401–1000)
• Extensive	(> 1000)

CT CORONARY ANGIOGRAPHY

High-resolution (16-slice or higher) CT scanners are capable of acquiring noninvasive contrast coronary angiograms *(5,6)*. This technology is evolving very rapidly. It can be anticipated that new generations of equipment will have higher temporal and spatial resolution and emit lower radiation dose.

Hybrid PET/CT systems are very attractive in clinical cardiology because of the potential of combined acquisition of

- Myocardial perfusion
- Left ventricular global and regional function
- Coronary artery calcium
- Cardiac and coronary anatomy
- Coronary angiography

State-of-the-art 16- or 64-slice multidetector CT systems have high spatial slice resolution (0.5–0.75 mm) and high temporal resolution (330–420 ms rotation times). Data acquisition takes 10–20 s. Phasic modulation of X-ray current during data acquisition allows for reduced radiation exposure and ECG-triggered acquisition during diastole. An important practical requirement is a heart rate slower than 65 bpm. Thus, most patients may require pretreatment with IV beta-blocking medication.

CT imaging permits high-resolution assessment of the morphology of the heart, that is, coronary anatomy, cardiac chamber sizes, and CAC. After IV injection of contrast, the entire coronary artery tree can be visualized. An important advantage is that not only the coronary artery lumen is visualized but also the coronary artery vessel wall. Under optimal conditions, the maximum spatial resolution of a CT angiogram is $0.4 \times 0.4 \times 0.4$ mm, which is still less than that of invasive coronary

Table 12-4
Advantages and Problems of Invasive Coronary Angiography

Advantages	*Problems*
• High resolution	• Arterial access
• Complete arterial tree	• Endoluminal space only
• Plaque visualization	• Eccentric remodeling not visualized
• PCI during same procedure	• Iodinated contrast load
	• Procedural risks
	• Insignificant disease

PCI, percutaneous coronary intervention.

Table 12-5
Advantages and Problems of Noninvasive CT Coronary Angiography

Advantages	Problems
Venous access	Coronary artery motion
Short procedure time	Limited temporal resolution
Coronary anatomy/anomalies	Missed coronary artery segments
Luminal stenoses	Overlying calcium, metal stents
Visualization vessel wall	Slow and regular heart rate required
Plaque composition (calcified and soft)	Iodinated contrast load
High negative predictive value	Radiation exposure

angiography (Table 12-4). The sensitivity of noninvasive CT coronary angiography under optimal conditions (high-quality studies, interpretation by expert readers, and appropriately selected patients) exceeds 95%. However, in practice, study quality may be suboptimal for various reasons (Table 12-5). A consistent observation in numerous clinical studies has been the high negative predictive value. Thus, an unequivocally normal CT coronary angiogram virtually excludes significant coronary artery disease. Consequently, one of the future clinical contributions of CT coronary angiography may be the reduction of the number of patients with normal invasive contrast coronary angiograms.

One can anticipate that with increasing use of CT coronary angiography, a greater number of patients with intermediate severity lesions will be identified. Radionuclide stress imaging will then be necessary to determine the pathophysiologic significance of such lesions (7,8).

CT COREGISTRATION FOR TARGETED IMAGING

Experimental research efforts currently focus on the development of means to visualize molecular aspects of the atherosclerotic process and of ischemic remodeling (9).

Radiolabeled substrates are being developed that target atherosclerotic plaques, myocardial and vascular matrix metalloproteinase activity, angiogenesis, inflammation, hypoxia and apoptosis, and others.

These radiopharmaceuticals are "hot-spot" agents. In contrast to conventional "cold-spot" agents, such as myocardial perfusion agents, where the abnormality, manifested as decreased tracer uptake, can be localized because the normal myocardium is visualized, with hot-spot imaging, anatomic landmarks are absent. Only with the use of hybrid imaging, that is, combined hot-spot radionuclide and CT imaging, will it be possible to anatomically localize the precise uptake site of targeted tracers.

At the time of this writing, it is not possible to predict the exact role of hybrid imaging in the future. CT technology is in full and rapid development. Appropriate clinical paradigms will have to be defined for stand-alone and/or combined hybrid noninvasive imaging procedures. Nuclear cardiologists with their experience of shaping the clinical role of radionuclide imaging, based on clinical research and cost-effectiveness analyses, are well positioned to play a leading role in the development and growth of cardiovascular CT and hybrid imaging. There is substantial potential for a complementary role of CT imaging with PET and/or SPECT.

REFERENCES

1. Shaw LJ, Berman DS, Bax JJ, Brown KA, Cohen MC, Hendel RC, Mahmarian JJ, Williams KA, Ziffer JA (2005). Computed tomographic imaging with nuclear cardiology. *J Nucl Cardiol* 12:131–142. Available at http://www.asnc.org/ — Menu:ManageYourPractice:Guidelines&Standards. (accessed May 2007).
2. Massood Y, Liu YH, Depuey G, Taillefer R, Araujo LI, Allen S, Delbeke D, Anstett F, Peretz A, Zito MJ, Tsatkin V, Wackers FJTh (2005). Clinical validation of SPECT attenuation correction using x-ray computed tomography-derived attenuation maps: multicenter clinical trial with angiographic correlation. *J Nucl Cardiol* 12:676–686.
3. Bateman TM, Heller GV, McGhie AI, Friedman JD, Case JA, Bryngelson JR, Hertenstein GK, Moutray KL, Reid K, Cullom SJ (2006). Diagnostic accuracy of rest/stress ECG-gated Rb-82 myocardial perfusion PET: comparison with ECG-gated Tc-99m Sestamibi SPECT. *J Nucl Cardiol* 13:24–33.
4. Raff GL, Gallagher MJ, O'Neill WW, Goldstein JA (2005). Diagnostic accuracy of noninvasive coronary angiography using 64-slice spiral computed tomography. *J Am Coll Cardiol* 46: 552 557.
5. Onuma Y, Tanabe K, Nakazawa G, Aoki J, Nakajima H, Ibukuro K, Hara K (2006). Noncardiac findings in cardiac imaging with multidetector computed tomography. *J Am Coll Card* 48:402–406.
6. Achenbach S (2005). Current and future status on cardiac computed tomographic imaging for diagnosis and risk stratification. *J Nucl cardiol* 12: 703–713.
7. Rispler S, Keidar Z, Ghersin E, Roguin A, Soil A, Dragu R, Litmanovicj D, Frenkel A, Aronson D, Engel A, Beyar R, Israel O (2007). Integrated single-photon emission computed tomography and computed tomography coronary angiography for the assessment of hemodynamically significant coronary artery lesions. *J Am Coll Cardiol* 49:1059–1067.
8. Goldstein JA, Gallagher MJ, O'Neill WW, Ross MA, O'Neil BJ, Raff GL (2007). A ramdomized controlled trial of multislice coronary computed tomography for evaluation of acute chest pain. *J Am Coll Cardiol* 49:863–871.
9. Bengel FM (2006). Atherosclerosis imaging on the molecular level. From bench to imaging. *J Nucl Cardiol* 13:111–118.

13 Display and Analysis of Planar Myocardial Perfusion Images

The display and nomenclature of nuclear cardiology images has been standardized. The analysis of nuclear cardiology images should follow a systematic approach and sequence as outlined in ref. *(1)*. Planar myocardial perfusion imaging is currently rarely performed as the routine imaging methodology. Planar imaging is often the last resort for patients who are claustrophobic, cannot lie still, or who are too heavy for the SPECT imaging table. However, with the increasing use of bariatric surgery, there is a need to evaluate these markedly obese candidates preoperatively. Planar imaging may find increasing use in this patient population. It should be appreciated that good quality planar perfusion images contain similar diagnostic information as SPECT images. Moderate to large myocardial perfusion abnormalities are usually well visualized on planar images. We believe that it is useful for the practicing nuclear cardiologist to have some experience with the analysis of planar images. Moreover, the rotating projection images of a SPECT study are also planar images. They often reveal perfusion abnormalities that can be confirmed on reconstructed slices.

Key Words: Display planar perfusion images, Breast markers, Nomenclature.

DISPLAY OF PLANAR IMAGES

For interpretation, planar stress–rest myocardial perfusion images are best displayed on computer screen side-by-side, that is, either paired view-by-view (**Fig. 13-1**) or paired side-by-side (**Fig. 13-2**) as a complete three-view study. For planar images, a linear gray scale is preferred over color display.

From: *Contemporary Cardiology: Nuclear Cardiology, The Basics*
By: F. J. Th. Wackers, W. Bruni, and B. L. Zaret © Humana Press Inc., Totowa, NJ

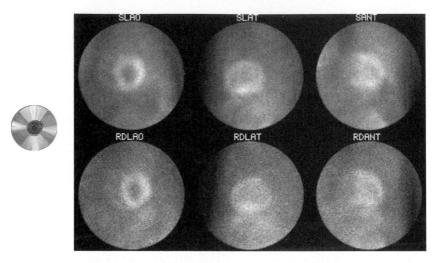

Fig. 13-1. Planar exercise Tl-201 images in view-by-view display. Exercise (S) images on top rest, (R) images on the bottom. There is mildly increased lung uptake and a reversible anteroseptal myocardial perfusion defect.

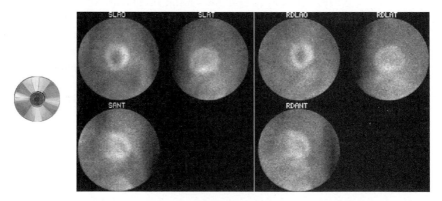

Fig. 13-2. Same planar exercise Tl-201 images as in fig 12-1 in side-by side display. Exercise (S) images on the left; rest (R) images on the right.

Breast Markers

To recognize breast tissue attenuation, simultaneous display of breast markers may be useful (**Fig. 13-3**).

ANALYSIS OF PLANAR IMAGES

Nomenclature and segmentation of planar myocardial perfusion imaging has been standardized in ref. *(1)* and are shown in **Figs. 13-4** and **13-5**.

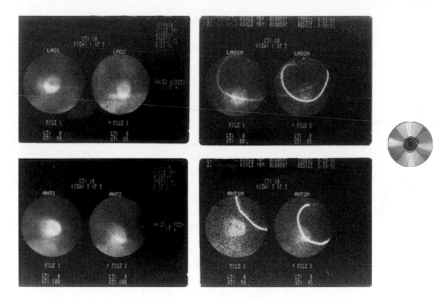

Fig. 13-3. Planar Tl-201 images (left) with breast markers (right).

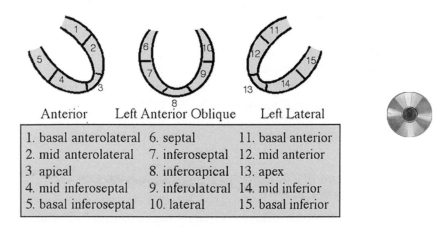

Anterior   Left Anterior Oblique   Left Lateral

1. basal anterolateral	6. septal	11. basal anterior
2. mid anterolateral	7. inferoseptal	12. mid anterior
3. apical	8. inferoapical	13. apex
4. mid inferoseptal	9. inferolateral	14. mid inferior
5. basal inferoseptal	10. lateral	15. basal inferior

Fig. 13-4. Standardized segmentation and nomenclature for planar myocardial perfusion images. (Reproduced with permission from ref 1).

Quantitative Analysis

A number of validated commercial and noncommercial software packages were previously available for quantification of planar myocardial perfusion [(CEQUAL) *(2)*, University of Virginia *(3)* and Yale University *(4)*]. Because of the current predominance of SPECT imaging in clinical practice, these software packages are no longer further developed or available.

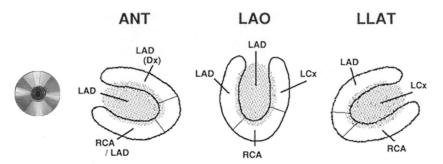

Fig. 13-5. Assignment of coronary artery territories on planar myocardial perfusion images. The shaded areas represent the projection of activity emanating from the facing walls overlying the left ventricular cavity. (LAD= left anterior descending coronary artery; Dx= diagonal coronary artery; LCx= left circumflex coronary artery; RCA= right coronary artery).

The basic principles of planar quantification are similar for each of these software packages. Raw planar projection images are corrected for differences in background activity on rest and stress images by the application of interpolative background subtraction.

Normalized relative radiotracer uptake in the background-subtracted left ventricular images is subsequently compared quantitatively with normal data files. Relative radiotracer uptake on planar images can be displayed in different ways *(2–4)*. In our laboratory, we prefer the display of circumferential count distribution profiles *(4)*. The size of myocardial perfusion defects can be expressed as percent of the total potentially visualized normal LV.

Example of Quantification of Planar Images

Figures 13-6 to **13-8** show representative screen captures of quantification of exercise-delayed Tl-201 images of a patient with a reversible anteroseptal defect (shown above), using software developed in our laboratory *(4)*.

Conservative Interpretation

As mentioned before, planar myocardial perfusion imaging is often performed in the worst possible candidates for radionuclide imaging, that is, the very obese and/or uncooperative patients. It is prudent to interpret images in these patients with a great deal of conservatism. Only unequivocal abnormalities should be reported. Many studies will be of suboptimal quality and nondiagnostic.

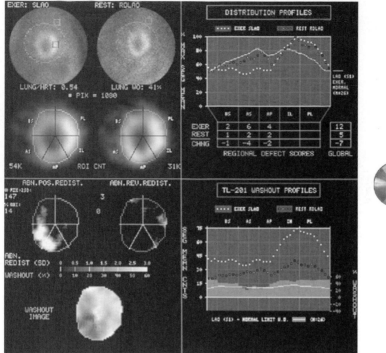

Fig. 13-6. Quantification of left anterior oblique (LAO) images of the planar Tl-201 images shown in fig. 12-1 and 12-2.

The top left panel shows raw LAO images with an elliptical region of interest (ROI) for interpolative background subtraction and small square ROIs for lung/heart (HRT) ratio calculation.

Lung/HRT ratio is abnormal at 0.54. Below in the same left top panel are the resulting background-corrected LAO images. On the top right are circumferential count profiles (exercise= white dots and rest=black dots) for quantification of defect size, displayed against the lower limit of normal Tl-201 uptake (white curve). Defect reversibility is quantified in the septal area (exercise defect 12 and rest defect is 5). The lower right panel shows a graphic display of regional Tl-201 washout. Tl-201 washout is low in septal region.

The lower left panel shows functional images. In the top left image (ABN.POS.REDISTR.) the background-corrected exercise image is subtracted pixel-by-pixel from the background-corrected rest image. The difference between the two images (=defect reversibility) is displayed as positive values in the septal area. To the right of this image (ABN.REV.REDISTR)the rest image is subtracted from the exercise image. If reverse redistribution was present this would show as positive values. The bottom image displays Tl-201 washout on a pixel-by-pixel basis. The darker area in the inferoseptal region indicates low washout.

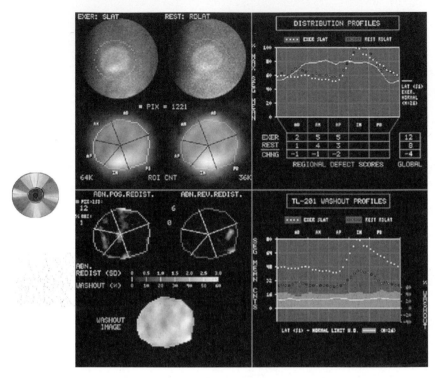

Fig. 13-7. Quantification of left lateral (LAT) images of the planar Tl-201 images shown in fig. 12-1 and 12-2. The same quantification method described in figure 12-6 is used. A large fixed anterior wall defect is present.

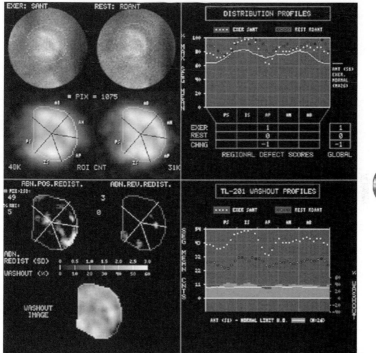

Fig. 13-8. Quantification of anterior (ANT) images of the planar Tl-201 images shown in fig. 12-1 and 12-2. The same quantification method described in figure 12-6 is used. Except for a small apical defect, no quantifiable myocardial perfusion defect is present. Summary of quantitative analysis of 3 planar Tl-201 images (Fig. 12-6 to fig. 12-8): Abnormal Tl-201 exercise-redistribution images with abnormally increased lung uptake after exercise and a large partially reversible anteroseptal myocardial perfusion defect.

REFERENCES

1. DePuey GV (ed.) (2006). *Imaging Guidelines for Nuclear Cardiology Procedures*. Available at http://www.asnc.org/—Menu:ManageYourPractice:Guidelines &Standards (accessed June 2007).
2. Garcia E, Maddahi J, Berman D, et al. (1981). Space/time quantification of thallium-201 myocardial scintigraphy. *J Nucl Med* 22:309–317.
3. Watson DD, Campbell NP, Read EK, Gibson RS, Teates CD, Beller GA (1981). Spatial and temporal quantitation of plane thallium myocardial images. *J Nucl Med* 22: 577–584.
4. Wackers FJTh, Fetterman RC, Mattera JA, Clements JP (1985). Quantitative planar thallium-201 stress scintigraphy: a critical evaluation of the method. *Semin Nucl Med* 15:46–66.

14 Display and Analysis of Planar Equilibrium Radionuclide Angiocardiography

The simplest and most reproducible methodology for quantifying LVEF and that has stood the test of time is ERNA. Accurate and reproducible serial measurement of left ventricular function is very important for patients undergoing chemotherapy. Another important clinical application is in the selection of patients who are considered candidates for placement of an internal cardiac defibrillator (ICD).

Key Words: Display planar ERNA images, Interpretation planar ERNA images, Nomenclature.

The display and nomenclature of nuclear cardiology images has been standardized. The analysis of nuclear cardiology images should follow a systematic approach and sequence as outlined in ref. *(1)*.

DISPLAY OF PLANAR ERNA IMAGES

It is standard that multiple views are displayed simultaneously in cine or movie format *(2)*. Multiple view planar ERNA images are best displayed simultaneously on computer screen as endless loop movies. For planar ERNA images, a linear gray scale is preferred over color display. The best speed to display ERNA movies is 8–10 frames/s.

To be able to appreciate the morphology and function of the entire heart and great vessels, the gains of gamma camera should be set such that a normal heart occupies about one-third to one-fourth of the FOV **(Fig. 14-1)**.

From: *Contemporary Cardiology: Nuclear Cardiology, The Basics*
By: F. J. Th. Wackers, W. Bruni, and B. L. Zaret © Humana Press Inc., Totowa, NJ

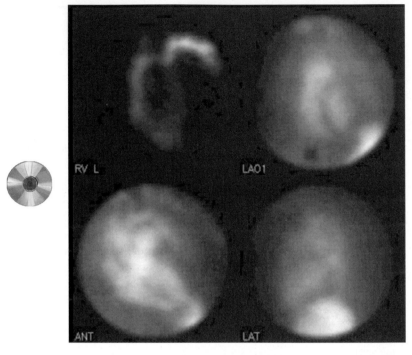

Fig. 14-1. Simultaneous movie display of planar ERNA images in left anterior oblique (LAO), anterior (ANT) and left lateral (LAT) views. In addition ECG-gated first pass angiocardiography for assessment of the right ventricle is displayed on the top left. The gains of the gamma camera were appropriately tuned so that the heart occupies about 1/3 of the field of view (**movie**).

INTERPRETATION

The interpretation of ERNA images should follow a systematic approach *(2)*.

Inspection of Overall Quality of Images, Efficiency of Red Cell Labeling

1. Size of the heart, RV and LV
2. Size and contraction of right atrium
3. Size and contraction of RV
4. Size of pulmonary artery
5. Size and contraction of left atrium
6. Size and contraction of LV
7. Size and morphology of ascending and descending aorta

Interpretation of ERNA images is, with the exception of EF, largely based on visual analysis (**Figs. 14-2** and **14-3**). The overall quality

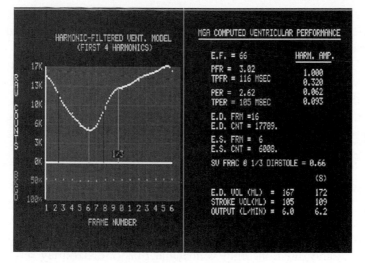

Fig. 14-2. Computer screen capture of normal ERNA. The left ventricular volume curve (left) shows a normal appearance. There is some counts drop-off in the last frame due to respiratory heart rate variability. On the right are quantitative results of volume curve analysis. Left ventricular ejection fraction (E.F.) is normal at 66%. End diastolic counts (E.D.) counts (CNT) are excellent (17,789), ensuring good statistical reliability. Peak filling rate (PFR) is normal at 3.82 ED volumes/s. The ED volume (VOL) is at the upper limit of normal at 167 ml.

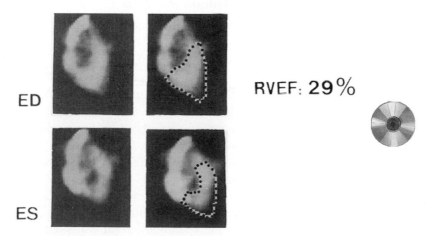

Fig. 14-3. Processed ECG-gated first pass angiocardiography. The end diastolic (ED) and end systolic (ES) frames are shown and the manually drawn regions of interest. RVEF is abnormal at 29%.

of study is determined by adequate labeling of red blood cells, the patient's weight, and counts emanating from the cardiac chambers and the ECG gating.

Although high labeling efficiency is important, free Tc-99m-pertechnetate usually is trapped in the thyroid gland and stomach mucosa and does not interfere with image interpretation.

Suboptimal quality ERNAs are frequently a problem in very obese patients in whom scattered photons significantly degrade image quality.

Chamber Size and Myocardial Thickness

High quality multiple view ERNAs contain considerably more clinically useful information than LVEF alone. One can qualitatively assess the relative size of various chambers, assuming that the same camera and magnification is used for all studies. As in most patients, the RV is normal in size and function, right ventricular diastolic size may serve as a reference for assessment of the relative size of the other cardiac structures. On a normal study, the RV is usually somewhat larger than the LV. The size of the ventricles should be compared in end-diastole.

The presence or absence of marked left ventricular hypertrophy can be estimated by qualitative assessment of the thickness of the septum, which is well delineated by the right and left ventricular blood pool. In severe left ventricular hypertrophy, a thick photopenic halo also may surround the left ventricular blood pool.

Regional Wall Motion Analysis

Complete evaluation of regional wall motion requires acquisition of multiple good quality projections or views.

LEFT VENTRICLE

On the anterior view, there is substantial overlap of right ventricular and left ventricular blood pool. Hence, only the anterior, lateral, and apical segments of the LV can be analyzed without inference due to superimposed structures on the anterior view.

On the LAO view, the lateral, inferolateral, inferoapical, and septal segments can be evaluated. It must be noted, however, that this projection produces substantial left ventricular foreshortening. Septal excursions may be minimized as major systolic motion occurs perpendicular to the FOV. Contraction of the apex and lateral walls are best evaluated in this view. An important view is the right side decubitus left lateral view. This projection shows the long axis of the LV with excellent delineation of both the entire anterior wall and inferobasal wall.

RIGHT VENTRICLE

Regional wall motion analysis of the RV is difficult even on multiple projections because of (i) the overlap with LV blood pool activity on the anterior projection, (ii) the foreshortening of right ventricular motion and atrial blood pool overlap on the LAO projection, and (iii) the superimposition and overlap of the LV on the left lateral projections.

Global and regional wall motion of the RV is best evaluated on the anterior ERNA view or from an ECG-gated first pass study acquired in the anterior or right anterior projection.

ATRIA

The size and contraction of the right atrium is best evaluated on the anterior view during ventricular systole. The right atrium forms the left lower border of the cardiac image.

The left atrium is best evaluated on the left lateral view during ventricular systole. Because of overlying structures and surrounding radioactivity, frequently, no sharp outline of the left atrium can be seen.

Contraction of the atria can be recognized as a change in count density during the cardiac cycle, out of phase with ventricular contraction.

GREAT VESSELS

The great vessels, the pulmonary artery and ascending and descending aorta, can be evaluated as well. Only qualitative assessments, such as dilation of the pulmonary artery, dilation and tortuosity of the ascending, aortic arch, and/or descending aorta, can be made.

NON-CARDIAC FINDINGS

ERNA studies should be analyzed also for non-cardiovascular abnormalities. For example, particularly in cancer patients, there may be marked enlargement of the spleen. This may affect the normalization of the images and make distinct visualization of the heart difficult. Moreover, a hot spleen should be avoided when choosing the background ROI for calculating LVEF.

Statistical Accuracy of EF

Accuracy of calculated RVEF and LVEF is importantly dependent on count statistics. This is also dependent on the value of EF.

We use the following rule of thumb:

If LVEF is normal (>0.50), at least 5000 counts are required in the background-corrected LV end-diastolic ROI.

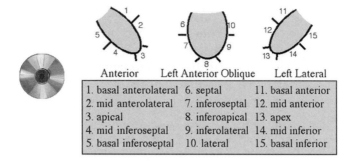

Anterior	Left Anterior Oblique	Left Lateral
1. basal anterolateral	6. septal	11. basal anterior
2. mid anterolateral	7. inferoseptal	12. mid anterior
3. apical	8. inferoapical	13. apex
4. mid inferoseptal	9. inferolateral	14. mid inferior
5. basal inferoseptal	10. lateral	15. basal inferior

Fig. 14-4. Standardized segmentation and nomenclature for planar equilibrium ventriculography (Reproduced with permission from ref 1).

If LVEF is moderately abnormal (<0.40) at least 20,000 counts are required in the background-corrected end-diastolic LV ROI.

Nomenclature ERNA

Nomenclature and segmentation of planar ERNA imaging has been standardized *(1)* (**Fig. 14-4**).

REFERENCES

1. DePuey GV (ed) (2006). *Imaging Guidelines for Nuclear Cardiology Procedures*. Available at http://www.asnc.org/Menu:Manage Your Practice: Guideline & Standards.
2. Wackers FJTh (1996). Equilibrium radionuclide angiocardiography. In: Gerson MC (ed.) *Cardiac Nuclear Medicine*, 3rd Edition, McGraw Hill Inc, New York, NY.

15 Display and Analysis of SPECT Equilibrium Radionuclide Angiocardiography

Although SPECT ERNA is not routinely performed in many laboratories, the gamma cameras used for the acquisition of SPECT myocardial perfusion imaging can, without modification, be used for the acquisition of gated blood pool images. In tomographic cine display, various cardiac structures may be analyzed without overlap, which allows for improved assessment of cardiac morphology and function, particularly of the right heart. The display and nomenclature of SPECT ERNA are essentially similar to that recommended for SPECT myocardial perfusion imaging.

Key Words: Display SPECT ERNA images, Three dimensional rendering, Right ventricular function.

Display of ERNA SPECT should include at a minimum:

1. Rotating planar projection images
2. Movie display of selected multiple ECG-gated slices: vertical long axis, short axis, and horizontal long axis, as well as (optional) 3-D display of cardiac chambers
3. Left ventricular volume curve
4. Optional: planar LAO view

Interpretation of SPECT ERNA images should follow a similar systematic approach and employ QC as described for SPECT myocardial perfusion imaging.

From: *Contemporary Cardiology: Nuclear Cardiology, The Basics*
By: F. J. Th. Wackers, W. Bruni, and B. L. Zaret © Humana Press Inc., Totowa, NJ

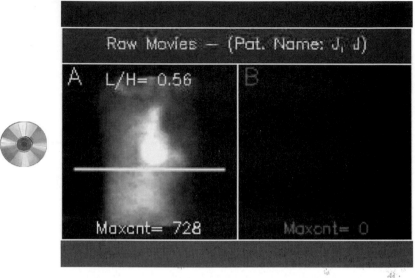

Fig. 15-1. Rotating planar blood pool projection images of a normal patient **(movie)**.

1. Inspection of rotating planar projection images
2. Analysis of movie display of reconstructed tomographic short axis, vertical, and horizontal long axis slices
3. Inspection of ED and end systolic regions of interest
4. Inspection of LV volume curve
5. Optional: analysis of planar LAO view in movie display

The rotating images (Fig. 15-1) should be inspected for

1. Overall quality of images (evidence for free Tc-99m-pertechnetate in thyroid or/and stomach?)
2. Motion by patient, and effectiveness of motion correction, if applicable
3. Count density in cardiac structures and spleen
4. Relative size of RV and LV and great vessels

DISPLAY OF SPECT ERNA

Reconstructed SPECT slices should be displayed using the same tomographic planes and format as is standard for SPECT myocardial perfusion images **(Fig. 15-2)**. Temporal and spatial smoothing should be used.

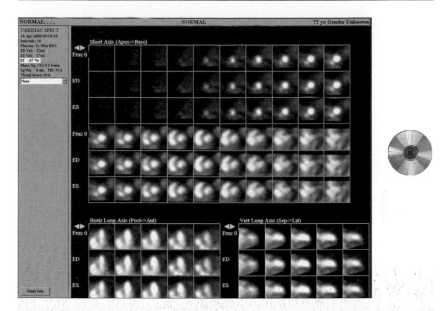

Fig. 15-2. Cine display of the reconstructed SPECT ERNA slices in the short axis (top), horizontal long axis (bottom left) and vertical long axis (bottom right) cuts of the normal patient shown in Fig. 15-1. The end diastolic (ED) and end systolic (ES) images are shown, as well as a 16-frame cine display. By visual inspection the right and left ventricles are normal in size and contraction (4D MSPECT display) **(movie)**.

Cine display of tomographic ERNA slices is done on computer screen with preferably gray scale or monochromatic color setting **(Fig. 15-3)**. Because of potentially marked differences in count density during the cardiac cycle, as well as the great difference in count density between blood pool and background, multicolor scale display makes reliable analysis of regional motion difficult.

Chamber sizes, global contraction, and regional wall motion may be evaluated from cine display of multiple short-axis and long-axis slices.

Several commercial software packages provide 3-D displays of the cardiac chambers with shaded surface or/and wire frame displays or volume-rendered displays **(Fig. 15-4)**. In movie display, regional wall motion can be appreciated relative to the static end-diastolic surface of the ventricle. The 3-D images are best displayed in multiple views and may be rotated under user control.

Regional wall motion of ventricular segments can be graded as
• Normal
• Hypokinetic (mild or severe)
• Akinetic/dyskinetic

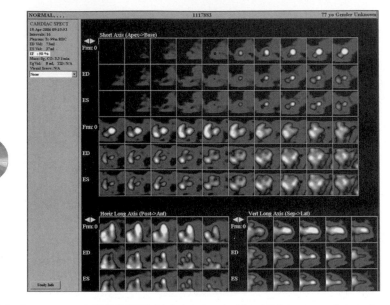

Fig. 15-3. Same normal SPECT ERNA images as in Fig. 15-2 in monochromatic color. (4D MSPECT display) **(movie)**.

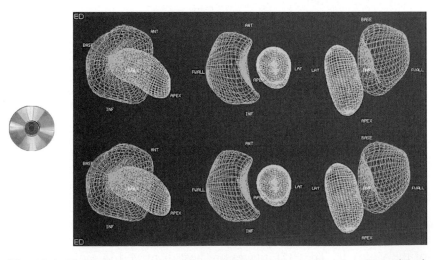

Fig. 15-4. Three-dimensional rendering SPECT ERNA in Figs 1-4. Right (blue) and left (pink) ventricular blood pool surfaces are displayed in "wire mesh" or "bird cage" mode. Top: End diastolic frames in anterior view (left), in left anterior oblique view (middle), and in cranial long axis view (right). Bottom: same views in cine display. Regional wall motion is normal (Cedars Sinai BPGS display) **(movie)**.

ERNA SPECT allows for description of the relative sizes of the cardiac chambers. As in adult cardiac patients, the RV is usually of normal size, the RV may be used as a reference for size. Enlargement of the LV can be identified and should be described.

Left Ventricular Ejection Fraction

Movie display of ERNA SPECT slices allows for visual estimation of global left ventricular function similar as done for planar ERNA. This should serve as crude QC measure for calculated LVEF. LVEF is determined using automated or semi-automated software packages using count-based 3-D volume rendering (1–6).

Before accepting a computed value for LVEF, the ventricular regions of interest should be reviewed (**Figs. 15-5** and **15-6**). Next, the contour of the left ventricular volume curve should be inspected. The volume curve should start and finish at the same (end-diastolic) level of counts or volume. A drop-off in the last frame of the cycle is acceptable and is due to physiologic variation of sinus rhythm. Because of lack of atrial overlap, ERNA-derived LVEF is slightly higher (about 0.5 EF units) than that computed from planar ERNA.

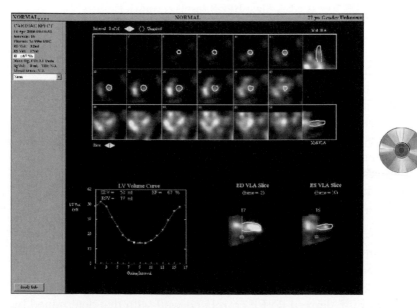

Fig. 15-5. Left ventricular volume curve of the normal images shown in Figs 15-1 to 15-3. The regions of interest used for calculation of LVEF are shown in cine for the short axis slices and mid ventricular horizontal (HLA) and vertical long axis (VLA) slices. LVEF is 67% and end diastolic volume is 51 ml. (4D MSPECT display) **(movie)**.

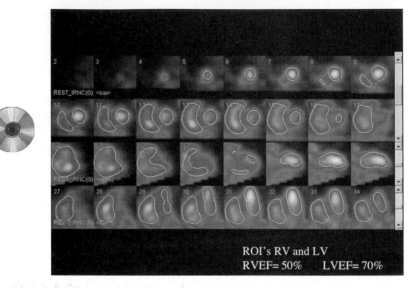

ROI's RV and LV
RVEF= 50%   LVEF= 70%

Fig. 15-6. Right ventricular and left ventricular regions of interest for calculating RVEF and LVEF of the same SPECT ERNA shown in Figs 15-1 to 15-5. Top two rows show short axis slices, 3rd row shows vertical long axis slices, and the 4th row shows the horizontal long axis slices. By the method shown, LVEF is 70% and RVEF 50% (Cedars Sinai BPGS display) **(movie)**.

Note that as long as ERNA SPECT software packages have not been thoroughly validated for calculation of LVEF, one still has the option to acquire one planar LAO view for calculation of LVEF in the conventional way (see Chapter 8). This may be prudent in particular in patients who had multiple previous planar studies with the purpose of monitoring LVEF during chemotherapy.

Figures 15-7 to **15-11** show an example of SPECT ERNA in a patient with ischemic cardiomyopathy.

Right Ventricular Ejection Fraction

Recently, algorithms have been described for computing RVEF from ERNA SPECT (**Figs. 15-6** and **15-11**) This is feasible because of the lack of superimposition of cardiac structures using tomography. ERNA SPECT-derived RVEF correlated well with that determined by MRI or electron beam CT (*7,8*). Similar to what is required for LVEF, one should review the accuracy of the right ventricular regions of interest, particularly whether the RV outflow tract is included. Finally, the shape of the RV volume curve should be inspected.

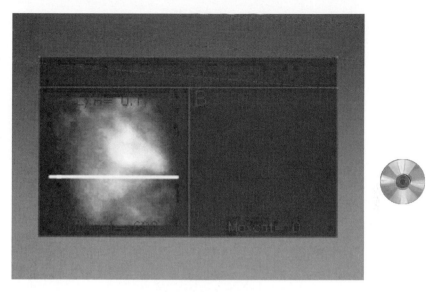

Fig. 15-7. Rotating planar blood pool projection images of a 71 yr old patient with severe ischemic cardiomyopathy **(movie)**.

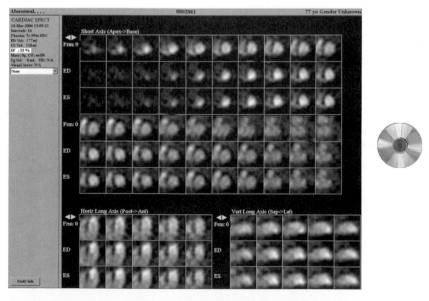

Fig. 15-8. Cine display of reconstructed SPECT ERNA slices of the patient shown in Fig. 15-7. The format is the same as in Fig. 15-2. By visual inspection, the right ventricle is normal in size and contraction. However, the left ventricle is enlarged and shows diffuse hypokinesis. (4D MSPECT display) **(movie)**.

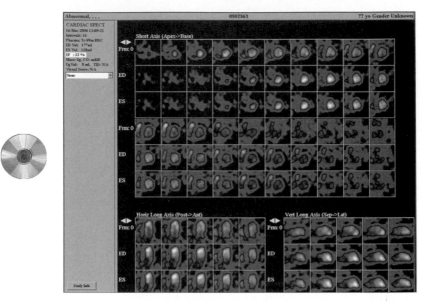

Fig. 15-9. Same abnormal SPECT ERNA images as in Fig. 15-6 in monochromatic color. (4D MSPECT display) **(movie)**.

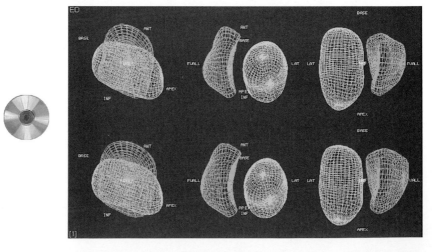

Fig. 15-10. Three-dimensional rendering of SPECT ERNA in Figs 15-8 and 15-9. The format is the same as in Fig. 15-4. Right ventricular contraction is normal, left ventricular contraction shows diffuse hypokinesis with inferoseptal dyskinesis at the apex. (Cedars Sinai BPGS display) **(movie)**.

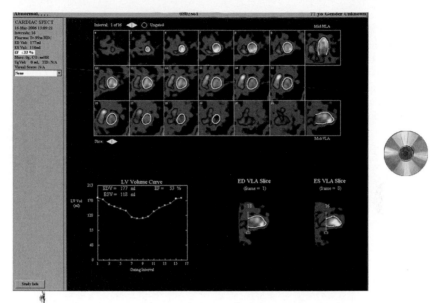

Fig. 15-11. Left ventricular volume curve of SPECT ERNA shown in Figs 15-8 and 15-9. The regions of interest used for calculation of LVEF are shown in cine for the short axis slices and mid ventricular horizontal (HLA) and Vertical long axis (VLA) slices. LVEF is severely depressed at 33%, and the end diastolic volume is large at 177 ml. (4D MSPECT display) **(movie)**.

REFERENCES

1. Bartlett ML, Srinivasan G, Barker WG, Kitsiou AN, Dilsizian V, Bacharach (1996). Left ventricular ejection fraction: comparison of results of planar and SPECT gated blood pool studies. *J Nuc Med* 37: 1795–1799.
2. Groch MW, DePuey EG, Belzberg AC, Erwin WD, Kamran M, Barnett CA, Hendel RC, Spies SM, Ali A, Marshall RC (2001). Planar imaging versus gated blood-pool SPECT for assessment of ventricular performance: a multicenter study. *J Nucl Med* 42: 1773–1779.
3. Van Kriekinge SD, Berman DS, Germano G (1999). Automatic quantification of left ventricular ejection fraction from gated blood pool SPECT. *J Nucl Cardiol* 6: 498–506.
4. Vanhove C, Franken PR, Defrise M, Momen A, Everaert H, Bossuyt A (2001). Automatic determination of left ventricular ejection fraction from gated blood-pool tomography. *J Nucl Med* 42: 401–407.
5. Daou D, Harel F, Helal BO, Fourme T, Colin P, Lebtahi R et al. (2001) Electrocardiographically gated blood pool SPECT and left ventricular function: comparative value of 3 methods for ejection fraction and volume estimation. *J Nucl Med* 2001; 42: 1043–1049.
6. Nichols K, Humayun N, De Bondt P, Vandenberghe S, Akinbobye OO, Bergmann SR (2004). Model dependence of gated blood pool SPECT ventricular function measurements. *J Nucl Cardiol* 11: 282–292.

7. Nichols K, Saouaf R, Ababneh AA, Barts RJ, Rosenbaum MS, Groch MW et al. Validation of SPECT equilibrium radionuclide angiographic right ventricular parameters by cardiac magnetic resonance imaging. *J Nucl Cardiol* 2002;9: 153–160.

8. Clements IP, Brinkmann B, Mullan BP, O'Connor MK, Breen JF, MCGregor CGA. Operator-intercative method for simultaneous measurement of left and right ventricular volumes and ejection fraction by tomographic electrocardiography-gated blood pool radionuclide ventriculography. *J Nucl Cardiol* 2006; 13: 50–63.

16 Artifacts and Technical Problems in Cardiac Imaging

When interpreting nuclear cardiology images, one should always consider the possibility of artifacts or other technical problems that may interfere with image quality. Artifacts are not unexpected in conventional SPECT imaging. During the process of external detection of relative low-energy photons emanating from inside the body, tissue attenuation, noncardiac uptake, and motion may distort images.

Key Words: Recognition and correction of artifacts, Low counts, Patient motion, Sinogram, Inferior attenuation, Attenuation correction, Misregistration, Breast attenuation, Non cardiac radiotracer uptake, Reconstruction and processing, Misalignment, Quantification errors, Filtering, ECG gating, Myocardial thickening, Misregistration PET/CT, Red blood cell labeling, Left ventricular volume curve, Calculation LVEF, LVEF and fixed and variable ROI.

Examples of artifacts and other problems and their recognition and correction are discussed in this chapter and on the computer disk that accompanies this book.

Various artifacts and problems will be addressed in a logical temporal sequence as one might encounter them in the course of interpreting nuclear cardiology images.

SPECT MYOCARDIAL PERFUSION IMAGING

Rotating Images

Inspection of the rotating planar projection images (**Fig. 16-1**) is always the first step of interpretation, because these images may provide important clues for problems or artifacts to be anticipated during analysis of reconstructed SPECT images.

From: *Contemporary Cardiology: Nuclear Cardiology, The Basics*
By: F. J. Th. Wackers, W. Bruni, and B. L. Zaret © Humana Press Inc., Totowa, NJ

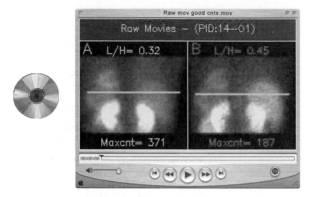

Fig. 16-1. Cine display of rotating planar projection images. In this, and all following movies of projection images, the stress study is on the left and the rest study on the right. The horizontal white line serves as a reference mark and is placed by the technologist approximately at the level of the left ventricular apex. The most convenient display speed for inspecting these images is at 10 frames/second. The lung/heart ratio (L/H) is displayed, as is the maximal count density/pixel within the left ventricle. Studies with less than 100 maximal counts are of suboptimal quality. The rotating projection images should always be viewed before analysis of reconstructed tomographic slices. The images should be inspected for patient motion, breast shadow, and overall quality. **(movie)**

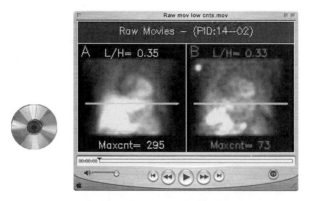

Fig. 16-2. Cine display of rotating planar projection images. The count density of the rest study as measured by maximal count/pixel within the left ventricle is low (73 counts). The stress study in contrast has excellent count density. One can expect the reconstructed tomographic slices of the rest study to be of suboptimal quality. **(movie)**

Low Counts (Figs. 16-2 to 16-4)

One of the most important parameters affecting image quality is count density. Low-count density can be suspected readily from the visual appearance of the rotating planar projection images. Low-count

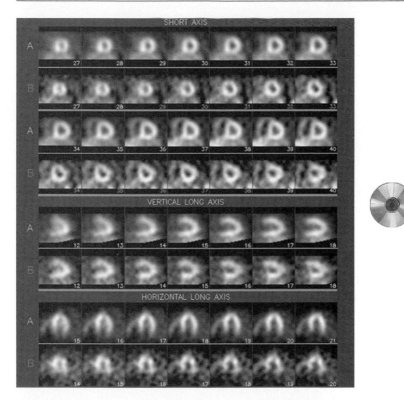

Fig. 16-3. Reconstructed SPECT slices of the raw projection data shown in Figure 16-2. The display of reconstructed slices in this and other images follows ASNC standards. The short axis (SA) slices are displayed on top, the vertical long axis (VLA) slices in the middle and the horizontal long axis (HLA) slices on the bottom. The rows marked with "A" show the stress images and rows marked with "B" show rest images. The SA slices are displayed from apex (#27) to base (#40); the VLA slices are displayed from septum (#12) to lateral wall (#18); the HLA are displayed from inferior wall (#15) to anterior wall (#21). The suboptimal quality of the low-count rest images can be appreciated in comparison to the good quality stress images.

studies have an overall "noisy" appearance, and the heart is poorly visualized (**Figs. 16-2** to **16-4**). Software developed in our laboratory displays maximal counts/pixel in the LV on the rotating images screen.

Good quality SPECT images (**Fig. 16-4**) usually have >150 maximal counts/pixel in the heart. Low-count studies are often caused by patient obesity. It is helpful if the imaging worksheet for technologists contains information about patient weight, chest circumference, and bra size.

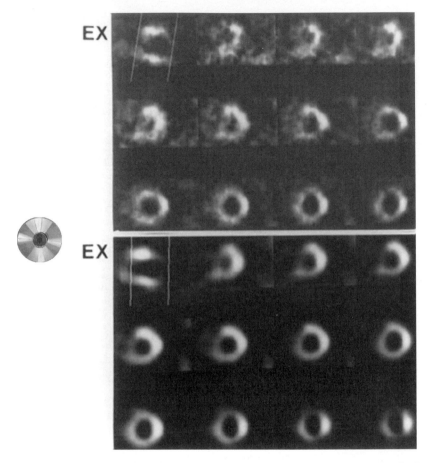

Fig. 16-4. Reconstructed SPECT slices of a patient with an anteroseptal and apical myocardial perfusion defect. The top study was acquired with Thallium-201 and is of suboptimal quality due to relatively low counts (max 87 cnts/pixel). The study was repeated with Tc-99m Sestamibi (bottom). This study is of excellent quality with high count density (256 counts/pixel).

Low-count-density SPECT studies can be avoided in two ways: by increasing the injected dose and by increasing imaging time. One can use patient weight or chest circumference as a guide for increasing these parameters (see Chapter 6, p. 82-83). Another practical method for avoiding low-count studies involves the acquisition of a short (e.g., 15 s) "scout" planar image prior to the start of SPECT acquisition. By comparing total counts in this image to "usual" count density in other patients, one may identify the potential for a low-count study ahead of time and make appropriate adjustments. This preventive QA method is particularly recommended for Tl-201 SPECT imaging.

Low Counts

Recognition
  Record count rate prior to start of acquisition in planar scout
    image
Preventive Measure
  Adjust dose according to weight/chest circumference
  Adjust acquisition time according to weight/chest
    circumference
Corrective Measure
  Repeat imaging with longer imaging times

Motion (Figs. 16-5 to 16-20)

Patient motion may be up-and-down (y-axis) or sideways (x-axis). Motion in the z-axis is difficult to identify and to correct for. In addition to motion caused by the patient, there may be a gradual change in position of the heart itself within the chest, for example, upward creep after good exercise effort. Inspection of rotating planar projection images is important for the recognition of patient motion **(Figs. 16-5** to **16-19)**.

A simple and commonly used method for identifying patient motion or upward creep consists of the use of a horizontal reference line on the computer screen (as shown in Figs 16-1 and 16-2). Using such a line as a fixed reference, for example, at the level of the apex, up-and-down motion of the heart can be readily recognized.

Another more sophisticated method involves the generation of a sinogram **(Fig. 16-5)**, in which each horizontal row of pixels represents the summed counts of an entire projection image on the x-axis. Motion can be recognized by "breaks" in the smooth sinusoid pattern of inhomogeneous activity. A modification of the sinogram is the linogram in which each vertical column represents summed counts of the cardiac activity.

Most vendors supply motion correction software. Motion correction software does not always correct appropriately and must be used judiciously. Prevention of motion is the most effective way to avoid artifacts. One should take time to instruct patients about the importance of remaining still on the table and use straps or hand holds to facilitate this.

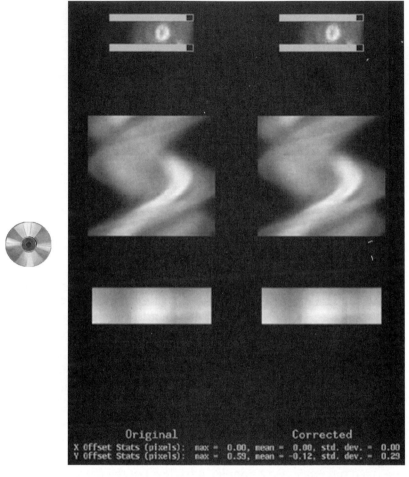

Fig. 16-5. Normal sinogram. The simplest method to recognize patient motion is the horizontal reference line as shown in Fig. 15-1. The sinogram as shown is this figure is another method. A normal sinogram shows smooth and continuous curves (sinusoids) of activity. Projecting all activity in one projection image on the x-axis creates this image. Due to the rotating motion of the gamma camera, the location of projected counts at each stop moves in a sinusoid pattern. In this image, the brightest activity are counts from the heart. As can be seen, there are no breaks in the sinusoid pattern, indicating no patient motion. On the bottom, the x and y offsets are shown. In the absence of significant motion, only minor corrections are made.

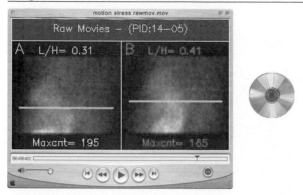

Fig. 16-6. Cine display of rotating planar projection images of a patient who moved during acquisition of the SPECT study. The heart can be seen "bouncing" on the left stress images, indicating marked patient motion. The stress study is not motion corrected. This can be concluded as image itself is not moving. The rest study is apparently motion corrected as the projection images are moving up and down while rotating. **(movie)**

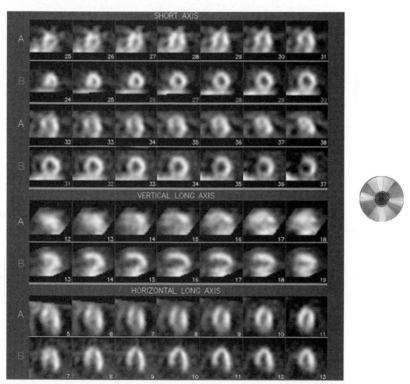

Fig. 16-7. Reconstructed slices of the study in Fig. 16-6. The motion-corrected rest study appears normal. However, the stress study shows marked distortion of the normal morphology of the heart in short axis slices and vertical and horizontal long axis slices. The stress study is uninterpretable.

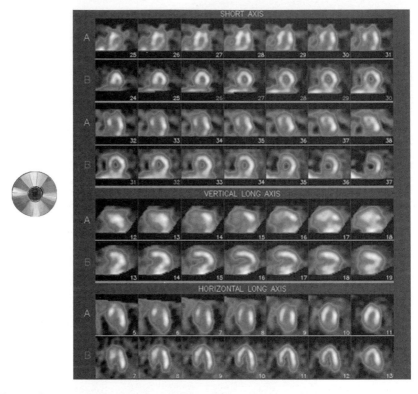

Fig. 16-8. Same figure as in 6-7 in colour.

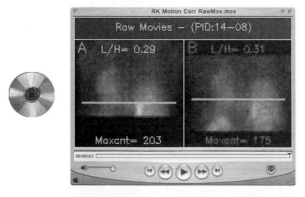

Fig. 16-9. Cine display of rotating planar projection images of the same study as in Figs 16-6–16-8. Motion correction is applied to both the stress and rest studies. Note the up-and-down motion of the projection images due to correction in the y-axis. Although there is still some motion of the heart after correction, it is significantly less. **(movie)**

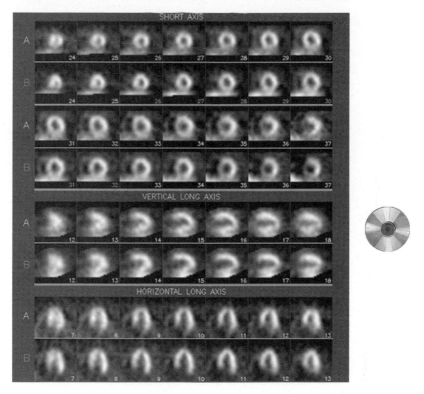

Fig. 16-10. Motion-corrected reconstructed slices of the study in Figs 16-6 to 16-8. The quality of the stress study is markedly improved. The motion-corrected stress study shows a very small reversible inferoapical defect. This is a good example of successful motion correction.

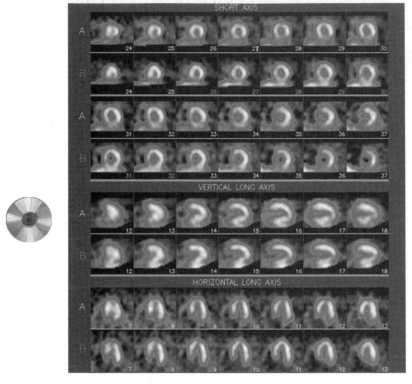

Fig. 16-11. Color images of the reconstructed slices shown in Fig. 16-10.

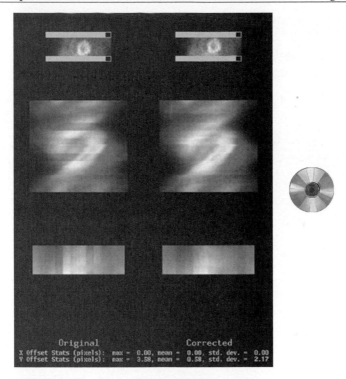

Fig. 16-12. Sinogram (original and motion corrected) of the patient study shown in Figs 16-6 to 16-11. The corrected sinogram is by no means normal but greatly improved compared to the original one. The x and y offset of pixels is shown in the bottom.

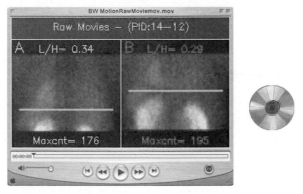

Fig. 16-13. Cine display of rotating planar projection images of another patient who moved during acquisition of the SPECT study. The heart can be seen "bouncing" on the left stress images, indicating marked patient motion. In addition to up-and-down motion, there is also marked sideways motion in the anterior position. The stress study is not motion corrected as the image itself is not moving. The rest study is apparently motion corrected as the projection images are moving up and down while rotating. **(movie)**

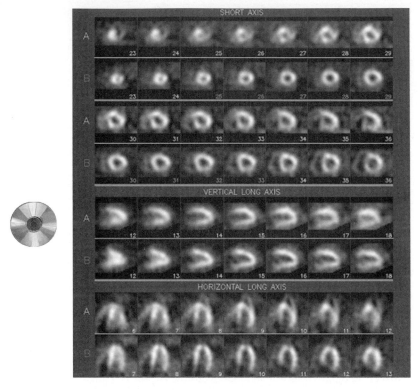

Fig. 16-14. Reconstructed slices of the study in Fig. 16-13. The motion-corrected rest study appears relatively normal. However, the stress study shows marked distortion of the normal morphology of the heart in short axis slices and vertical and horizontal long axis slices. The stress study is uninterpretable.

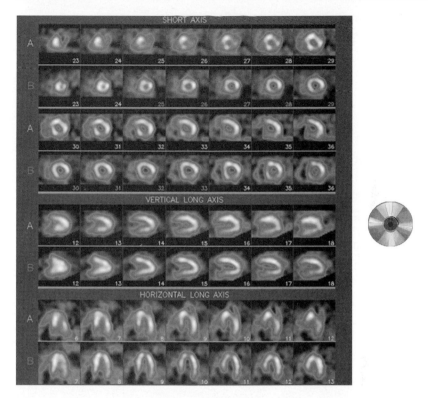

Fig. 16-15. Same images as in Fig. 16-14 in color.

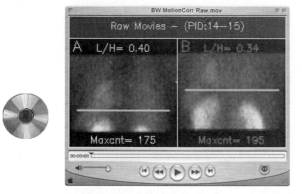

Fig. 16-16. Cine display of rotating planar projection images of the same study as in Figs 16-13 to 16-15. Motion correction is applied to both the stress and rest studies. Note the up-and-down motion of the projection images due to correction in the y-axis. Although the up-and-down motion of the stress study is less, the sideways motion is still present. On the rest image motion-correction was effective. **(movie)**

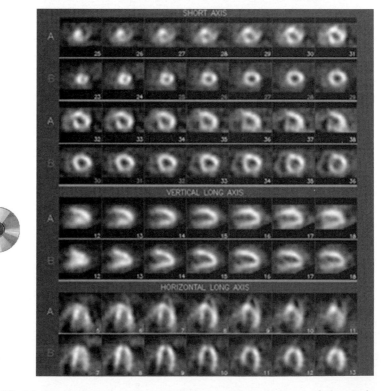

Fig. 16-17. Motion-corrected stress and rest reconstructed slices of the study shown in Figs 16-13 to 16-15. Motion correction was not successful on the stress study. There is still marked distortion of normal morphology. The study remains uninterpretable. The rest study is successfully corrected for motion.

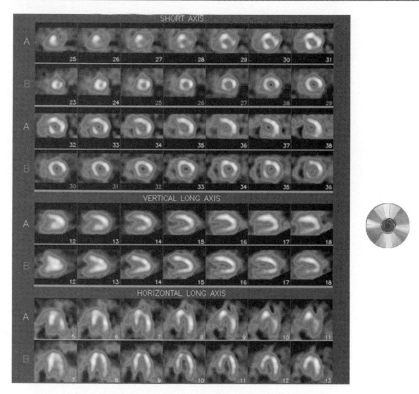

Fig. 16-18. Same images as in Fig. 16-16 in color.

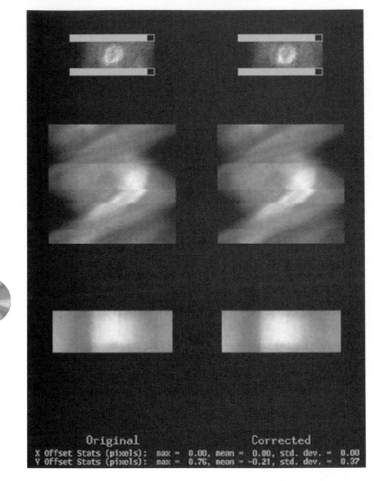

Fig. 16-19. Sinogram (original and motion-corrected) of the stress study shown in Figs 16-13 to 16-18. The corrected sinogram is still markedly abnormal. The x and y offset of pixels is shown in the bottom. The computer algorithm erroneously did not make correction for x-axis offset.

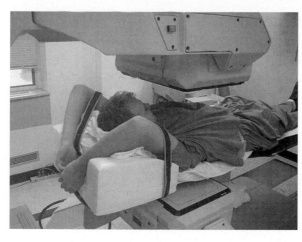

Fig. 16-20. For many patients it is difficult to keep still with the arms extended over the head. Velcro straps may be helpful in making this position more tolerable.

Patient Motion

Recognition
   Horizontal reference line
   Sinogram
   Linogram
Preventive Measure
   Explain the importance of not moving to patients and the need
      not to fall asleep (snore)
   Position patient in comfortable position
   Immobilize arms with Velcro straps
   Delay stress imaging till 10–15 min after exercise to avoid
      upward creep
Corrective Measure
   Apply motion correction software
   Repeat imaging after better patient instruction and better
      immobilization with straps (Figs 16-20)

Inferior Attenuation (Figs. 16-21 to 16-40)

SPECT imaging is performed with the patient in the supine position. In this position, the dome of the left hemidiaphragm may attenuate photons emanating from the inferior wall of the LV. Diaphragmatic attenuation can be suspected when the inferior wall *suddenly* disappears when going from LAO to left lateral angles on the rotating planar projection images (**Figs. 16-21** to **16-40**).

Diaphragmatic attenuation can be demonstrated by acquiring two planar left lateral images: one with the patient *supine* and one with the patient on the *right side decubitus* position *(1–3)* (**Fig. 16-25**). Inferior attenuation is present when the left-lateral right decubitus is normal, or less abnormal, and the supine image shows an unequivocal inferior wall defect. This occurs in about one-quarter of patients.

Inferior attenuation usually results in fixed myocardial perfusion defects suggesting infarction. ECG-gated SPECT has been very helpful in differentiating inferior attenuation from scar: if regional wall motion and thickening is normal in a region with a fixed inferior defect, the defect is very likely caused by attenuation *(4)*.

Inferior attenuation can be avoided by performing SPECT imaging in a different position: right side decubitus (**Fig. 16-25**), upright sitting, and prone (**Fig. 16-32**). In many centers, imaging is repeated in prone position if inferior attenuation is suspected.

Nevertheless, these methods have only limited utility: patients with inferior attenuation may also have coronary artery disease.

The only effective methodology to deal with non-uniform attenuation artifacts is to acquire images with AC devices *(5,6)*.

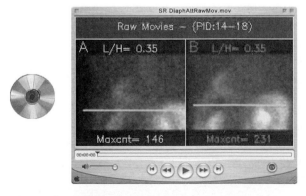

Fig. 16-21. Rotating planar projection images of a patient with inferior attenuation. Note how the inferior wall suddenly disappears on the stress and rest left lateral projection images. (**movie**)

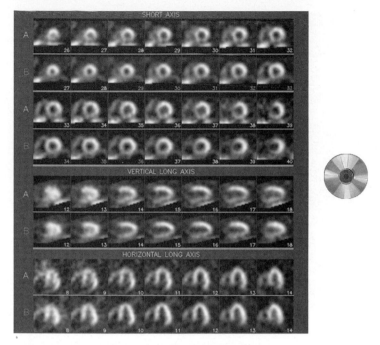

Fig. 16-22. Reconstructed tomographic slices of the images shown in Fig. 16-21. A fixed inferior myocardial perfusion defect is present.

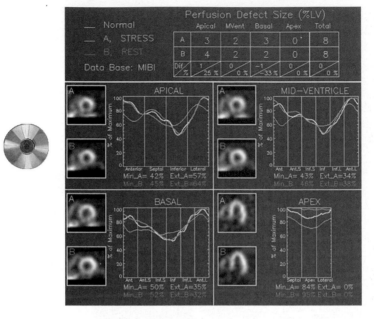

Fig. 16-23. Quantification of the SPECT slices in Fig. 16-22. The yellow curves represent the count distribution on the stress images and the red curves represent the rest images. The white curves represent the lower limit of normal radiotracer distribution. The stress and rest curves are below the lower limit of normal in the inferolateral walls in the apical, midventricular sand basal short axis slices. Note that the yellow and red curves are virtually identical, indicating a fixed myocardial perfusion abnormality due to either scar or attenuation. In the table on top the results of computer quantification are shown. The total stress and rest defect size is moderate and involves 8% of the left ventricle.

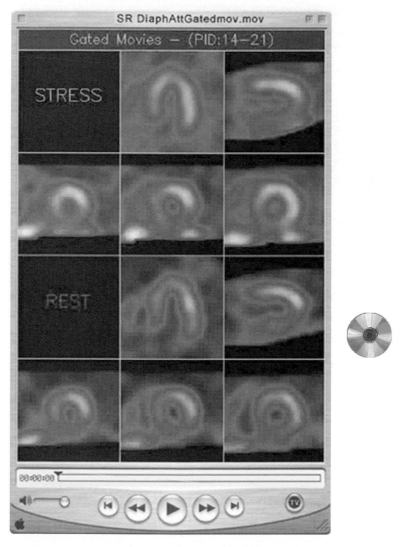

Fig. 16-24. Movie display of ECG-gated SPECT of images shown in Fig. 16-22. Note that the wall motion and thickening of the inferior wall (location of fixed defect) is normal. This suggests that the fixed defect may be artifactual and due to attenuation. **(movie)**

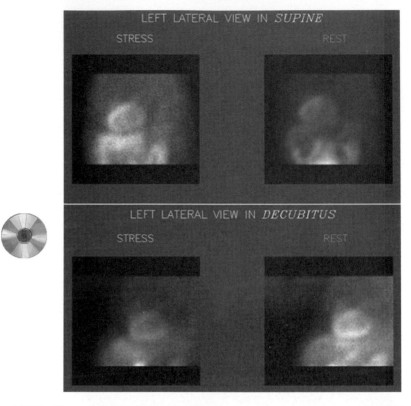

Fig. 16-25. Planar left-lateral images of the patient whose reconstructed SPECT images were shown in Fig. 16-22. Planar images were acquired in supine position (top) and in right side decubitus position (bottom). One can appreciate that the planar images on the bottom are normal with good visualization of the inferior wall, whereas on the supine images, in the position that SPECT was acquired, the inferior wall is practically absent due to attenuation. The constellation of findings on rotating images, gated images and planar images all confirm the presence of inferior attenuation.

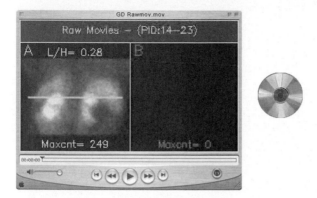

Fig. 16-26. Rotating planar projection images of another patient with inferior attenuation. Note again how the inferior wall suddenly disappears on the stress left lateral projection images. **(movie)**

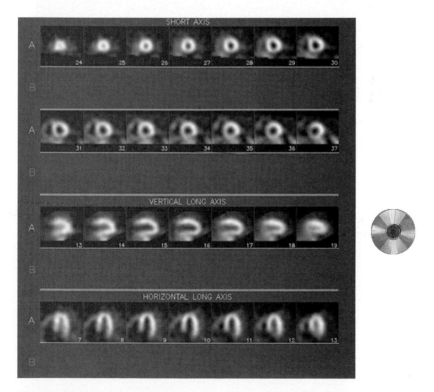

Fig. 16-27. Reconstructed tomographic slices of the images shown in Fig. 16-26. Mild decreased uptake in the inferior wall is noted.

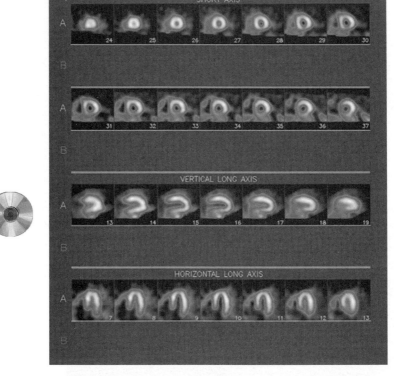

Fig. 16-28. Same images as in Fig. 16-27 in color. The decreased uptake in the inferior wall is better appreciated.

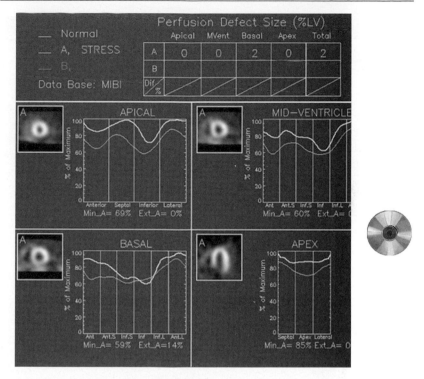

Fig. 16-29. Quantification of the SPECT slices in Fig. 16-27. A small basal inferior wall perfusion defect is present

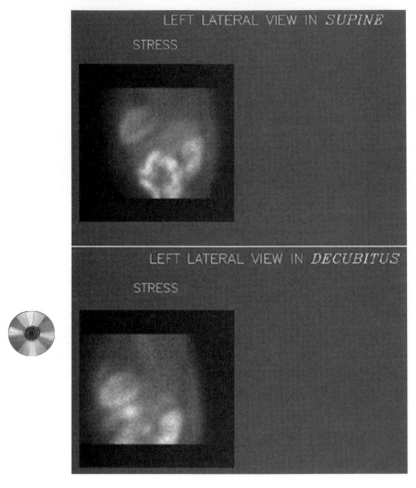

Fig. 16-30. Planar left lateral images of the patient in Fig. 16-27. In supine position, there is inferobasal defect, which is not present on the image acquired in the right side decubitus position. This suggests the presence of inferior attenuation.

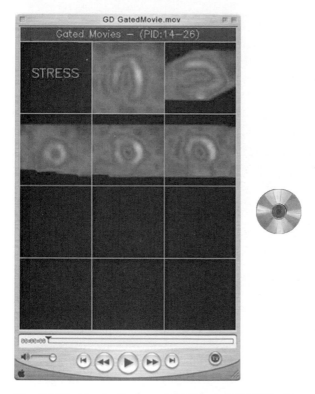

Fig. 16-31. Movie display of ECG-gated SPECT of images in Fig. 16-27. Note that wall motion and wall thickening of the inferior wall are normal. This suggests that the small inferobasal defect may be due to attenuation. **(movie)**

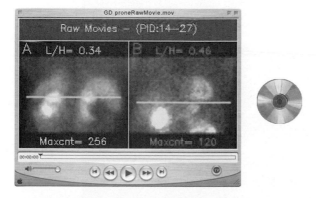

Fig. 16-32. Rotating planar projection images of the patient, whose images were shown in Figs 16-26 to 16-30. The patient had repeat imaging in prone position. The supine stress images are displayed on the left; the prone stress images are displayed on the right. Note that because of the different patient position the images rotate in opposite directions. **(movie)**

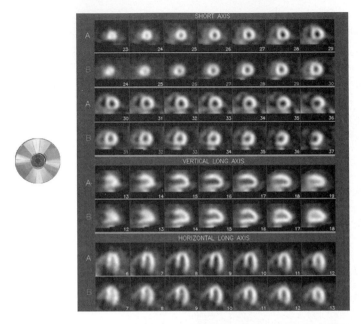

Fig. 16-33. Reconstructed tomographic slices of the images in Fig. 16-32. The stress **supine** images are shown in rows "A"; whereas the **prone** images are shown in rows "B". The small inferior defect present on the supine images is not present on the prone images.

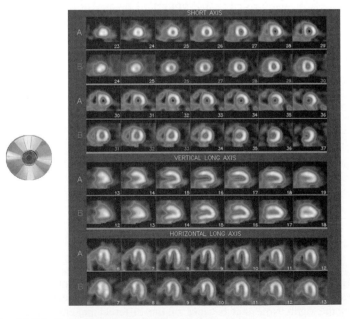

Fig. 16-34. Same images as in Fig. 16-33 in color.

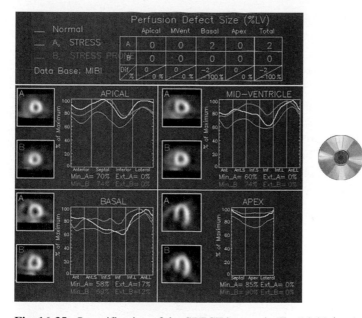

Fig. 16-35. Quantification of the SPECT images in Fig. 16-33 (supine and prone). The yellow curves represent the circumferential count distribution profiles on the **supine** images, whereas the red curves represent that on the **prone** images. It can be appreciated that in the mid ventricular and basal slices inferior attenuation is significantly less in prone position than in supine position.

INFERIOR ATTENUATION

Recognition
 Compare planar left lateral images in supine and right side
  decubitus position
 Normal regional wall motion and thickening on gated SPECT
Preventive Measure
 Imaging in prone, upright, or right side decubitus position
Corrective Measure
 Attenuation correction

Attenuation Correction (AC) and Errors, Misregistration (Figs. 16-36 to 16-41)

For non-uniform tissue AC, sealed radioisotope sources or X-ray CT can be used to generate transmission maps for the correction of emission images. Defects due to soft tissue attenuation (diaphragm or breast) can be corrected using this technology. Using sealed sources, emission and transmission images are perfectly aligned, because they were acquired simultaneously. However, using X-ray CT systems, misalignment or misregistration may occur because emission and transmission images are acquired sequentially. Artifacts due to such misalignment are predictable *(7)*. Artifactual defects may occur particularly in the (antero-)lateral wall of the LV. When the emission image is misaligned with the CT image and the heart is positioned too much to the left, that is, over the left lung, the attenuation algorithm will "conclude" that there is less attenuation of the lateral wall than of the rest of the heart. Consequently, the lateral wall undergo less mathematical correction. The ultimate image will consequently show a lateral wall defect (**Fig. 16-41**).

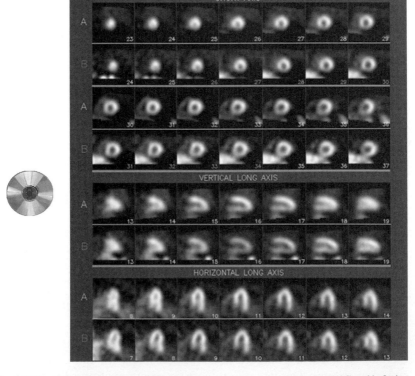

Fig. 16-36. Stress (A) and rest (B) reconstructed slices showing a small fixed inferior defect. Supine and right-side decubitus planar left lateral images suggested attenuation of the inferior wall. Inferior wall thickening on gated SPECT was normal.

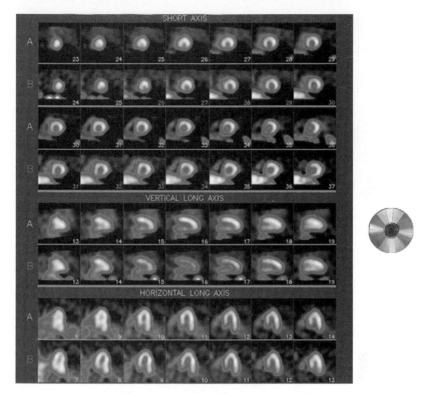

Fig. 16-37. Same images as in Fig. 16-36 in color.

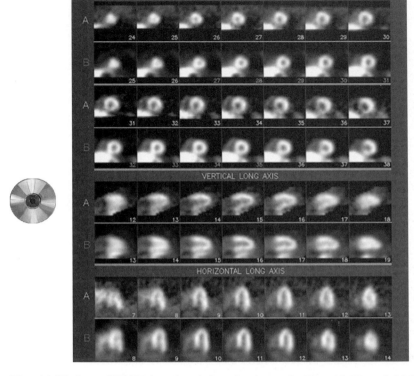

Fig. 16-38. Rest SPECT imaging (of study shown in Figs 16-37 and 16-38) was performed with X-ray CT attenuation correction. Shown are the uncorrected images in rows "A" and attenuation-corrected images in rows "B". On the attenuation-corrected images in B radiotracer distribution is more homogeneous. There is no longer an inferior wall defect.

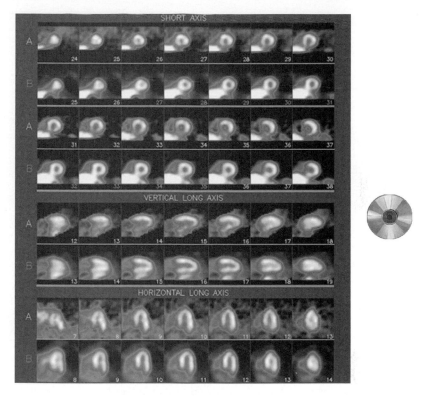

Fig. 16-39. Same images as in Fig. 16-38 in color.

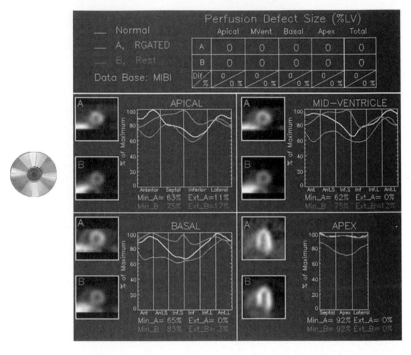

Fig. 16-40. Quantification of the images in Figs 16-39 and 16-40. The yellow curves (A) represent the circumferential count distribution profiles of the **uncorrected** images, whereas the red curves (B) represent that of the **attenuation-corrected** images. It can be appreciated that radiotracer distribution is more homogeneous after attenuation correction.

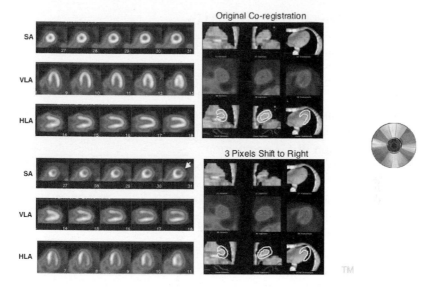

Fig. 16-41. Effect of misregistration of x-ray CT attenuation map and Tc-99m Sestamibi SPECT emission images. Top: Original images with correct coregistration. Bottom: Same image data with intentional 3-pixel misregistration. Right: Attenuation-corrected tomographic slices. Left on top: Single-slice CT attenuation map in coronal (left), sagittal (middle), and transaxial (right) views. Left middle: Emission images SPECT images. Left bottom: Fusion of CT and emission images. Automatically generated outlines of the left ventricle are shown in yellow. The attenuation-corrected tomographic slices on top left are normal. Some slight overcorrection of the inferior wall may be present. On the bottom images, the emission images are intentionally shifted 3 pixels to the left. The lateral wall of the emission image is now in the left lung of the CT image. The attenuation correction algorithm applied substantially less mathematical correction to the lateral wall. The corrected tomographic slices bottom-left show an artifactual anterolateral defect due to erroneous correction.

MISREGISTRATION ATTENUATION MAP

Recognition
  Defect not present on non-attenuation-corrected images, in
    particular of the anterolateral wall
Preventive Measure
  Simultaneous acquisition emission/transmission data
  Shorten duration of CT acquisition
  QC of fusion images of emission and transmission images for
    alignment
Corrective Measure
  Software that allows for shifting of emission and transmission
    images until well aligned

Breast Attenuation (Figs. 16-42 to 16-47)

When interpreting SPECT images of women, the rotating planar
projection images should always be scrutinized for breast attenuation.
In some obese men upper chest attenuation may also occur (**Figs. 16-42
to 16-47**).

On rotating images, the breast can be recognized as a round shadow
that moves over the heart in the LAO and lateral positions. It is helpful
if the technologist records information about chest circumference and
bra size on the imaging worksheet.

In contrast to the serious interpretative problems one can have on
planar images due to breast attenuation, breast attenuation on *SPECT*
images is often not a significant problem. Most of the time, only a
mild fixed anterior defect may be present. *Because of possible change
in position of the breast on rest and stress images, the defect is not
necessarily fixed.* Again analysis of regional wall motion on ECG-
gated SPECT has been shown to be helpful in recognizing breast
artifacts *(4)*.

Nevertheless, these methods have only limited utility: patients
with anterior attenuation may also have coronary artery disease.
The only effective methodology to deal with non-uniform attenuation artifacts is to acquire images with attenuation-correction
devices *(5,6)*.

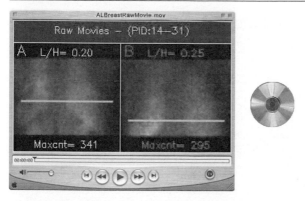

Fig. 16-42. Rotating planar projection images of a patient with large breasts. Chest circumference was inch and bra cup size. Note that both the right and left breasts can be seen as shadows that move over the screen. The left breast almost completely eclipses the heart. **(movie)**

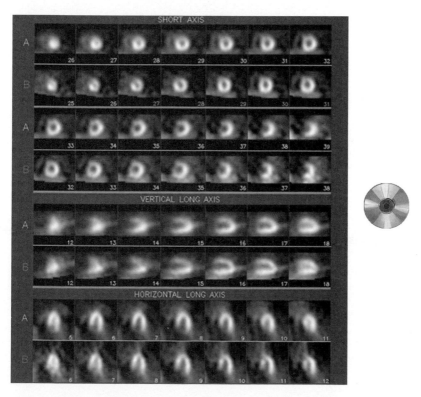

Fig. 16-43. Reconstructed tomographic slices of the images in Fig. 16-42. A moderate fixed anterior wall defect can be noted on the stress and rest images on short axis and vertical long axis slices. The "streaks" at the apex on the horizontal long axis slices may be due to breast tissue.

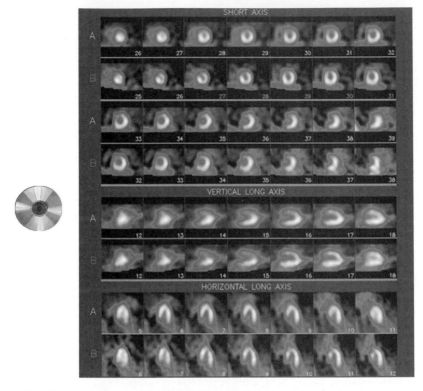

Fig. 16-44. Same images as in Fig. 16-43 in color.

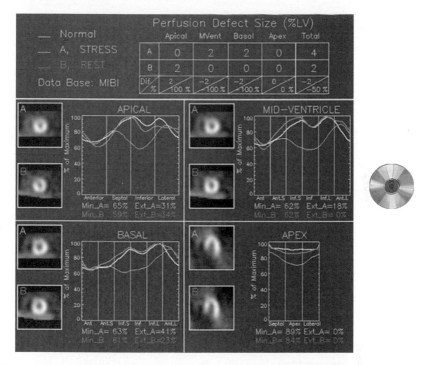

Fig. 16-45. Quantification of the SPECT slices in Figs 16-43 and 16-44. A small anterolateral defect is present on the apical, midventricular and basal slices. Some minor defect reversibility is quantitatively present

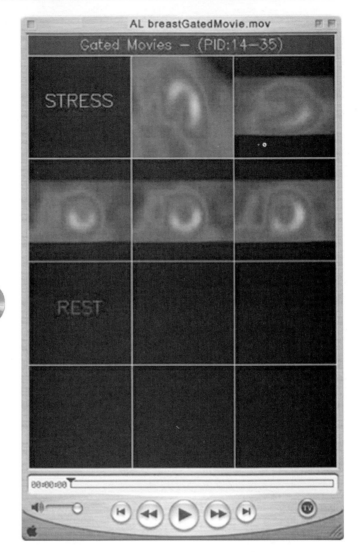

Fig. 16-46. Gated SPECT movie of the slices shown in Figs 16-43 and 16-44. Regional wall motion and thickening is normal in the area of the apparent defect. **(movie)**

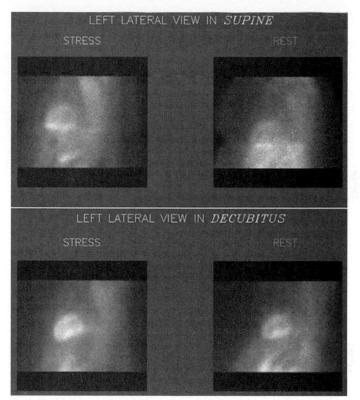

Fig. 16-47. Planar supine (top) and right side decubitus (bottom) left lateral images of the same patient. The right side decubitus images are normal because in this position the breast moves to the middle of the chest. The supine images, the position in which the SPECT images were acquired, show attenuation of the anterior wall by breast tissue. The constellation of findings on the rotating images, these planar images and gated SPECT movie, suggest that breast attenuation may be responsible for the anterior defect. This patient had normal coronary arteries on coronary angiography.

BREAST ATTENUATION

Recognition
   Shadow on rotating images
   Normal regional wall motion on gated SPECT
Preventive Measure
   None
Corrective Measure
   Attenuation correction

Non-Cardiac Radiotracer Uptake (Figs. 16-48 to 16-54)

The rotating images should not only be analyzed for motion and attenuation but also for other non-cardiac radiotracer uptake that may be of significance for the interpretation of the study. One should routinely watch for non-cardiac uptake in the axilla, mediastinum, breasts, lungs, and elsewhere as such uptake may represent malignancies (**Figs. 16-48** to **16-54**).

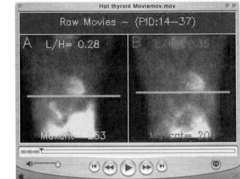

Fig. 16-48. On these rotating planar projection images, one can note in the top of the field of view radiotracer uptake is the thyroid gland. This is most likely due to suboptimal labeling of the radiopharmaceutical. Free Tc-99m-pertechnetate accumulates in thyroid gland and mucosa of the stomach. (**movie**)

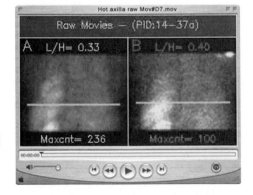

Fig. 16-49. The rotating planar projection images show on the rest study intense radiotracer uptake in the right axilla. One should attempt to understand the cause for such a finding. This is important, as radiotracer uptake in the axilla could indicate malignancy in an axillary lymph node. The uptake then is usually present on both the stress and rest images. The intensity of uptake, and presence in the rest study only, suggests contamination of skin or gown with radiotracer is a more likely cause. One should try to clarify this finding by discussion with the nuclear medicine technologist. (**movie**)

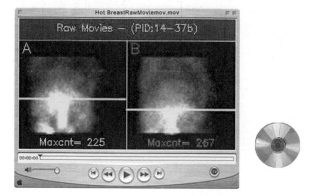

Fig. 16-50. On the rotating images, abnormal radiotracer uptake can be noted in both breasts. This is always an abnormal finding that should be reported. It is feasible that the woman is lactating, has a bilateral infection, or may have a malignancy. **(movie)**

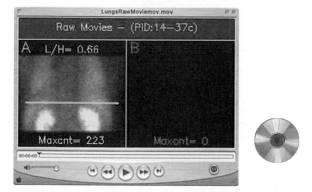

Fig. 16-51. The rotating stress images show markedly increased pulmonary uptake of radiotracer. This image pattern, seen in conjunction with a reversible myocardial perfusion abnormality, may be a marker of transient ischemic left ventricular dysfunction and is a predictor of poor outcome. On the images the heart is clearly enlarged and this patient may have chronic congestive heart failure. **(movie)**.

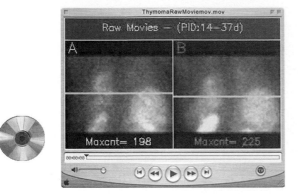

Fig. 16-52. The rotating planar projection images show clearly abnormal radio-tracer uptake to the right side of the heart. This abnormal finding was mentioned in the report. The patient was later found to have a thymoma. (**movie**).

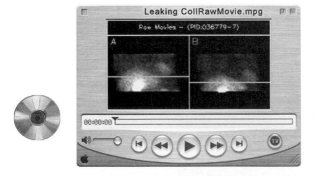

Fig. 16-53. Rotating stress (A) and rest (B) planar projection images. During the rotation of the stress images a bright "glow" appears on the top of the images in the anterior positions. This is most likely due to "leaking" radioactivity from outside the field of view between the mounted collimator and the gamma camera detector head. The technologist must investigate the cause of this artifact by surveying the patient's gown, neck and arms for contamination or extravasation of injected dose. It is also possible that the collimator is not mounted correctly on the camera head. This is potentially dangerous because the collimator could fall off and injure the patient. If the collimator is mounted correctly, one can purchase lead guards that cover the slit between the collimator and camera, and this will avoid this artifact from recurring. (**movie**).

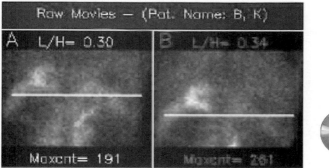

Fig. 16-54. During rotation of these planar projection images, several unusual photopenic areas are noted at the level of the heart and below the heart. On closer inspection, these appear to be located in the right liver lobe and both kidneys. These patient had known multicystic disease of the kidneys and liver. **(movie).**

RECONSTRUCTED TOMOGRAPHIC SLICES

Correct Orientation of Tomographic Axis and Alignment of Slices (Figs. 16-55 to 16-58)

Incorrect Orientation of Tomographic Axis (Figs. 16-59 to 16-62)

The first step in reconstruction of tomographic images is to create tomographic slices that are oriented along the anatomical axis of the body, resulting in transverse, coronal, and sagittal slices.

Since the heart is positioned in the chest at an angle to the body axis, interpretation of conventional coronal, transverse, and sagittal slices is difficult, because the walls of the heart are cut tangentially. Therefore, tomographic cuts through the heart must be re-oriented according to the anatomical axis of the *LV*.

Two conceivable mistakes can be made: (i) The selection of long axis is not precisely along the anatomical axis of the heart and (ii) The orientations of the selected axis in the stress and rest images are not parallel. These errors can be relatively easily recognized since the slices "do not look" like usual images. Although the eye usually may be able to deal with slight deviations in slicing, quantification of images and inspection of bull's eye display alone can lead to incorrect conclusions.

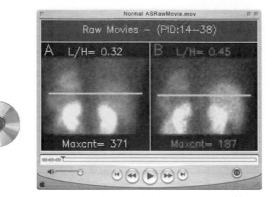

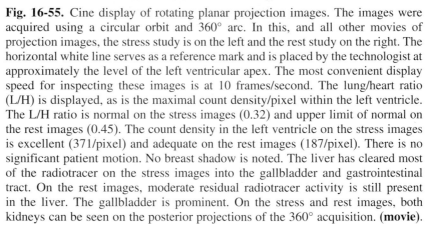

Fig. 16-55. Cine display of rotating planar projection images. The images were acquired using a circular orbit and 360° arc. In this, and all other movies of projection images, the stress study is on the left and the rest study on the right. The horizontal white line serves as a reference mark and is placed by the technologist at approximately the level of the left ventricular apex. The most convenient display speed for inspecting these images is at 10 frames/second. The lung/heart ratio (L/H) is displayed, as is the maximal count density/pixel within the left ventricle. The L/H ratio is normal on the stress images (0.32) and upper limit of normal on the rest images (0.45). The count density in the left ventricle on the stress images is excellent (371/pixel) and adequate on the rest images (187/pixel). There is no significant patient motion. No breast shadow is noted. The liver has cleared most of the radiotracer on the stress images into the gallbladder and gastrointestinal tract. On the rest images, moderate residual radiotracer activity is still present in the liver. The gallbladder is prominent. On the stress and rest images, both kidneys can be seen on the posterior projections of the 360° acquisition. **(movie)**.

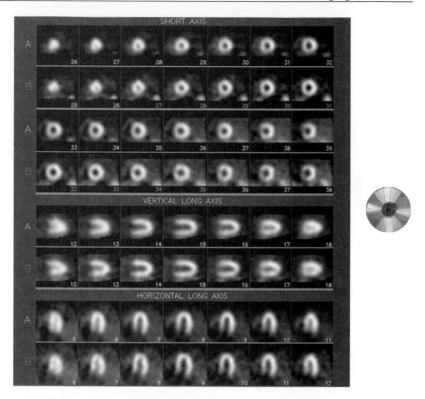

Fig. 16-56. Reconstructed SPECT slices of the raw projection data shown in Fig. 16-55. The display of reconstructed slices in this and other images adheres to ACC/AHA/ASNC/SNM standards for display of tomographic images. The short axis (SA) slices are displayed on top, the vertical long axis (VLA) slices in the middle, and the horizontal long axis (HLA) slices on the bottom. The rows marked with "A" show the stress images and rows marked with "B" show rest images. The SA slices are displayed from apex (#26 and 25) to base (#39 and 38); the VLA slices are displayed from septum (#12) to lateral wall (#18); and the HLA are displayed from inferior wall (#5 and #6) to anterior wall (#11 and #12). This is an example of normal SPECT images.

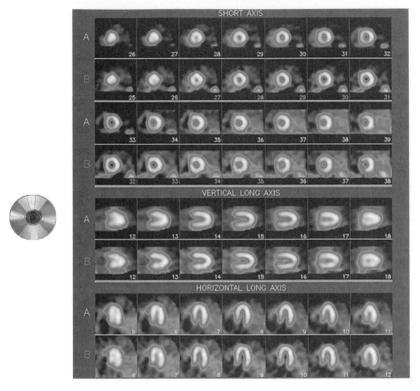

Fig. 16-57. Same images as in Fig. 16-56 in color.

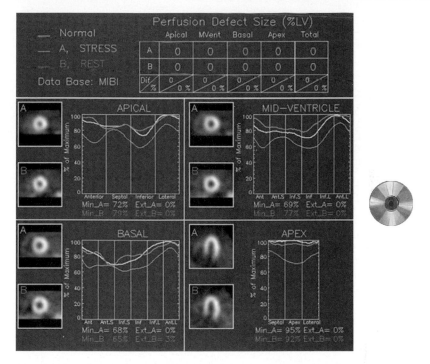

Fig. 16-58. Quantification of the SPECT slices in Figs 16-56 and 16-57 using circumferential count distribution profile analysis. The yellow curves represent the count distribution on the stress images and the red curves represent the rest images. The white curves represent the lower limit of normal radiotracer distribution (mean − 2 SD). The stress and rest curves are within the lower limit of normal in the apical, mid-ventricular, and basal short axis slices. The apical segment is quantified from a mid horizontal axis slice and is normal as well. In the table on top, the results of computer quantification are shown. No defects are quantified. These are quantitatively a normal SPECT images.

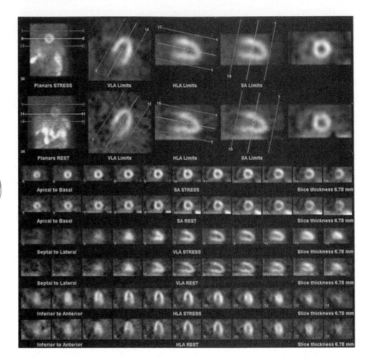

Fig. 16-59. Correct slicing To obtain tomographic slices of the heart perpendicular to the anatomic axis of the left ventricular limits of slicing (red lines) and direction of long axis (green lines) must be chosen on transverse and sagittal body slices. Correct limits of slicing ensure that tomographic slices of the entire heart are obtained. Most important for the generation of cardiac slices that meet standards of tomographic display is the selection of the anatomical axis of the left ventricle by the technologist. The figure shows **correct selection** of the angles of slicing and of limits of slicing. This results in SPECT images of the heart that meet standards of display. Short axis slices should be circular with the right ventricle at the same level at the left. The vertical long axis images should show a horseshoe with the closed tip pointing to the right. The anterior and inferior wall should be of approximately equal length. The inferior wall should be parallel to the lower border of the image. The horizontal long axis image should show a horseshoe configuration with the closed tip pointing upward. The right ventricle is to the left. The septum in the middle should be one-half to three-fourth of the lateral wall. This is achieved by correct selection of angles of slicing.

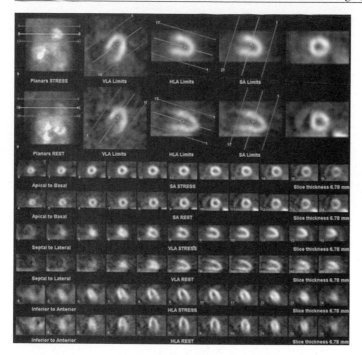

Fig. 16-60. Incorrect slicing (vertical) In this example, the angle of the anatomical long axis of the left ventricle as a direction for slicing is incorrectly selected for the **stress verticall long axis limits**. The angles for the rest images are correct. The incorrect angles result in nonstandard stress slices of the left ventricle. This is best appreciated in the horizontal long axis slices. The stress images are at an unusual angle and point to the left. The stress vertical long axis slices are apparently foreshortened compared to the rest slices. Some of the short axis slices have an elliptical rather than circular shape

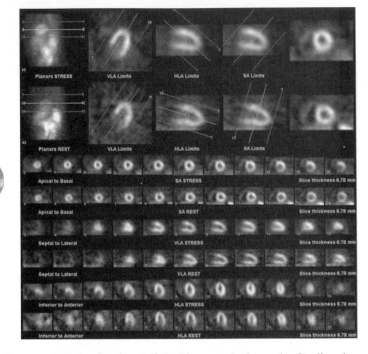

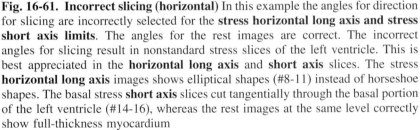

Fig. 16-61. Incorrect slicing (horizontal) In this example the angles for direction for slicing are incorrectly selected for the **stress horizontal long axis and stress short axis limits**. The angles for the rest images are correct. The incorrect angles for slicing result in nonstandard stress slices of the left ventricle. This is best appreciated in the **horizontal long axis** and **short axis** slices. The stress **horizontal long axis** images shows elliptical shapes (#8-11) instead of horseshoe shapes. The basal stress **short axis** slices cut tangentially through the basal portion of the left ventricle (#14-16), whereas the rest images at the same level correctly show full-thickness myocardium

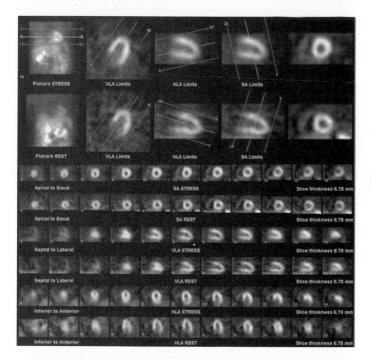

Fig. 16-62. Incorrect slicing (short axis) In this example the angles for direction for slicing are incorrectly selected for the stress horizontal long axis and stress short axis limits. The angles for the rest images are correct. The incorrect angles for slicing result in nonstandard stress slices of the left ventricle. This is best appreciated in the horizontal long axis and short axis slices. The stress horizontal long axis images show elliptical shapes (#7-9) instead of horseshoe shapes. The basal stress SA slices cut tangentially through the anteroseptal basal portion of the left ventricle (#14-16), whereas the rest images at the same level still show full-thickness myocardium

Fig. 16-63. The tomographic slices of this SPECT study were not aligned correctly. All stress slices should be moved one position to the right to match the rest study. This patient has a relatively small fixed inferolateral basal defect, as can be appreciated in the vertical and HLA slices. Because of the misalignment of slices, one could erroneously conclude that the defect is partially reversible

INCORRECT AXIS ORIENTATION

Recognition
  Inspect anatomical appearance of reconstructed slices
  Compare anatomical appearance of slices in stress and rest
    studies
Preventive Measure
  Appropriate training of technologist with understanding of
    anatomy and technology
Corrective Measure
  Repeat processing with correct axis selection

Misalignment of Slices on Display (Figs. 16-63 to 16-67)

Interpretation of stress–rest SPECT slices consists of comparison
of myocardial perfusion pattern in stress and rest reconstructed slices.
In order for comparison to be valid, slices must be well aligned,
that is apical and basal slice selections must match. Misalignment in

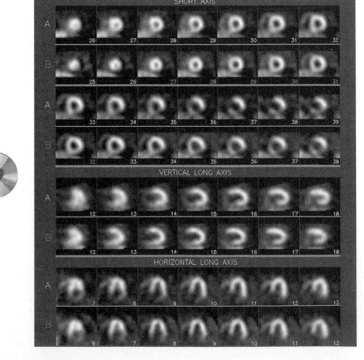

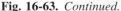

Fig. 16-63. *Continued.*

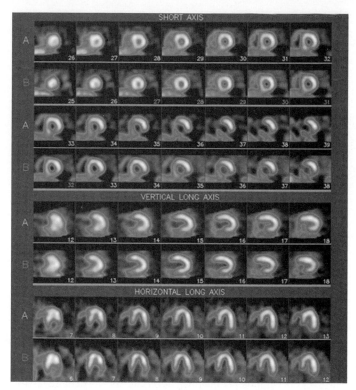

Fig. 16-64. Same images as in Fig. 16-63 in color.

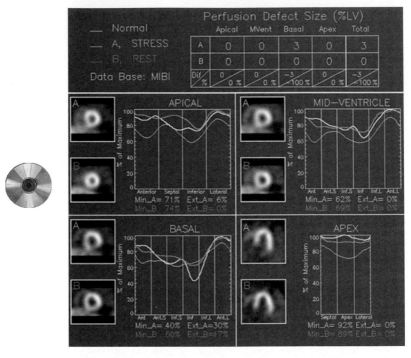

Fig. 16-65. Quantification of the stress and rest SPECT slices in Figs 16-63 and 16-64. Because of misalignment, quantification shows a small reversible inferolateral basal defect

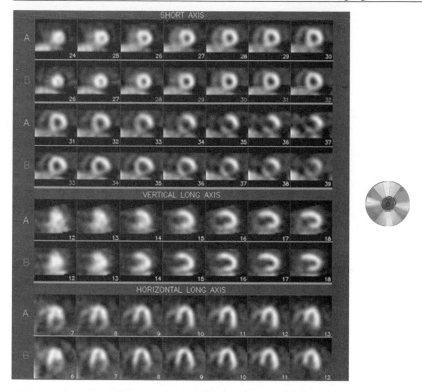

Fig. 16-66. Same SPECT study as in Figs 16-63 and 16-64 with correct alignment. The inferolateral basal defect appears fixed

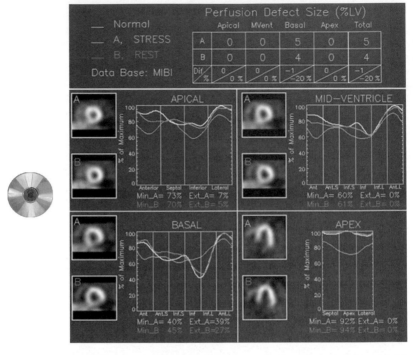

Fig. 16-67. Quantification of the stress and rest SPECT slices in Fig. 16-66. Because of correct alignment, quantification shows a small fixed inferolateral basal defect (5% of left ventricle). The defect reversibility suggested in Fig. 16-65 was erroneous

display may lead to misinterpretations, for example, erroneous transient ventricular dilation or erroneous defect reversibility. Mistakes can be avoided by careful inspection of the arrangement of reconstructed stress and rest slices on display, for example, the first apical slices showing left ventricular cavity and first slice showing membranous septum should be well aligned. Nevertheless, it may not always be possible to align images; in markedly abnormal studies with true transient dilation of the LV, it may not be possible to make a match.

Misalignment

Recognition
    Careful inspection of match at apex and base of reconstructed
        stress and rest slices
Preventive Measure
    Appropriate training of technologist. The written procedure
        protocol should provide instruction on how to align images

Corrective Measure
Repeat processing with correct comparative display of slices

Intense GI Uptake (Figs. 16-68 to 16-75)

Using Tc-99m-labeled agents, intense GI uptake of radiopharmaceutical can be a serious problem, generally after pharmacological stress and on resting images. This is particularly true if "hot" extracardiac activity is present immediately adjacent to the heart, that is, the inferior wall.

Intense uptake *at a distance* from the heart, that is, gallbladder and lower intestines, usually do not cause much problem unless a very hot organ is present within the selected block for backprojection and reconstruction. This may result in the so-called northern light artifact.

Measures to reduce the amount of GI activity are inconsistently effective. Low level of exercise may decrease splanchnic uptake. Drinking a large amount of fluid may help to move radioactivity through the GI tract.

Intense GI activity immediately adjacent to the heart may cause interpretive problems in several ways:

1. Superimposition of activity on the inferior left ventricular wall and making analysis of inferior wall impossible.
2. Scattering of photons into the left ventricular inferior wall: a fixed inferior defect may appear reversible.
3. Back projection and filtering artifact resulting in erroneous defects *(8)*.

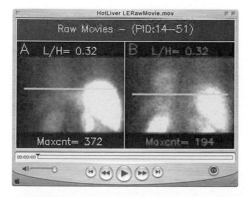

Fig. 16-68. Adenosine stress and rest rotating projection images of a female patient. During adenosine infusion, the patient was supine on the imaging table. One can appreciate intense radiotracer uptake in the liver. Technical problems during filtered backprojection may be anticipated. **(movie)**

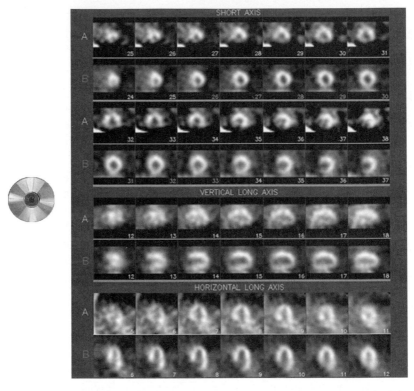

Fig. 16-69. Reconstructed tomographic slices of the images in Fig. 16-68. The rest images are of acceptable quality. However, the stress images are of suboptimal quality with substantial background noise. There is an inferior wall defect on the stress images that is not present at rest. Because of intense liver uptake adjacent to the heart, one should be concerned about a filtered backprojection artifact. It is conceivable that the filter suppressed image data in the inferior wall of the heart in the presence of the hot liver.

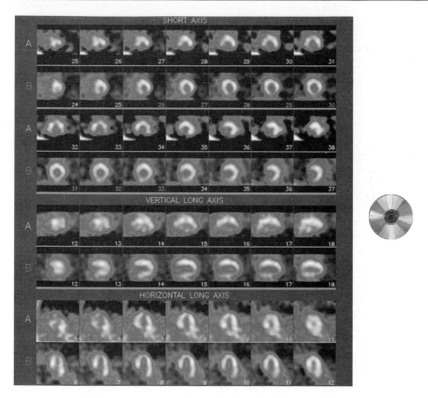

Fig. 16-70. Same images as in Fig. 16-69 in color.

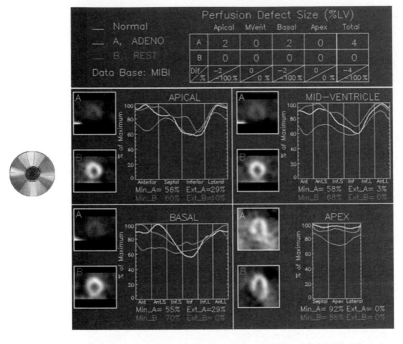

Fig. 16-71. Quantification of the images in Figs 16-69 and 16-70. The circumferential profiles show an inferior defect that is reversible at rest. Because of intense adjacent liver uptake, one should be concerned about the possibility of a filtered backprojection artifact. It is conceivable that the filter suppressed image data in the inferior wall of the heart in the presence of the hot liver.

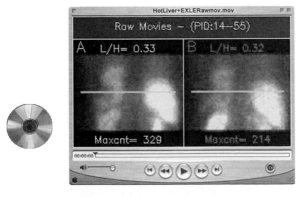

Fig. 16-72. Rotating projection images of the same patient as in Figs 16-68 to 16-71. Since the first study was considered potentially artifactual, adenosine stress test was repeated with simultaneous low-level (Bruce 1) treadmill exercise. On the repeat stress images, liver uptake is markedly less compared to that in Fig. 16-68. The breast shadows are now better recognizable (movie).

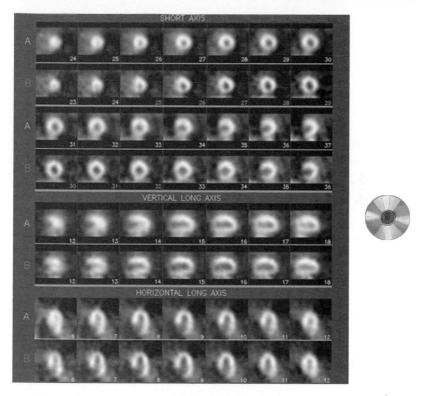

Fig. 16-73. Reconstructed tomographic slices of the images in Fig. 16-72. The stress images are of much better quality than those in Fig. 16-69. A small inferior myocardial perfusion defect is present after stress and at rest.

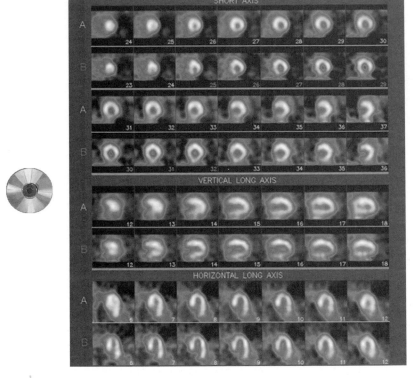

Fig. 16-74. Same images as in Fig. 16-73 in color.

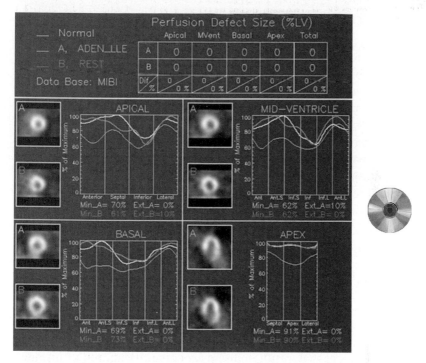

Fig. 16-75. Quantification of the images in Fig. 16-73 and 16-74. The small inferior defect is not quantifiable against the Sestamibi normal database and probably due to inferior attenuation.

GASTROINTESTINAL UPTAKE

Recognition
  On reconstructed slices
Preventive Measure
  Ingestion of a large amount of fluid before imaging
    (inconsistent result)
  Low level exercise during injection
Corrective Measure
  Wait until radioactivity has moved down the intestinal tract
    and repeat imaging
  Ingestion of large amount of fluid

Quantification Errors (Figs. 16-76 to 16-84)

Image quantification may be a great help for consistency in interpretation. However, when used in an uncritical way, it also may lead to errors. It is important that visual analysis of reconstructed slices and image quantification are considered together. Information from visual and quantitative analysis should be concordant. Inappropriate selection of slices may result in discordant quantification. For instance, inclusion of too many basal slices (of a normal study) may result in quantification of an erroneous septal defect, whereas inclusion of too few basal slices (e.g., of a study with a septal defect) may result in an erroneously normal study by quantification.

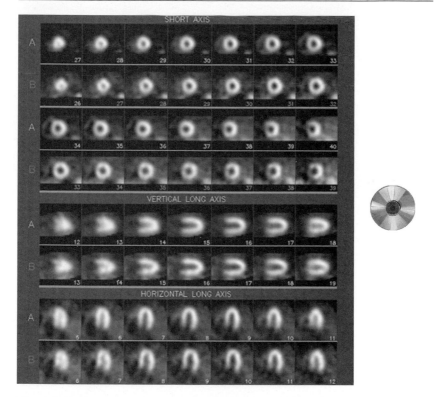

Fig. 16-76. Errors can be made in the process of image quantification. In this normal SPECT study, the technologist selected erroneously too many basal slices. Slices selected for quantification are indicated in color. Of the stress study slices #28-40 and of the rest study slices #27-39 were included for quantification. It can be appreciated that the membranous septum is present in the last two basal slices.

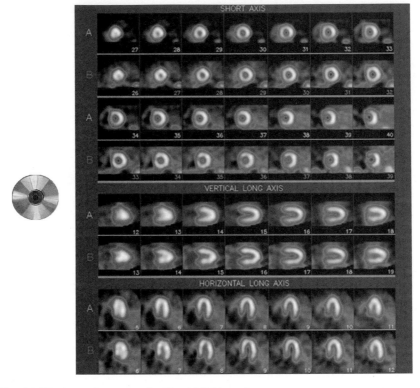

Fig. 16-77. Same images as in Fig. 16-76 in color.

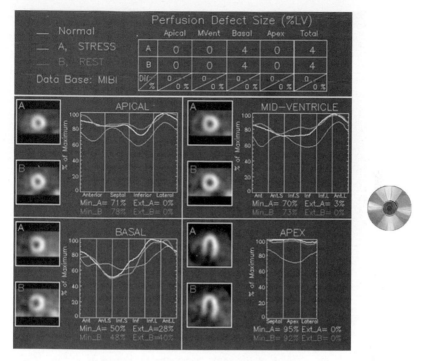

Fig. 16-78. Quantification of the tomographic images in Figs 16-76 and 16-77. Because of the inclusion of too many basal slices, a small fixed basal septal defect is quantified. This is in error and represents the membranous septum. Correct quantification of these images is shown in Fig. 16-58.

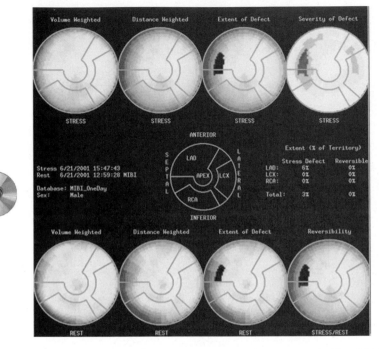

Fig. 16-79. Bull's eye display of the same reconstruction error as in Fig. 16-78. An erroneous septal defect (6%) is present in the LAD territory.

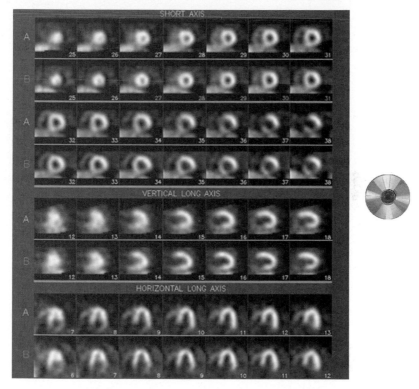

Fig. 16-80. Reconstructed SPECT images with a fixed inferolateral basal myocardial perfusion defect (slices #34-36). The technologist attempting not to include the membranous septum included too few basal slices. Slices selected for quantification are indicated in color. Only slices #27-31 were included for quantification. It can be appreciated that the basal defect is not included.

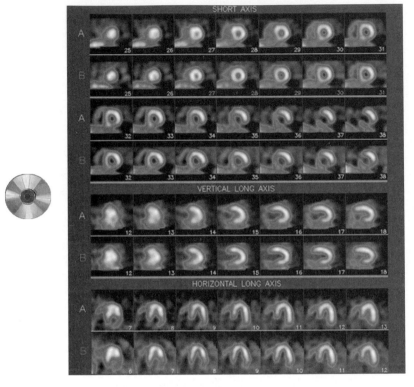

Fig. 16-81. Same images as in Fig. 16-80 in color.

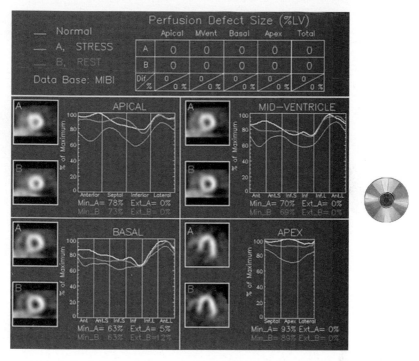

Fig. 16-82. Quantification of tomographic images in Figs 16-80 and 16-81. Because of the inclusion of too few slices, the basal defect is not quantified and quantitatively the study is normal.

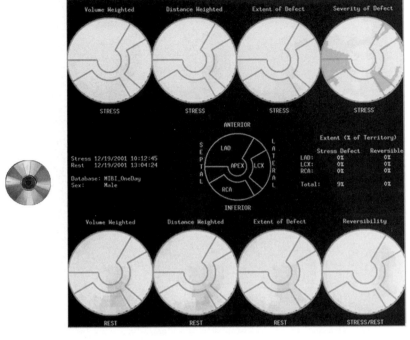

Fig. 16-83. Bull's eye display of the same reconstruction error as in Fig. 16-82. No defect is displayed.

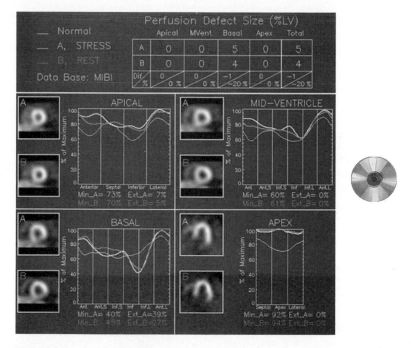

Fig. 16-84. Correct quantification of tomographic images in Figs 16-80 and 16-81. A small fixed inferolateral basal defect is quantified.

QUANTIFICATION ERRORS

Recognition
    Integrate visual interpretation of images with results of
        quantification
Preventive Measure
    Understand limitations of quantitative program
Corrective Measure
    Repeat processing and quantification
    Integrate other clinical and imaging information in final
        interpretation

Filtering Errors (Figs. 16-85 to 16-90)

Filtering is applied to remove noise from the images and "make them look better." The low-pass Butterworth filter is currently considered standard for cardiac SPECT imaging. Of the two variables of this filter, "order and cutoff," only the Nyquist frequency cutoff is to be considered.

No true standardization exists for filter settings, only general guidelines. There is no standardization of the effect of a given filter cutoff value using filters provided by different vendors. It is recommended that one check with the vendor for preferred cutoff values. Furthermore, images with different imaging characteristics require different filter cutoffs. For example, images acquired using different imaging protocols, images acquired with high dose or low dose, images with significant or little extra cardiac activity may need a different filter cutoff each.

Nevertheless, using the equipment available in an imaging facility, one should develop *standard filter settings* for images acquired with routinely used protocols to achieve reproducible image quality.

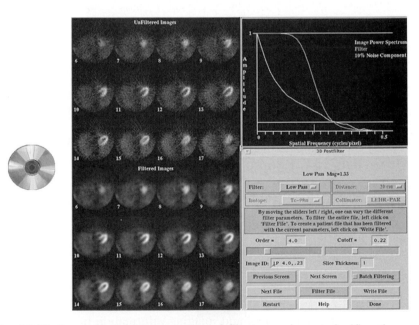

Fig. 16-85. Inconsistent or incorrect use of filters may impact significantly on image quality. The left panel shows unfiltered transverse axis SPECT images (top) and filtered images (bottom). A low-pass Butterworth filter is used. The right panel shows the image power spectrum (green curve) that is characteristic for an individual image. High frequencies generally represent "noise," whereas low frequencies represent "signal" and presumably true image components. The filter (orange curve) is characterized by order, that is, slope of the curve, and most importantly by the cutoff. The selection of the cutoff level determines how much noise is suppressed and how smooth or blurred the filtered image will look. The filter used for these images is standard in our laboratory and has an order of 4.0 and cutoff of 0.22.

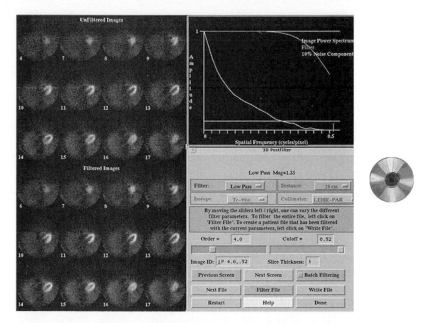

Fig. 16-86. The filter used for the images in the left panel (bottom) has an order of 4.0 and cutoff of 0.52. The orange curve is moved to the far right. Basically all noise is left into the images by the filter. The unfiltered and filtered images look similar in quality.

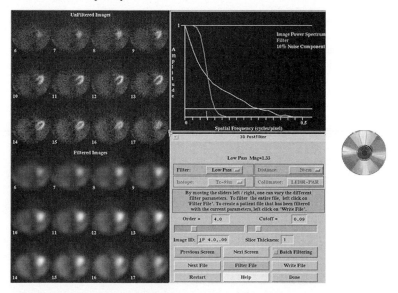

Fig. 16-87. The filter used for the images in the left panel (bottom) has an order of 4.0 and cutoff of 0.09. The orange curve is moved to the far left. The filter has suppressed all noise. The filtered images are extremely blurred with loss of image detail.

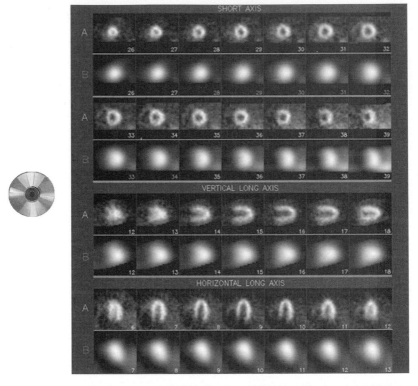

Fig. 16-88. Reconstructed tomographic slices of the normal SPECT study shown in Fig. 16-56. The images in rows "A" were filtered with a high cutoff value (0.52), whereas the images in rows "B" were filtered with a low cutoff value (0.09). The results of using the appropriate filter cutoff (0.22) are shown in Fig. 16-56.

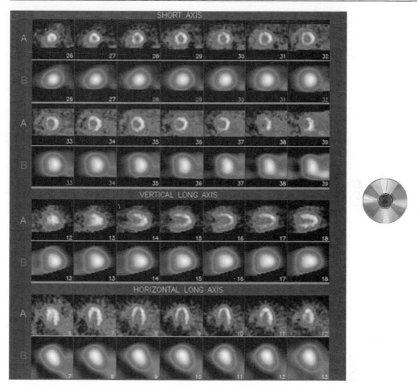

Fig. 16-89. Same images as in Fig. 16-88 in color.

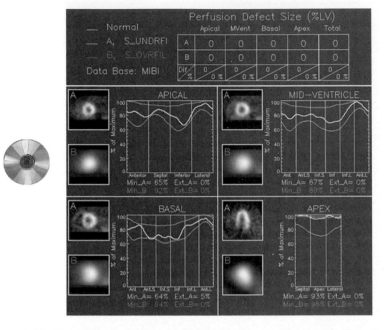

Fig. 16-90. Quantification of the tomographic slices in Fig. 16-88. The circumferential profile of the heavily smoothed images is smooth and almost a straight line. The circumferential count profile of the underfiltered images shows considerably greater noise and approaches in some segments the lower limit of normal. Although both curves of this example are within the normal range, one can appreciate that circumferential count profiles of low-count and unfiltered images fall outside the normal reference range due to "noise" and create false-positive defects.

FILTERING ERRORS

Recognition
Inspection of reconstructed stress. Images should not be
exceedingly blurred or noisy.
Preventive Measure
Appropriate training of technologists. The written procedure
protocol with standard filter selection
Corrective Measure
Repeat processing of slices with appropriate filter selection

Synchronization Error ECG-Gated SPECT
(Figs. 16-91 to 16-97)

The validity of information gained from ECG-gated SPECT depends on a regular heart rate and appropriate synchronization with the

ECG. This is a much-ignored aspect of QC of gated-SPECT imaging (**Figs. 16-91** to **16-97**).

The occurrence of irregular heart rate results in missed data during image acquisition and may lead to errors in calculation of ejection fraction and display of cardiac function. A gated-SPECT study acquired with only eight frames per cardiac cycle is more likely to be corrupted

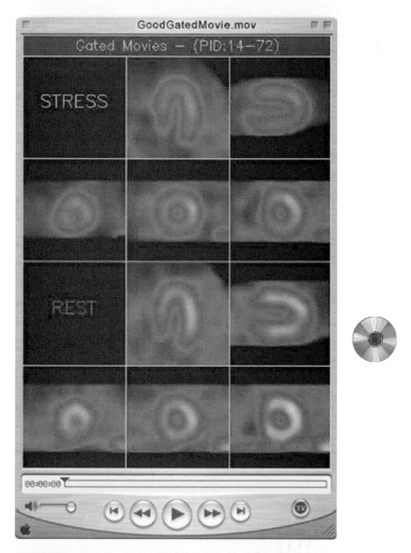

Fig. 16-91. Sixteen-frame ECG-gated SPECT movie. This is a good quality study. There is gradual change in color from diastole to systole (blue to white). Regional wall motion and wall thickening are normal (movie).

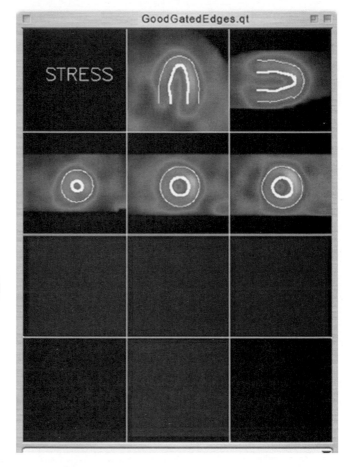

Fig. 16-92. ECG-gated SPECT movie. Display of computer-derived endocardial edges for calculation of left ventricular EF.

by arrhythmias than a study acquired with 16 frames per cycle. Pacemaker spikes may also cause inappropriate gating and artifacts.

ECG-gating error may be suspected from the inspection of the rotating planar projection images. If an arrhythmia occurred at a certain time point during SPECT acquisition, one or more planar projection images may contain less total counts than others may. This may result in "flashing" (darker images) during the movie display. This can also be displayed graphically *(9)*.

ECG-gating error may also be suspected from movie display of reconstructed slices. Normally, there is a gradual change in color from systole (brightest color) to diastole (darkest color). If significant

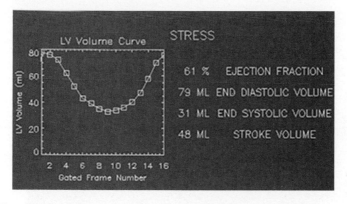

Fig. 16-93. Sixteen-frame left ventricular volume curve of Figs 16-91 an 16-92. The left ventricular volume curve is derived from the sum of volumes determined on the basis of number of voxels within the endocardial boundaries of each individual SA slice and the apical cap. The volume curve shows a physiologic shape and thus credible EF. End diastolic and end systolic volumes are shown as well.

irregular heart rate occurred, the ED frame is abruptly darker than the preceding frames.

One can also inspect the morphology of the left volume curve. The volume curve should start and end at approximately the same ED volume and display a well-defined systolic nadir. When heart rate during acquisition is significantly irregular, the volume curve is distorted.

As the visual appearance of motion and contraction on gated SPECT is due to the greater count recovery during cardiac contraction due to partial volume effect, it is more appropriate to inspect myocardial-thickening curves *(10)*. In the absence of arrhythmias, myocardial

$\blacktriangleright$

Fig. 16-94. Three-dimensional myocardial thickening profile. The left ventricular volume curve in Fig. 16-93 is based on computer-derived edges and volumes. The visual impression of cardiac contraction is based on improved count recovery when partial volume effect is operational during the cardiac cycle. To judge the quality of an ECG-gated SPECT study, in particular to recognize technical gating problems, inspection of the count recovery or thickening curves is more appropriate. The figure shows families of thickening curves for apical, mid-ventricular and basal SA slices, and the apex (horizontal log axis slice). The y-axis shows counts normalized to ED. The three-dimensional display shows the increase in count in ES and decrease in ED as circumferential profiles from anterior (A), septum (S), inferior (I), and lateral (L) wall. In a gated SPECT study with good ECG-synchronization, the thickening profiles start and end at the same count level. Thickening curves can thus be used as an easy method to recognize technical ECG-gating problems.

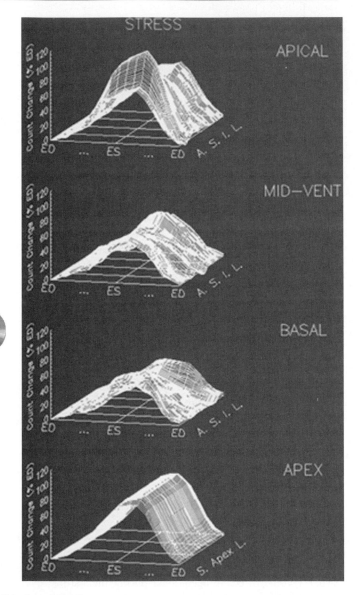

Fig. 16-94. *(continued).*

counts at both ends of the thickening curve, ED, are the similar. In case of irregular heart rate, counts at the end of the thickening curve are lower than those at the beginning of the curve.

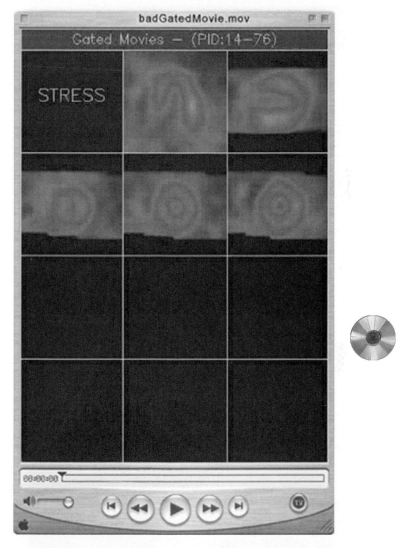

Fig. 16-95. ECG-gated SPECT movie. The "jerky" motion of the movie should raise the suspicion of a technical ECG-gating problem. There appears to be an abrupt transition at ED (movie).

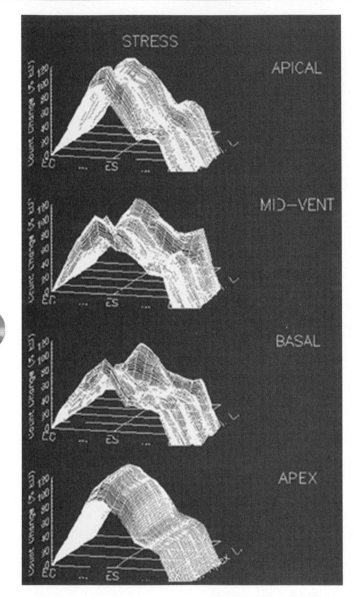

Fig. 16-96. Three-dimensional myocardial thickening profile of the gated SPECT study shown in Fig. 16-95. In contrast to the thickening profiles shown in Fig. 16-94, the counts in ED at the end of the cardiac cycle fall below count values in ED at the beginning of the cardiac cycle. This is due to heart rate variability and may invalidate calculation of EF. Quality control for ECG-gating problems is often ignored.

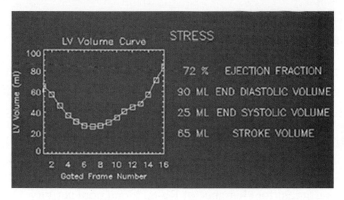

Fig. 16-97. Sixteen-frame LV volume curve of the ECG-gated SPECT study shown in Figs 16-95 and 16-96. The volume curve does not have a "physiological appearance." It is uncertain which of the two points for ED should be used for calculation of EF. The validity of the calculation of EF can be questioned. Note: In contrast to Fig. 16-96 where end diastolic counts are lower in frame #16 than in frame #1, in this geometrically derived curve end diastolic volume in frame #16 is larger than that in frame #1. A plausible explanation for these discordant data is that both curves are derived from different parameters (true counts vs. mathematically derived edges).

ECG-GATING PROBLEMS

Recognition
   Flashing on display of rotating planar projection images
   Flashing on display of gated-SPECT movie
   Curve displaying in each frame of projection images
   LV volume curve
   Thickening curve
Preventive Measure
   Do not acquire ECG-gated SPECT in patients with irregular
      heart rate
Corrective Measure
   None

PET IMAGING

   Although in general, image quality with PET imaging is remarkably better than with SPECT imaging, suboptimal quality studies occur as well.

Delay of PET Acquisition After Rb-82 Infusion

According to standard PET protocol (Table 11-1) acquisition of PET images should be delayed by about 90–120 s after the start of Rb-82 infusion to allow for clearance of cardiac blood pool activity. In patients with normal cardiac output, the delay is relatively short, 90 s. In patients with depressed left ventricular function, the delay is extended to 120 s.

Figure 16-98 shows Rb-82 PET images in an obese patient with severely compromised right ventricular function due to hypoventilation syndrome. Because of slow right ventricular inflow, the standard delay of 90 s was insufficient for clearance of Rb-82 blood pool activity. Only after a longer delay of 210 s were acceptable Rb-82 images obtained (**Fig. 16-99**).

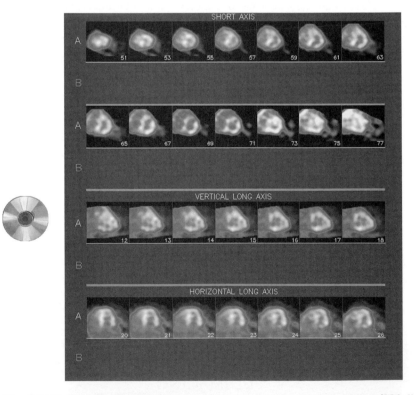

Fig. 16-98. Rest Rb-82 PET images in a 27 year old markedly obese (332 lb, 151 kg) male with hypoventilation syndrome, hypertension, and diabetes mellitus. The images were acquired after the standard delay of 90 s after start of Rb-82 infusion. The images are of poor quality due to persistent blood pool activity.

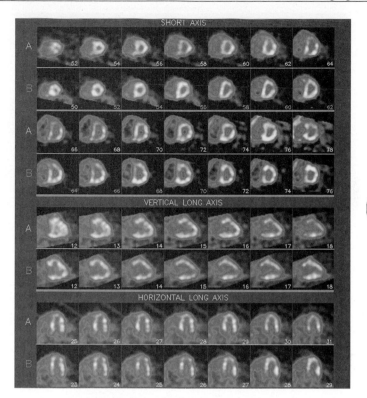

Fig. 16-99. Repeat stress (A)-rest (B) Rb-82 PET images in the patient shown in Fig. 16-98. PET acquisition was delayed for 210 s after start of Rb-82 infusion. Although the images are still of suboptimal quality, they are better than in Fig. 16-98. It can be appreciated that the heart is enlarged, particularly the right ventricle, which is hugely dilated and showed very poor contraction. The poor quality and persistent blood pool activity in Fig. 16-98 can be explained by very sluggish inflow into the right heart due to severe right ventricular dysfunction.

Misregistration of PET Emission and CT Transmission Images

Co-incidence PET imaging is subject to twice the attenuation problems of SPECT imaging. Therefore, AC is an absolute necessity for PET imaging. State-of-the-art PET–CT cameras use CT images to scan and the PET images are acquired sequentially of each other. An important aspect of QA of PET imaging is verification of accurate coregistration. **Figures 16-100** to **16-103** show an example of misregistration of CT scan and PET images resulting in a marked image artifact.

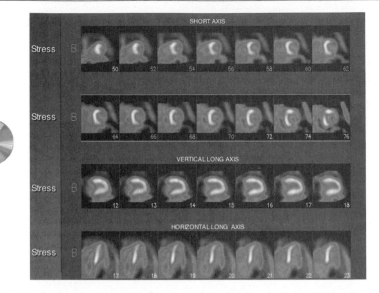

Fig. 16-100. Stress Rb-82 PET/CT images of a 53-year-old male with atypical chest pain. The images show a large lateral wall defect. It was noted that the patient moved during the CT scan.

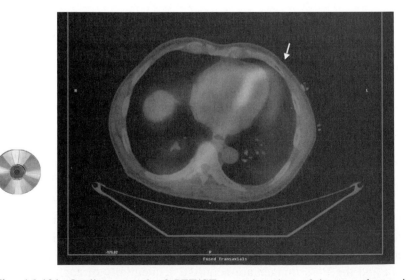

Fig. 16-101. Quality control of PET/CT coregistration of images shown in Fig. 16-100. The fusion image of 16-slice CT scan and Rb-82 perfusion image (yellow-red) shows marked misregistration. The patient apparently moved to the right on the table during the acquisition of the CT scan. The lateral wall of the Rb-82 image is positioned over the left lung (arrow).

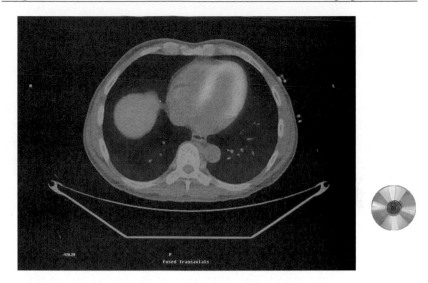

Fig. 16-102. Repeat CT scan of the patient in Fig. 16-100. The emission image data are the same as in Fig. 16-100. The fusion image shows correct coregistration of CT scan and RB-82 emission image (yellow-red), which is appropriately within the CT border of the heart.

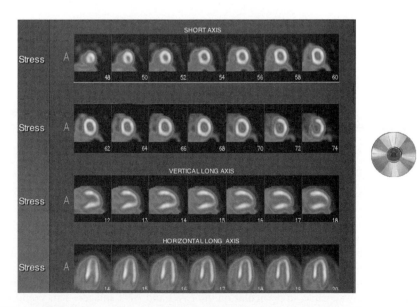

Fig. 16-103. Same stress Rb-82 PET/CT image data of Fig. 16-100, processed after correct coregistration with CT scan. The stress Rb-82 PET images are entirely normal.

PLANAR MYOCARDIAL PERFUSION IMAGING

Breast Attenuation

Breast attenuation is a serious problem with planar myocardial perfusion imaging. This is in marked contrast to SPECT imaging. In planar imaging, only three projections images are acquired. Breast attenuation defects may make images that are affected uninterpretable; thus interpretation is then limited to the one or two remaining images, thereby seriously limiting the diagnostic yield of planar myocardial perfusion imaging *(2)* (**Figs. 16-104** and **16-105**).

The only planar image not likely to be affected by breast attenuation is the left-lateral right side decubitus image. With the patient lying on the right side, the left breast moves away from the heart and the anterior wall and inferior wall can be imaged without attenuation.

We have found that breast markers (small plastic tubing filled with radioisotope) that outline the contours of the breast are useful for recognizing breast attenuation *(1)*. However, although one may identify the presence of breast attenuation, one cannot exclude the presence of an ischemic myocardial perfusion defect as well.

In many laboratories, planar imaging is currently only performed in overweight patients who are too heavy for SPECT-imaging tables. In

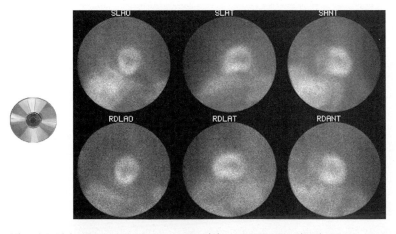

Fig. 16-104. Planar adenosine stress (S)-redistribution (RD) Tl-201 images of a patient with large breasts. There appears to be a reversible anterior wall defect on the LAO LAT images and anterior images (ANT). However, there are also large breast shadows visible, in particular on the LAO and ANT images. This could be a cause for anterior defects. Because the LAT images are acquired in right side decubitus position, breast attenuation is usually not a problem on these views. To interpret these images, the overlap of breast over the heart should be defined.

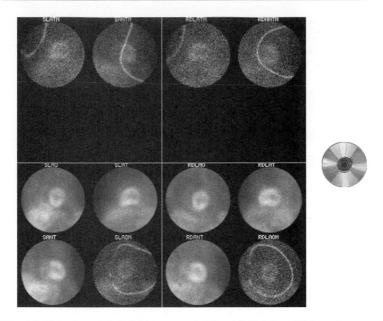

Fig. 16-105. Same Tl-201 images as in Fig. 16-104. In addition, there are images with radioactive line sources to mark the contours of the breast. The breast markers in the LAO views show that the left breast is indeed large and completely covers the entire heart in this projection. This will generally result in homogeneous attenuation and not in regional defects. The contour of the breast in the ANT view is across the base of the heart and does not match up with the mild anteroapical perfusion defect in this view. The breast markers in the LAT view confirm that the breast is not overlying the heart. Knowing the exact location of the contours of the breast relative to the heart and the observed perfusion defects is helpful in concluding that this patient most likely has a true anteroapical and lateral reversible myocardial perfusion defect.

these obese patients, it is our policy to be conservative in interpreting planar images in obese. Only *unequivocally*, abnormal features are reported as abnormal. More subtle inhomogeneities are presumed to be equivocal due to attenuation.

PLANAR IMAGING: BREAST ATTENUATION

Recognition
  Planar images with breast markers
Preventive Measure
  None
Corrective Measure
  None

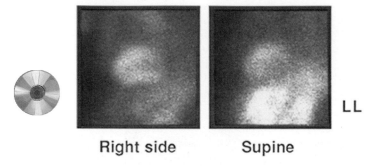

Right side   Supine

Fig. 16-106. Inferior attenuation by the left hemi-diaphragm occurs in about 25% of patients when imaging is performed in supine position. Diaphragmatic attenuation can be demonstrated by comparing two planar LAT images, one supine and another one with the patient in right side decubitus position. The figure shows an example of inferior attenuation. The supine LAT image (right) shows an apparent inferobasal myocardial perfusion defect. This defect is not present on a second LAT image (left) taken a few minutes later with the patient in right side decubitus position. The latter image is normal. Therefore, there is attenuation when the patient is supine.

Inferior Attenuation

As discussed under SPECT imaging, inferior attenuation is importantly dependent on imaging position. Steep 60° LAO and 90° left-lateral planar images, with patient in supine position during image acquisition, have high likelihood of inferior attenuation artifacts (**Fig. 16-106**).

However, a left-lateral planar image acquired with the patient in right side decubitus is not affected by inferior attenuation *(1)*.

PLANAR IMAGING: INFERIOR ATTENUATION

Recognition
    Inferior defect on supine steep LAO or left-lateral planar
        images
Preventive Measure
    Acquisition of left-lateral planar image with patient in right
        side decubitus position
Corrective Measure
    Repeat planar left lateral image with patient in right side
        decubitus position

EQUILIBRIUM RADIONUCLIDE ANGIOCARDIOGRAPHY

Zoom and Acquisition of Views

ERNA images allow for interpretation of the morphology and contraction of heart as well as large vessels. To obtain optimal results, ERNA studies should be acquired with appropriate zoom. The heart should not be too small or too large on the images. In addition to visualization of the right and LV, a good quality ERNA visualizes also the aortic arch and pulmonary artery *(11)*. Using a 13-inch diameter cardiac camera, the size of the heart should be about one-third to one-fourth of the diameter of the FOV (**Figs. 16-107** to **16-114**).

Three planar projection images should be acquired for complete evaluation of the heart: supine anterior, supine LAO, and right side decubitus left lateral.

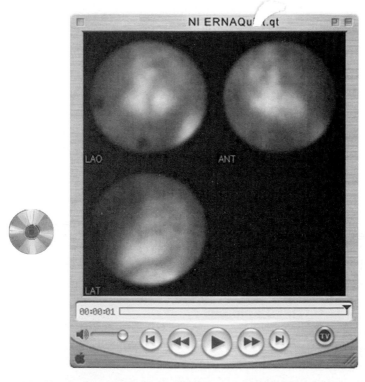

Fig. 16-107. Normal planar 3-view ERNA study. The zoom factor should be such that the heart occupies about one-third to ne-fourth of the field of view. All four chambers of the heart as well as great vessels should be visible. This is normal good quality study. The right atrium and right ventricle are normal in size and contraction. The left ventricle in slightly enlarged with normal regional wall motion. The great vessels are normal in shape. (**movie**)

Labeling Efficiency

Poor labeling of red blood cells may affect overall quality of ERNA images. However, free Tc-99m pertechnetate is usually trapped in thyroid gland, salivary glands, and stomach mucosa, and images may be of adequate interpretable quality. Poor quality of ERNA images is often due to body habitus. In overweight patients, scattering of low-energy photons may significantly degrade image quality. As the labeling of red cells is performed in vitro, there is a small chance of formation of small clumps of red blood cells. After injection of the radiolabeled red cells, the microclots may be trapped in the lungs and are visualized as multiple hot spots in the lungs *(12)*. These clots are of microscopic size and of no clinical consequence.

ECG-Gating Problems

The validity of information gained from ERNA studies depends importantly on regular heart rate and appropriate ECG-synchronization during acquisition *(9,11)*. ECG-gating problems may be suspected by "blinking" during movie display of ERNA. The blinking is due to low total counts in the last frame(s) of ERNA. For purpose of display, technologists may remove frames with low counts from the end the movie, resulting in display without blinking.

To assess the validity of image data and ejection fraction, one should inspect the generated left ventricular volume curve (Figs 16-108 and 16-109). The "drop-off" in counts at the end of the curve indicates irregular heart rate during acquisition. As long as the ejection part and end systole are not affected, calculated ejection fraction is accurate. An extreme example of heart rate irregularity is atrial fibrillation with wide range of R–R intervals. In the latter condition, an ERNA volume curve may have no well-defined end systole nadir. In the latter situation, LVEF cannot be calculated. In contrast, patients with atrial fibrillation and medically controlled heart rate may have a relatively narrow range of R–R intervals, and (average) LVEF can be calculated.

ERNA ECG-GATING PROBLEMS

Recognition
   Blinking on movie display of ERNA
   Left ventricular volume curve with drop-off
   Left ventricular volume curve without clear systolic nadir
Preventive Measure
   Acquire ERNA in patients with stable heart rate

Acquire ERNA in list mode and reformat data

Administer bolus of lidocaine IV unless contraindicated

Corrective Measure

Repeat ERNA acquisition when patient has regular heart rate

Reformat list mode image data with selection of narrow R–R
interval

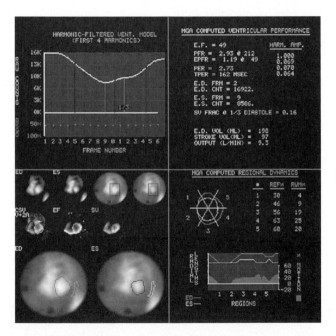

Fig. 16-108. Screen capture of processed data of the ERNA study shown in
Fig. 16-107. The bottom panel at the left shows the end diastolic and end systolic
regions of interest for calculation of EF, as well as the crescent-shaped background
region to the right of the left ventricular lateral wall. At the top in the same
panel, functional images are shown that may be used as guides for processing.
The top panel on the left shows the count-based left ventricular volume curve.
The curve has an appropriate physiologic shape. Diastolic filling appears to be
relatively slow. The top right panel shows calculated parameters. EF is calculated
to be low normal, 0.49. Early peak filling rate (EPFR) is 1.19 EDV per second.
The counts in the ED frame (FRM) are 16,922 counts, ensuring good statistical
reliability. The ED volume is enlarged at 198 ml. The bottom right panel shows
values for regional ejection fraction (REF). Overall, this study shows normal right
ventricular function. Slightly enlarged left ventricle with preserved low normal
EF and decreased diastolic function.

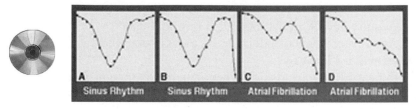

Fig. 16-109. Examples of count-based ERNA left ventricular volume curves in sinus rhythm and in atrial fibrillation. (A) Volume curve of a patient in sinus rhythm and perfect regular heart rate. After systole, the volume curve returns to a similar end diastolic counts level as at the beginning of the cardiac cycle. (B) Volume curve of a patient in sinus rhythm but irregular heart beats, either premature ventricular beats or marked respiratory variation. The last frames of the acquisition cycle were not always "filled" because of premature R-waves prematurely stopping the acquisition. This is reflected as a drop-off in counts at the end of the volume curve. (C) Volume curve of a patient in atrial fibrillation and medically controlled heart rate. The drop-off in counts at the end of the volume curve is more marked due to variation in R-R intervals. A systolic trough is discernable and an "average" EF can be calculated. (D) Volume curve of a patient in atrial fibrillation without control of heart rate. There is a wide variation in R-R intervals. Numerous acquisition sequences are prematurely stopped. The volume curve slopes down and does not show a clear end systolic through. EF cannot be calculated.

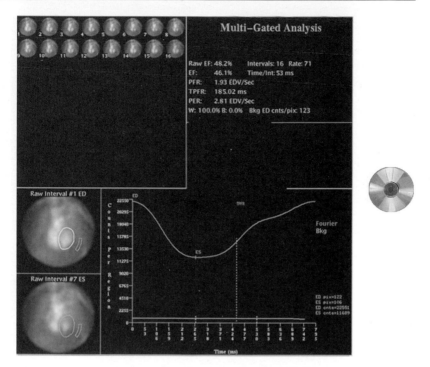

Fig. 16-110. This ERNA was processed using a fixed ROI. The two images on the bottom left show the end diastolic image and the end systolic image. The ROI drawn over the left ventricle in ED is also used in the ES image. The ROI for background is shown in blue. LVEF is calculated as 46%. Using a fixed left ventricular ROI, non-cardiac background activity is included in systolic counts and thus calculated LVEF is an underestimation of true LVEF.

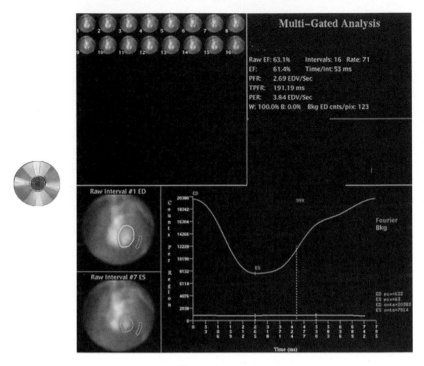

Fig. 16-111. Same ERNA as in Fig. 16-110. This time a variable ROI is used for calculation of LVEF. The ES ROI is smaller than the ED ROI and follows ES edges. The background ROI is placed in the same location as in Fig. 16-104. Thus, the only change is the ES ROI. Using a variable ROI LVEF is now 61%, which is the correct value for this patient.

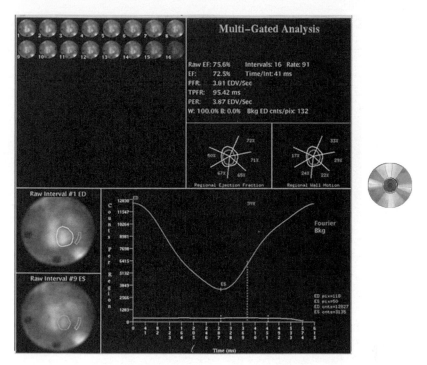

Fig. 16-112. Using correct processing parameters: Variable ROIs over the left ventricle and background ROI to the right of the lateral in diastole, LVEF in this patient is 72%. Note the green line under the orange volume curve, which represents the level of background counts.

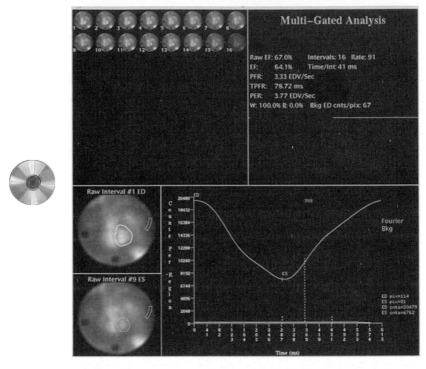

Fig. 16-113. Same ERNA as in Fig. 16-112. The same variable ROIs over the left ventricle are used as in Fig. 16-112. The background ROI is erroneously moved to the chest wall where background counts are lower. Note that the green background curve is lower than in Fig. 16-112. Using these ROIs, LVEF is calculated to be 64%, which is too low.

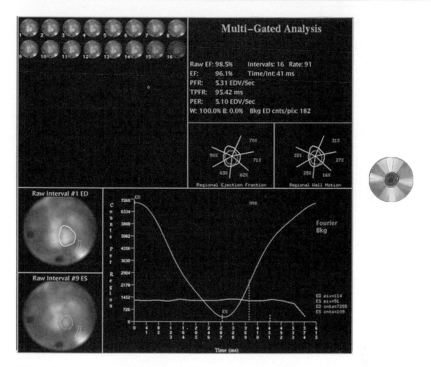

Fig. 16-114. Same ERNA as in Fig. 16-112. The same variable ROIs over the left ventricle are used as in Fig. 16-112. The background ROI is now erroneously moved to the spleen where background counts are higher. Note that the green background curve is substantially higher than in Fig. 16-112. Using these ROIs, LVEF is calculated to be 96%, which is too high.

Calculation of LVEF and Effect of Background Counts

LVEF is derived from end diastolic (ED) counts, end systolic (ES) counts, and background (BKG) using the formula:

$$\frac{(ED - BKG) - (ES - BKG)}{ED - BKG} = LVEF \tag{1}$$

For example, if BKG = 0, ED = 5000, and ES = 2000.

$$LVEF = \frac{5000 - 2000}{5000} = 0.60 \tag{2}$$

LVEF determined using the above number is generally too low compared to a "gold standard" such as angiographic LVEF.

To obtain an accurate value for LVEF, left ventricular counts must be corrected for background activity. The important effect of background subtraction is illustrated below:
If BKG = 500

$$LVEF = \frac{4500 - 1500}{4500} = 0.66 \tag{3}$$

If BKG = 900

$$LVEF = \frac{4100 - 1100}{4100} = 0.73 \tag{4}$$

These example calculations show clearly that the higher background counts, the higher is the derived LVEF.

Because of the important effect of background selection on LVEF, the appropriate placement of the ROI must always be checked before stating the value of LVEF in a final report.

Background subtraction in processing ERNAs has been standardized as follows:

- LAO view
- About 4 pixels off the lateral wall of the LV in ED
- A crescent-shaped ROI about 4 pixel wide
- About the height of the LV

Figs 16-110 and 16-111 illustrate the effect of fixed and variable left ventricular regions of interest on calculated LVEF. **Figs 16-112 to 16-114** illustrate the effect of background selection on calculated LVEF.

REFERENCES

1. Johnstone DE, Wackers FJTh, Berger HJ, Hoffer P, Kelley MJ, Gottschalk A, Zaret B (1979) Effect of patient positioning on left lateral thallium-201 images. *J Nucl Med* 20:183–188.
2. Wackers FJTh (1992) Artifacts in planar and SPECT myocardial perfusion imaging. *Am J Cardiac Imaging* 6:42–58.
3. DePuey EG, Garcia EV (1989) Optimal specificity of thallium-201 SPECT through recognition of imaging artifacts. *J Nucl Med* 30:441.
4. DePuey EG, Rozanski A (1995) Gated Tc-99m sestamibi SPECT to characterize fixed defects as infarct or artifact. *J Nucl Med* 36:952.
5. Hendel RC, Corbett JR, Cullom J, DePuey EG, Garcia EV (2002) The value and practice of attenuation correction for myocardial perfusion imaging: a joint position statement from the American Society of Nuclear Cardiology. *J Nucl Cardiol* 9:135–143.
6. Massood Y, Liu YH, Depuey G, Taillefer R, Araujo LI, Allen S, Delbeke D, Anstett F, Peretz A, Zito MJ, Tsatkin V, Wackers FJTh (2005) Clinical validation of SPECT attenuation correction using x-ray computed tomography-derived attenuation maps: Multicenter clinical trial with angiographic correlation. *J Nucl Cardiol* 12:676–686.
7. Chen J, Caputlu-Wilson SF, Shi H, Galt JR, Faber TL, Garcia EV (2006) Automated quality control emission-transmission misalignment for attenuation correction in myocardial perfusion imaging with SPECT-CT systems. *J Nucl Cardiol* 13:43–49.
8. King MA, Xia W, de Vries DJ, et al. (1996) A Monte Carlo investigation of artifacts caused by liver uptake in single photon emission computed tomography perfusion imaging with technetium-99m labeled agents. *J Nucl Cardiol* 3:18.
9. Nichols K, Dorbala S, DePuey EG, Yao SS, Sharma A, Rozanski A (1999) Influence of arrhythmias on gated SPECT myocardial perfusion and function quantification. *J Nucl Med* 40:924–934.
10. Shen MYH, Liu Y, Sinusas AJ, Fetterman R, Bruni W, Drozhinin OE, Zaret BL, Wackers FJTh (1999) Quantification of regional myocardial wall thickening on ECG-gated SPECT imaging. *J Nucl Cardiol J Nucl Cardiol* 6:583–595.
11. Wackers FJTh (1996) Equilibrium radionuclide angiocardiography. In: Gerson MC (ed.) *Cardiac Nuclear Medicine*, 3rd Edition. McGraw Hill Inc., New York, NY.
12. Benoit L, Wackers FJTh, Clements JP (1984) Clotting of Tc-99m labeled red cells. *J Nucl Med Tech* 12:59–60.

17 Nuclear Cardiology Reports

Until 1997, no standards for reporting results of nuclear cardiology studies existed. The ICANL was the first to publish standards and templates for optimal nuclear cardiology reports *(1)* (see also http://www.icanl.org). The reason for this publication was that peer review of numerous nuclear cardiology laboratories revealed that the form, content, and quality of nuclear cardiology reports were highly variable and frequently poor. A poor quality report is at best of little value to the referring physician and at the worst confusing, useless, and potentially harmful for patient care.

Key Words: Reporting standards, Reporting templates, Required elements in report.

The report of findings and interpretation is the final product of a nuclear cardiology procedure. The most important purpose of a nuclear cardiology report is to *clearly communicate* findings and clinical implications of stress tests and nuclear images to a referring physician. Thus, the report should help a referring physician in making clinical management decisions.

A referring physician is entitled to a clear conclusion: *normal or abnormal*, and if abnormal, how severely abnormal. The report may indicate, when appropriate, whether the risk for future cardiac events is low, moderate, or high. Certain imaging findings may have different clinical implications depending on the clinical context and results of stress testing. These nuances should be conveyed in an optimal report. If there were technical limitations to the study, they need to be stated and their impact on the final interpretation indicated. The second purpose of a report is to document the services provided for reimbursement purposes.

From: *Contemporary Cardiology: Nuclear Cardiology, The Basics*
By: F. J. Th. Wackers, W. Bruni, and B. L. Zaret © Humana Press Inc., Totowa, NJ

An adequate report should contain the following elements (*1–4*):

- Patient demographics (age, gender, and race) and ID number
- Date of study
- Summary of history
- Indication for study
- Type of stress and imaging test
- (Radio)pharmaceutical(s) and activity administered
- Stress findings, symptoms, and ECG changes
- Descriptive image interpretation
- Final impression integrating stress and imaging finding
- Original signature by the interpreter

An adequate final impression should contain the following elements:

- Quality of study. Suboptimal study quality must be mentioned
- Normal or abnormal result
- Description of perfusion abnormality (size, reversibility, severity, and location)
- Non-perfusion abnormalities (lung activity, transient LV dilation, and right ventricular visualization)
- Left ventricular function (global and regional)
- Non-cardiac radiotracer uptake

Nuclear cardiology studies should be interpreted and reported on the day of performance. Final reports must be completed, signed, and mailed on average within 2 working days. This is an important requirement for ICANL accreditation.

It is strongly recommended that abnormal test results be communicated directly to referring physicians on the day of performance of the test. This allows for a discussion of the results within the clinical context. Patients with markedly abnormal tests should not leave the imaging facility before the referring physician has been contacted.

Final reports must be hand-signed by the interpreter. Stamped signatures are not acceptable.

The following templates for standardization (**Fig. 17-1** to **17-3**) of nuclear cardiology reports were published by the ICANL.

These templates should be viewed as guidelines for form and content. Obviously, reports can be individualized to one's personal style and needs.

Standardization is also one of the prerequisites for the development of electronic reports (*5*). In **Figs. 17-4** and **17-5**, examples of *computer-generated reports* and a *dictated report* on the same patient are shown. Both reports contain all elements required in an optimized report. **Figure 17-6** is a sample dictated report on a ERNA study of a different patient.

Type of study:
MYOCARDIAL PERFUSION IMAGING WITH *(SESTAMIBI/ TETROFOSMIN/ THALLIUM)*
SPECT AT REST AND AFTER EXERCISE, AND GATED SPECT *(,AND RESTING FIRST PASS RADIONUCLIDE ANGIOGRAPHY)*.

History:
(e.g. 65-yr woman with known coronary artery disease and recurrent chest pain).

Indication:
(e.g. Evaluation for coronary insufficiency; risk stratification; evaluation of ischemia; evaluation of functional capacity; evaluation of myocardial viability).

Procedure:
The patient exercised on treadmill *(bicycle)* for a total of ___ minutes, reaching stage ___ of the *(Bruce; modified Bruce, etc.)* protocol, achieving an estimated workload of ____ METs. The heart rate was ___bpm at baseline, and increased to ___bpm at peak exercise, representing 85% *(or ___ %)* of age-predicted maximal heart rate. The blood pressure response was *(normal/ hypertensive/ hypotensive)*. Resting blood pressure was ___mmHg, and peak/nadir blood pressure was ____mmHg.
The patient *(did/ did not)* have chest pain/symptoms during the procedure.
The electrocardiogram *(did not show/ showed)* ST-segment changes diagnostic for ischemia *(describe appropriate changes)*.

The patient had myocardial perfusion imaging performed *(using a same day/ two day, dual isotope imaging protocol)*, with the injection of ___mCi of *(radiopharmaceutical)* at peak exercise, and the injection of ___mCi of *(radiopharmaceutical e)* at rest. Images were acquired by *(gated)* tomographic technique.

Findings:
The left ventricle was normal in size *(enlarged (degree of enlargement)/ LVH was present etc. Describe presence of transient dilation, if present. Describe increased post stress lung uptake, if present. Describe right ventricular abnormality, if present)*.
There were no myocardial perfusion defects *(if abnormal describe: e.g.: there was a large antero-apical, antero-lateral perfusion defect on stress images, that was partially reversible on the rest images)*. *Mention whether artifacts were noted or suspected as well*.
By gated SPECT *(or by first pass angiography)* resting *(post exercise)* global resting LVEF was *normal/ abnormal.* LVEF was calculated *(or visually estimated)* at ___%. Regional wall motion/thickening was normal, abnormal *(describe)*. *(If appropriate one can describe right ventricular function from the gated SPECT study)*.

IMPRESSION:
Normal *(or mildly abnormal, moderately abnormal, or markedly abnormal)* myocardial perfusion *(sestamibi/ tetrofosmin/ thallium-201)* SPECT imaging after *(excellent/ adequate/ fair/ submaximal)* exercise, showing a *(small/ moderate/ large)* area of [*anatomic location*] infarction with or without *(small/ moderate/ large)* amount of [*anatomic location*] ischemia.
[If considered pertinent add the following info:] The patients had *(yes or no)* symptoms. The stress ECG was *abnormal (describe)*. The hemodynamic response was *abnormal (describe)*. Resting RV and LV function was *(normal/ abnormal)*.

[Add additional pertinent information that addresses the clinical reason for performing the study, such as low/high risk study. If appropriate mention suboptimal quality of study because of e.g. patient's obesity, etc].

Fig. 17-1. Template for standard exercise SPECT myocardial perfusion imaging report.

Type of study:
MYOCARDIAL PERFUSION IMAGING WITH (*SESTAMIBI/ TETROFOSMIN/ THALLIUM)*
SPECT AFTER VASODILATION WITH ADENOSINE *(DIPYRIDAMOLE, DOBUTAMINE),* AND
GATED SPECT *(, AND RESTING FIRST PASS RADIONUCLIDE ANGIOGRAPHY).*

History: As in figure 1. *Clarify why pharmacological stress was indicated, i.e. inability to exercise.*

Indication: As in figure 1.

Procedure:
The patient had a maximal dose of 140 mcg/kg/min of adenosine infused *(state if the patient also performed low level exercise). (If dipyridamole, give total dose infused over 4 minutes) (If dobutamine give maximal dose in mcg/kg/min).* The heart rate was ___bpm at baseline, and was ___bpm at peak adenosine/dipyridamole infusion. *(For dobutamine state maximal heart rate as percent of target heart rate).* The blood pressure response was (*normal/ hypertensive/ hypotensive*). [If blood pressure response was abnormal state: Resting blood pressure was ___mmHg, and peak/nadir blood pressure was ___mmHg].
The patient (*did/ did not*) have chest pain/symptoms during the procedure.
The electrocardiogram did *(did not) show* ST-segment changes suggestive of ischemia (describe changes if appropriate).

Imaging procedure: As in figure 1

Findings: As in figure 1

IMPRESSION: As in figure 1

Fig. 17-2. Template for standard vasodilator/adrenergic stress SPECT myocardial perfusion imaging report.

Type of study:
EQUILIBRIUM RADIONUCLIDE ANGIOGRAPHY AT REST *(AND EXERCISE). (and gated first pass).*

History:
(e.g. 74-yr male with lung cancer)

Indication: (e.g.assessment of global right ventricular/ left ventricular systolic/ diastolic function, regional wall motion, chemotherapy).

Procedure:
The patient's red blood cells were labeled with ___mCi of Technetium-99m using the modified in vivo technique (using Ultratag etc). Imaging was performed at rest (and exercise) by planar technique in multiple views. *(By tomographic technique).*
(If study is acquired during exercise describe type of exercise, duration, hemodynamic response, symptoms and ECG).

Findings:
The right atrium was normal in size *(enlarged)*. The right ventricle was normal in size *(enlarged (degree of enlargement)*. Resting RVEF was ___%.
The pulmonary artery was normal in size *(dilated)*.
The left atrium was normal in size *(enlarged)*.
The left ventricle was normal in size *(enlarged (degree of enlargement)*. There was suggestion of left ventricular hypertrophy.
Regional wall motion was normal (*describe wall motion, paradoxical septal motion, hypokinesis (mild, moderate, severe), akinesis, or dyskinetic segments*).
Global resting LVEF was normal (*mildly, moderately, severely reduced*) at ___%. *(During exercise LVEF was ___ %)*
Resting end-diastolic volume was normal / *abnormal (i.e. mildly, moderately, severely enlarged)* at ___ mls.
Resting peak diastolic filling rate was normal *(abnormal)* at _____ end diastolic volumes/sec.

IMPRESSION:
Normal/ abnormal rest right ventricular function. Normal/abnormal resting left ventricular function.
(Normal/ abnormal LVEF response to exercise)
(Compare present assessment of LVEF to previous studies and comment)

Fig. 17-3. Template for standard equilibrium radionuclide angiocardiography report.

CARDIOVASCULAR NUCLEAR IMAGING AND EXERCISE LABORATORY

99 Main St., City, ST 99999   (999) 999-9999   Rev. 4/02

Patient

Clinical history: 60 year old white male with history of end stage ischemic cardiomyopathy. Admitted with chest pain, shortness of breath post car accident. CK/MB Troponin negative.

Indications: Angina Pectoris (ICD-9: 413.9); Other forms of chronic ischemic heart disease (ICD-9: 414.8)

Asso.'d factors: hypertension; smoking; hyperlipidemia; diabetes; known history of CAD; ICD

Chest pain class: atypical angina

Medications: Metformin, Losartan, Torsemide, Gabapentin, Potassium Chloride, Warfarin, Omeprazole, Allopurinol

Phys. Ex. - Heart: normal

- Lungs: normal

Weight: 280 lbs.   Height: 6 ft. 1 in.

Resting ECG: sinus rhythm; Q waves- V1-5; Non-specific ST-T wave changes

Pharmacological Stress with Adenosine

Technique: The patient underwent pharmacological stress with Adenosine at a maximum rate of 140 micrograms/kg/min. (Total dose= 79.8 mg)

Rest HR: 70 bpm   Peak HR: 82 bpm

Rest BP: 100/78 mm Hg   Endpoint BP: 100/70 mm Hg   RPP/1000: 8.2 (adequate > 25)

Symptoms: flushing

Termination: protocol

ECG Changes:

Fig. 17-4. *Continued.*

CARDIOVASCULAR NUCLEAR IMAGING AND EXERCISE LABORATORY

Nuclear Cardiology   99 Main St., City, ST 99999   (999) 999-9999   Rev. 4/02

Patient

SPECT Myocardial Perfusion Imaging Following Adenosine Vasodilation and at Rest w Tc-99m Sestamibi with Gated SPECT and Analysis of Regional Wall Motion

The patient was injected with Tc-99m Sestamibi at peak stress (32.1 mCi) and at rest (30.2 mCi) and was studied with gated tomographic perfusion imaging.

Findings: Lung Uptake: normal
                 RV Size: normal
                 LV Size: enlarged LV
                 Artifact: mild motion artifact

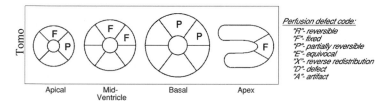

Perfusion defect code:
"R"- reversible
"F"- fixed
"P"- partially reversible
"E"- equivocal
"X"- reverse redistribution
"D"- defect
"A"- artifact

Tomo   Apical   Mid-Ventricle   Basal   Apex

Perfusion Imaging Interpretation

LV perfusion demonstrates: large mixed defect, predominantly scar

Gated SPECT interpretation: LVEF: 44 %
                                 Regional Wall Motion: Anteroapical akinesis

Stress Interpretation

Blood pressure response was normal. Chest pain was present. ECG changes were   nondiagnostic secondary to baseline ECG abnormality.

Final Interpretation

Abnormal SPECT imaging after vasodilation with adenosine showing an enlarged LV with a large anterolateral and apical scar with a small amount of apical lateral ischemia.   Global LVEF is depressed with anteroapical akinesis. Compared to previous studies there is no significant change.

Read by: _____
                 Frans J. Th. Wackers. M.D./ eit

Fig. 17-4. Sample of computer-generated report.

CARDIOVASCULAR NUCLEAR IMAGING
AND EXERCISE LABORATORY

| Nuclear Cardiology | 99 Main St., City, ST 99999 | (999) 999-9999 | Rev. 4/02 |

Patient

SPECT Myocardial Perfusion Imaging Following Adenosine Vasodilation and at Rest w Tc-99m Sestamibi with Gated SPECT and Analysis of Regional Wall Motion

The patient was injected with Tc-99m Sestamibi at peak stress (32.1 mCi) and at rest (30.2 mCi) and was studied with gated tomographic perfusion imaging.

Findings: Lung Uptake: normal
                 RV Size: normal
                 LV Size: enlarged LV
                 Artifact: mild motion artifact

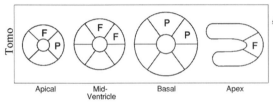

Perfusion defect code:
"R"- reversible
"F"- fixed
"P"- partially reversible
"E"- equivocal
"X"- reverse redistribution
"D"- defect
"A"- artifact

Perfusion Imaging Interpretation

LV perfusion demonstrates: large mixed defect, predominantly scar

Gated SPECT interpretation: LVEF: 44 %
                                 Regional Wall Motion: Anteroapical akinesis

Stress Interpretation

Blood pressure response was normal. Chest pain was present. ECG changes were   nondiagnostic secondary to baseline ECG abnormality.

Final Interpretation

Abnormal SPECT imaging after vasodilation with adenosine showing an enlarged LV with a large anterolateral and apical scar with a small amount of apical lateral ischemia. Global LVEF is depressed with anteroapical akinesis. Compared to previous studies there is no significant change.

Read by: _____

Frans J. Th. Wackers. M.D./ eit

Fig. 17-5. *Continued.*

DOE, JOHN
MRUN: 1234567   DOB: Dec-02-1941   Report Date: May-13-
2002
Cardiovascular Nuclear Imaging

Responsible Physician:
SMITH, JOHN   MD
CITY HOSPITAL
99 MAIN STREET
CITY, ST 99999

SPECT MYOCARDIAL PERFUSION IMAGING FOLLOWING ADENOSINE
VASODILATION AND AT REST WITH TC-99M SESTAMIBI WITH GATED
SPECT AND ANALYSIS OF REGIONAL WALL MOTION: 5/13/2002

CLINICAL HISTORY:
60 year old white male with history of end stage ischemic
cardiomyopathy. Admitted with chest pain and shortness of
breath after a car accident. Serial CK/MB and Troponin
were negative.

INDICATION:
Angina Pectoris; Chronic ischemic heart disease.

PROCEDURE:
The patient underwent pharmacological stress with
adenosine at a maximum infusion rate of 140
micrograms/kg/min (Total dose= 79.8 mg). Resting heart
rate was 70 beats per minute and increased to 78 beats per
minute at peak adenosine infusion. The blood pressure
response was normal: 100/78 mmHg at rest and 100/70 mmHg
at peak adenosine. The patient developed chest pain
during adenosine infusion. There were non diagnostic
electrocardiographic changes during vasodilatory stress.
The patient had a two-day imaging protocol and was
injected with 32.1 mCi of Sestamibi at peak adenosine
infusion and 30.2 mCi of Sestamibi at rest. Imaging was
performed by ECG-gated tomographic technique.

FINDINGS:
The lung uptake for this study was normal. The right
ventricle was normal in size. The left ventricle was
enlarged. Myocardial perfusion imaging demonstrated a
large fixed anterolateral and apical defect with small
reversiblity in the same area, in particular at the base.
Interpretation of this study was complicated by mild
motion artifact. By gated SPECT, global left ventricular
ejection fraction was moderately depressed at 44% with
anteroapical akinesis.

Fig. 17-5. Sample of dictated report on the same patient as in Fig. 16-4.

```
SMITH, JANE
MRUN: 0123456   DOB: JUL-22-1945  Report Date: NOV-19-2002

DIAGNOSTIC IMAGING CONSULTATION

        Responsible Physician:
            SMITH, JOHN  MD
            CITY HOSPITAL
            CITY, ST 9999
------------------------------------------------------------
--

EQUILIBRIUM RADIONUCLIDE ANGIOGRAPHY:  11/19/2002

CLINICAL HISTORY:
57 year old female presents with syncope, here for
cardiac
evaluation.

INDICATION:
Acute ischemic heart disease

PROCEDURE:
The patient's red blood cells were labeled with 32.1 mCi
of technetium using the Ultratag technique.  Imaging was
performed by the planar technique in multiple views.

FINDINGS:
The right atrium was normal in size.  The right ventricle
was normal in size.  Right ventricular function was
normal.  The left atrium was normal in size.  The left
ventricle was enlarged.  The left ventricular ejection
fraction was markedly depressed at 33%. End diastolic
volume was abnormal at 250 cc.  There was also dilation
of the aorta.  Regional wall motion was abnormal with
anteroapical-septal hypokinesis.

IMPRESSION:
Normal right ventricular function. Abnormal left
ventricular function with an enlarged left ventricle,
depressed LVEF, and anteroapical and septal regional wall
motion abnormality. This study is consistent with
ischemic cardiomyopathy.

I have reviewed the images and dictated/reviewed/or
edited the final
(signed)     Frans Wackers, MD
```

Fig. 17-6. Sample of dictated report on an ERNA study of a different patient.

REFERENCES

1. Wackers FJTh (2000). Intersocietal Commission for the Accreditation of Nuclear Medicine Laboratories (ICANL) position statement on standardization and optimization of nuclear cardiology reports. *J Nucl Cardiol* 7:397–400.
2. Cerqueira MD (1996). The user-friendly nuclear cardiology report: what needs to be considered and what needs to be included. *J Nucl Cardiol* 3:350–355.
3. Conzalez P, Canessa J, Massardo T (1998). Formal aspects of the user-friendly nuclear cardiology report. *J Nucl Cardiol* 5:365–366.
4. Hendel RC, Wackers FJT, Berman DS, Ficaro E, DePuey EG, Klein L et al. (2006). Reporting of radionuclide myocardial perfusion imaging studies. *J Nucl Cardiol* 13:e152–e157. Available at http://www.asnc.org/imageuploads/ ReportingRadionu-clideMPIStatement.pdf (accessed April 20, 2007).
5. Tilkemeier PL, Cooke CD, Ficaro EP, Glover DK, Hansen CL, McCallister BD (2006). American Society of Nuclear Cardiology information statement: standardized reporting matrix for radionuclide myocardial perfusion imaging. *J Nucl Cardiol* 13:e152–e171. www.asnc.org;menu:ManageYourPractice;Guidelines andStandards (accessed May 2007).

18 Remote Reading and Networking
Tele-Nuclear Cardiology

Remote interpretation of nuclear cardiology images by electronic means or "tele-nuclear cardiology" may be very useful for two reasons. It is not unusual at the present time for a nuclear cardiology laboratory to provide interpretation for one or more remote satellite imaging facilities *(1)*. These facilities operate generally under the same technical and medical directors but are geographically distant and may have their own local technical staff. On the other hand, even if there is only one laboratory, for reasons of competitiveness, an imaging facility may be required to provide service outside routine office hours. Under these conditions, it is very desirable to create a technical environment that allows for remote interpretation through tele-nuclear cardiology. Guidelines have been published that address procedures, QA, and security for tele-nuclear medicine *(2,3)*.

Key Words: Tele-nuclear cardiology, Local network, Web reading, HIPAA.

Tele-nuclear cardiology can be achieved in a number of ways as described in brief below. One has to consider various modes of electronic communication and transfer of image data.

Several media can be used to connect two remote locations. From slower to faster connectivity speed:

- By modem and regular phone line (56 k bps)
- Digital subscriber line (DSL) (1.5 M bps)
- Digital cable modem (10–100 M bps)
- T1 line (1 G bps)

From: *Contemporary Cardiology: Nuclear Cardiology, The Basics*
By: F. J. Th. Wackers, W. Bruni, and B. L. Zaret © Humana Press Inc., Totowa, NJ

One should also consider whether one intends to use a personal computer as a remote workstation or merely as a viewing terminal.

The electronic connection can be established:

1. Between a computer in the main nuclear cardiology laboratory and a remote computer in a satellite laboratory or
2. Between a computer in the main nuclear cardiology laboratory and a remote personal computer at the physician's home or a remote laptop computer while the physician is traveling.

Three practical options are to be considered.

First Option

The remote computer dials in through one of the above mentioned connectivity media with the digital environment in the main nuclear cardiology laboratory. Using window emulator software (e.g., X-Window Emulator or PC-Anywhere®), the physician can review processed image data. In this configuration, the home computer serves as a viewing terminal of the main computer in the laboratory.

Second Option

Once a connection with the main laboratory has been established, raw image data are downloaded through one of the above connectivity means to the remote workstation, which has all the processing and display software required for offline data processing, image viewing, and interpretation. In this configuration, the home computer becomes another workstation of the laboratory.

These two options are both somewhat cumbersome and in our view not optimal. The speed of access and of viewing using the first option may be relatively slow, but the physician does not have to (re)process any image data.

The speed of the second option depends largely on the quantity of data to be downloaded. For example, the downloading of complete data of an ECG-gated SPECT study may be very time consuming. Furthermore, the physician has to perform all data processing by him/her self.

Third Option

Web reading

We consider this the most practical solution. In fact, in our laboratory, we have used remote web reading routinely for over 10 years during evenings and weekends. Physicians on-call interpret nuclear cardiology images on our secure Internet website. Reconstructed and processed images are uploaded by a technologist from the nuclear medicine computer in the main laboratory to a dedicated website as simple compressed image files, for example, gif, tiff, jpeg, png, bmp, or mpeg cine files. One can also upload scanned files of technologists' worksheets, rest/stress ECGs, and other relevant written data. The website is accessed by the physician from a remote computer through the Internet and a commercial web browser. The physician can then either view the images on the website or download data to a personal computer. The advantage of "web reading" is its simplicity and speed of access. In our experience, even a regular phone line provides acceptable speed although high-speed Internet access is considerably more convenient. A minor disadvantage of this method is that the interpreter cannot (re)process images if he/she desires to do so. However, standardization of processing and display should make this unnecessary most of the time.

QUALITY ASSURANCE

As with every other procedure in radionuclide imaging, a number of QA issues should be considered for tele-nuclear cardiology.

The Integrity and Preservation of Images

It is conceivable, although rare, that during transfer of raw or processed images, corruption of data occurs. Also too much compression of images for uploading to the website may deteriorate image quality. These potential problems should be evaluated by empirical testing of a number of different compressed file formats. Original image data should be compared qualitatively and quantitatively to the digitally transferred data on the receiving computer.

Speed

The speed of access and the speed of viewing individual images are extremely important in clinical practice. For example, if it takes longer than 45–60 s to download or display one single image, the entire process of remote reading becomes extremely tedious. In particular, if multiple patient studies are to be interpreted, reasonable speed is crucial.

Security

Patients confidentiality and security has become extremely important with the new Health Insurance Portability and Accountability Act (HIPAA) regulations. Incoming and outgoing patient data must be encrypted and should be accessible only by authorized users with username and password and must be in compliance with HIPAA regulations.

What is HIPAA?

The Health Insurance Portability and Accountability Act (HIPAA) of 1996 (August 21), Public Law 104-191, that amends the Internal Revenue Service Code of 1986; also known as the Kennedy–Kassebaum Act.

Title II includes a section, Administrative Simplification, requiring

1. Improved efficiency in healthcare delivery by standardizing electronic data interchange and
2. Protection of confidentiality and security of health data through setting and enforcing standards

More specifically, HIPAA calls for

1. Standardization of electronic patient health, administrative, and financial data
2. Unique health identifiers for individuals, employers, health plans, and health care providers
3. Security standards protecting the confidentiality and integrity of "individually identifiable health information," past, present, or future

For more information see http://www.hipaadvisory.com

Tele-medicine can be viewed as communication of PHI between "business associates." The HIPAA business associate standard mandates that business associates who may receive, use, obtain, create, or have access to PHI are required to sign an agreement that will ensure that the business associate will safeguard and protect the integrity and confidentiality of the PHI.

Quality of Remote Display

To have diagnostic quality images, the remote display monitor should have the similar resolution and quality of display as those of the computers in the main nuclear cardiology imaging facility (e.g., 1024×768 resolution and true color).

LOCAL COMPUTER NETWORK

When there are multiple gamma cameras in a nuclear cardiology imaging facility, a LAN is useful for making daily operation easier and more efficient. The images acquired on different acquisition computers are transferred through the LAN to a central computer for either central processing and/or for central display in a reading room.

Typical hardware components of a LAN:

- Main computer with network software and Ethernet card
- Hub
- Router
- RJ45 cables for inter-computer connections
- Firewall for protection from intrusion from outside

STORAGE

Storage of digital image data (raw and/or processed data) is of clinical importance as it allows for comparison of a recent patient study with previous studies of the same patient. Raw image data may be transferred from the acquisition computers through the LAN to a central computer that serves as storage device. For easy access to previous studies, it is advisable to store relatively recent (<3 years) data online for a limited number of years. For long-term storage image, data can be stored on optical disks and/or tapes. Obviously, retrieval of data from optical disks, and in particular from magnetic tape, takes considerably more time than online retrieval. In our laboratory, all data are doubly backed up in storage. For storage of large volumes of digital data, storage on jukebox and raid library is an optimal solution. For accreditation by the ICANL, it is a requirement that one submits digital data retrieved from storage.

REFERENCES

1. Bateman TM, Cullom J, Case JA (1999). Wide area networking in nuclear cardiology. *J Nucl Cardiol* 6: 211–218.
2. Parker JA, Wallis JW, Jadvar H, Christian P, Todd-Pokropek A (2002). *Society of Nuclear Medicine Procedure Guideline for Telenuclear Medicine*. Available at http://interactive.snm.org/docs/pg_ch15_0403.pdf (accessed May, 2007).
3. Parker JA, Wallis JW, Jadvar H, Christian P, Todd-Pokropek A (2002). Procedure guideline for telenuclear medicine1.0. *J Nucl Med* 43:1410–1413.

19 Quality Assurance

Ongoing quality assurance (QA) is a vital component for the optimal functioning of a laboratory. All equipments, including imaging and nonimaging equipment, must be checked regularly to ensure proper functioning. In addition to the technical QA of equipment, it is recommended that a program is in place that periodically assesses the quality of technologists and interpreting staff.

Key Words: Quality control, Quality assurance, Continuing quality improvement, Acceptance testing, Gamma camera quality control, Field uniformity (integral/ differential), Jaszczak phantom.

The following are some common definitions used in quality assurance:

Quality Control (QC): Assessment of the proper performance of instrumentation.

Quality Assurance (QA): Assessment of all variables that are involved in the overall functioning of the laboratory.

Continuing Quality Improvement (CQI): Process of repeatedly setting new targets for improved performance of one of aspects of QA.

Standard QC protocols of imaging and nonimaging equipment are described in great detail in the 2006 Imaging Guidelines for Nuclear Cardiology Procedures *(1)*.

CAMERA QUALITY CONTROL

Acceptance Testing

QA starts the moment a new gamma camera has been purchased. Acceptance testing (Table 19-1) must be performed before using the equipment for clinical imaging. The assistance of a health physicist with experience in nuclear medicine imaging will be very useful. The results of acceptance testing will be the baseline for future regular QA testing.

From: *Contemporary Cardiology: Nuclear Cardiology, The Basics*
By: F. J. Th. Wackers, W. Bruni, and B. L. Zaret © Humana Press Inc., Totowa, NJ

Table 19-1
Acceptance Testing of New Gamma Camera

- Physical inspection for shipping damages and mechanical functioning
- Camera/computer interface
- Intrinsic and extrinsic uniformity, each detector head (flood source)
- Spatial resolution and linearity, each detector head (bar phantom)
- Extrinsic uniformity and spatial resolution (3-D Jaszczak phantom optional)
- Trial patient acquisition, procession, and display

One must refer to the manufacturer's instruction for specific acquisition details and recommended frequencies of QC. Table 19-2 lists some important items for camera QC. The following subsections discuss the individual items.

Comments

COLLIMATOR INTEGRITY

Collimators are a critical component of the imaging system. Collimators should be inspected daily, or whenever damage is suspected, by technologists for visual signs of surface damage (marks or indentations). The proper functioning of patient safety mechanisms, such as touch pads or contact sensors, should be tested routinely *(2)*.

Table 19-2
Gamma Camera QC

QC	Frequency
Collimator integrity	Daily
Uniformity (low count)	Daily (2–6 million counts)
Energy peaking	Daily
Linearity	Weekly
Center of rotation	Monthly
High-count uniformity and calibration	Monthly (30 million counts)
Preventive maintenance	6 months
Very high-count uniformity and calibration	Annual (100 million counts)
Phantom	Optional (uniformity and resolution)
Preventive maintenance	6 months

Uniformity and Calibration

HIGH-COUNT UNIFORMITY

A high-count-uniformity flood (30 million counts) is acquired either monthly or quarterly, depending on the manufacturer's recommendations. A very high-count calibration with 100 million counts is performed annually. The high-count-uniformity flood is stored and used for correction of camera nonuniformity (calibration). A high-count-uniformity flood should be done both for each type of collimator used and for each isotope commonly used in the laboratory. However, it should be noted that on some older systems (over 10 years old), only one high-count-uniformity flood is capable of being stored. In these cases, by necessity, only one uniformity flood is applied to the different isotopes acquired. Although this is not ideal, storing one uniformity flood is an inherent limitation of the older imaging systems. Cameras less than 10 years old usually require a separate high-count-uniformity flood for each isotope. Check with the manufacturer for details.

High-count uniformity floods can be done extrinsically or intrinsically similar to the daily floods (see under "daily uniformity"). It is usually recommended to acquire extrinsic floods to correct for irregularities of the collimator.

As the required number of counts for these high-count floods is very high (30 million counts), they are often acquired over night and analyzed in the morning. For a multiple-headed camera system, it may take a number of hours to acquire the uniformity flood.

DAILY UNIFORMITY

Daily uniformity or floods (2–6 million counts) is performed to monitor the stability of the gamma camera system. They are not used for corrections. Just as with extrinsic floods, it is recommended that one visually inspects the image for hot and cold areas indicating nonuniformity. Daily percent uniformity should be recorded in a log. If any problems with the uniformity are noted, camera service should be called in immediately (**Figs 19-1** to **19-3**).

QC of daily uniformity flood can be done extrinsically (preferred) or intrinsically. Extrinsic uniformity refers to the spatial-dependent sensitivity of the camera with a specific collimator mounted. Intrinsic uniformity refers to the spatial-dependent sensitivity of the camera without a collimator.

An extrinsic flood is usually done with a Co-57 sheet source or a fillable flood source with Tc-99m, Tl-201, or any other isotope used in the laboratory. The source is placed directly on the detector's collimator. If the Co-57 source is new, there may be contamination

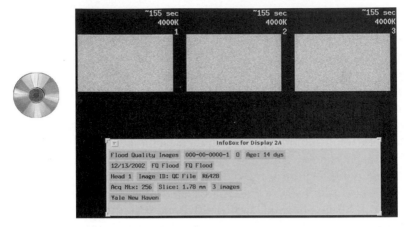

Fig. 19-1. Example of daily floods (approx 4,000,000 counts) of a triple-head gamma camera. All three heads are well-tuned and show good uniformity.

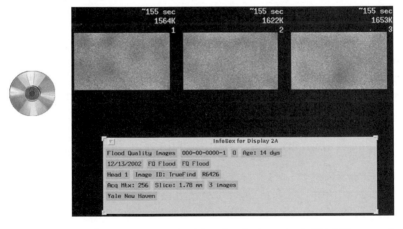

Fig. 19-2. Example of uncorrected daily floods (approx 1,500,000 counts) of a triple-head gamma camera. Non-uniformity is noted of for each head. This was less than 5% and could be corrected for clinical use.

from Co-56 and Co-57 (with higher energy than Co-57). To avoid erroneous nonuniformities, it is suggested to position the sheet source at about 30 cm distance from the collimator. A static image is acquired and then analyzed for uniformity. Each vendor may have different acquisition parameters, and one should check with the manufacturer for specific recommendations. Most systems have an automatic program for analyzing the static image for percent uniformity. Again, each manufacturer will have different uniformity tolerance limits. It is recommended that one always visually inspect the image for hot and cold areas, indicating nonuniformity. A daily log should be kept to

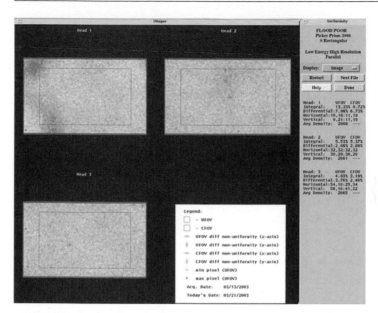

Fig. 19-3. Daily floods of a triple-head camera. The center field of view (CFOV) is marked by the red-lined rectangle in the center of the usable field of view (UFOV). The small circles and squares indicate pixels used for uniformity calculations. Head 1 has marked non-uniformity. Head 2 has minor non-uniformity. Head 3 shows good uniformity. For head 1 integral uniformity of the UFOV is 13.3% and that of the CFOV is 9.7%. Both should be less than 5%. The vendor of this camera recommends that the calculation of integral uniformity is used rather than of differential uniformity. For head 2 UFOV and CFOV uniformity is marginal at 5.53% and 5.37%. The area of non-uniformity can clearly be appreciated in the upper middle-half of the UFOV. Gamma camera service should be called to correct the problem before a patient can be imaged with this camera.

record the percent uniformity daily. This allows one to look for slow drifts in the uniformity.

Intrinsic floods are done with a Tc-99m point source with small volume (0.5 mL) and low activity ($100 - 200\,\mu$Ci) acquired with the collimator off the gamma camera detector head. The source is placed at a distance of at least five times the diameter of the detector FOV. A static image is acquired and then analyzed for uniformity.

> Two parameters are used to measure and document flood uniformity:
> **Integral uniformity:** This is a global parameter that measures contrast over an extended area of the detector and is expressed

as percentage [100% × (maximum − minimum)/maximum + minimum].

Differential uniformity: This is a regional parameter that measures contrast over a small neighborhood. The measurement is performed using a 5 × 1 pixel area in both the X and Y directions and is expressed as percentage [100% × largest deviation (maximum − minimum)/(maximum + minimum)].

Both percentages must be ≤ 5%, preferably around 3%.

Maximum = maximal count found in any pixel within the specified area; minimum = minimal count found in any pixel within the specified area.

ENERGY PEAKING

On many newer model cameras, energy peaking is done automatically with the daily flood. Even if the computer program performs the analysis, one must check that the peak is within specified limits. A pulse height analysis (PHA) or digital read out should be checked daily to make sure that the peak is centered. The peak should be recorded daily to watch for drifts in the peak.

If peaking is not an automated part of the daily flood setup, one should check the peak manually. All systems provide a visual display of the PHA and will allow adjusting the peak as necessary. Service should be notified of any drifts in the peak. Incorrect peaking, either too high or too low, may affect field uniformity as shown in **Fig. 19-4.**

LINEARITY

Linearity is more commonly known as "acquiring a bar flood." A bar phantom (phantom with variously sized lead bars) is placed on the collimator, and the Co-57 sheet source is placed on top of the phantom. A static image is acquired and visually inspected to make sure all of the bars are visible and that they are straight. Any "waviness" of the lines should be reported to service immediately (**Figs. 19-5 and 19-6**).

3-D TOMOGRAPHIC PHANTOM

This phantom consists of a lucite cylinder (8.5 × 7.32 inches, volume 6.9 L) that can be filled with water in which a small amount of radioisotope is dissolved. The phantom contains six sets of triangularly arranged solid rods of different thickness (ranging from 4.8 mm to 12.7 mm) and six solid spheres of different diameters

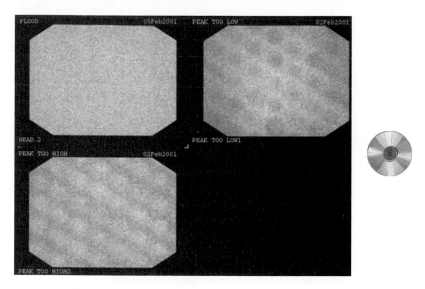

Fig. 19-4. Example of the effect of energy peaking on field flood uniformity. By peaking either too low (upper right) or too high (lower left) relative to the energy peak marked non-uniformity results which may affect clinical imaging.

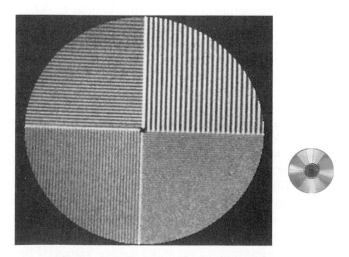

Fig. 19-5. Bar phantom. All lines are straight, indicating appropriate linearity. The bar phantom can also be used as a quick check on resolution. In the phantom shown, the lines in 3 of 4 quadrants are well separated and visible. Even smallest bars can be made out as a linear pattern although they are not clearly separated. For daily QC it is important to document *and record* gradual changes in camera performance.

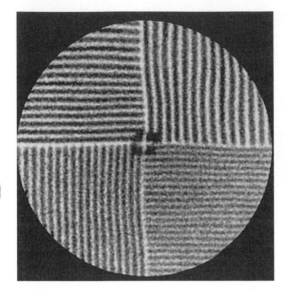

Fig. 19-6. Bar phantom showing wavy poor linearity. Nevertheless resolution is apparently not affected. The gamma camera needs to be tuned-up by the vendor's maintenance service.

(9.5–31.8 mm). SPECT acquisition of the phantom is performed to determine uniformity and the ability of the imaging system to detect cold lesions. On the reconstructed tomographic images of the phantom, one determines the smallest rods and smallest sphere that can be detected. It is recommended that this phantom is imaged for QA at acceptance testing and annually (**Figs. 19-7** and **19-8**).

CENTER OF ROTATION

This measures the alignment error between the electronic matrix of the detector and the mechanical center of rotation (COR). Depending on manufacturer recommendations, the COR should be tested monthly or quarterly. To assess COR offset, SPECT acquisition of a Tc-99m point source is performed. The half-width full-maximum of the reconstructed image of the point source is measured and analyzed to make sure that the COR has not drifted. Each manufacturer will have different acquisition parameters and different acceptable values. If the COR is not within the recommended range, the gamma camera should not be used, and service must be called immediately. COR errors can cause serious image artifacts. In general, COR offset should not exceed 2 pixels using a 64 × 64 matrix. COR offset affects image resolution and causes image blurring (**Figs. 19-9** and **19-10**).

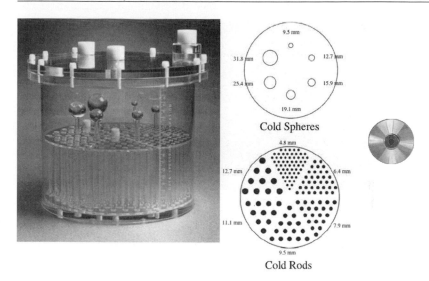

Fig. 19-7. Three-dimensional phantom (Deluxe Jaszczak Phantom™) for SPECT quality control. The cold spheres vary in diameter from 4.8 to 12.7 mm. The cold rods vary in thickness from 9.5 mm to 31.8 mm.

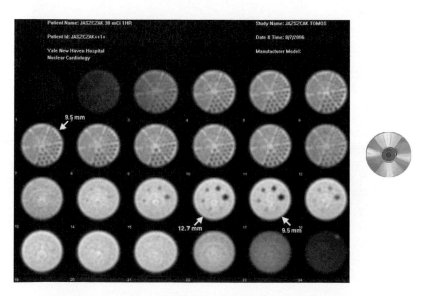

Fig. 19-8. Reconstructed SPECT slices of the 3D phantom shown in Fig. 19-7 filled with 30 mCi of Tc-99m. The smallest cold rods that can be resolved are 9.5 mm in diameter (arrow second row from top), whereas the smallest cold sphere that be discerned is between 9.5 and 12.7 mm in diameter (arrows second row from bottom).

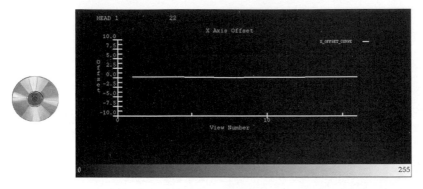

Fig. 19-9. Display of center-of rotation (COR) offset testing results. The offset is plotted against acquisition angles. The COR is within acceptable range.

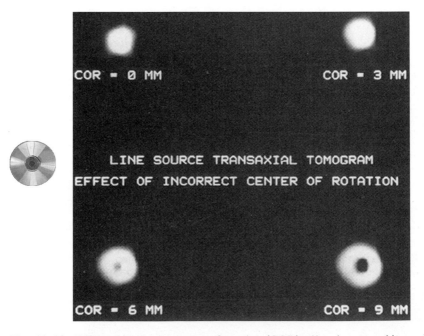

Fig. 19-10. Effect of increasing center of rotation (COR) offset (expressed in mm) on reconstructed image of a line source. The image is increasingly blurred by circular smearing with increasing COR offset. Ultimately, at 9 mm offset (about 4 pixels), the line source is reconstructed as a circle. COR offset results in loss of image resolution.

QUALITY ASSURANCE (QA) OF IMAGING EQUIPMENT WITH ATTENUATION CORRECTION (AC) DEVICES

AC devices require special QA checks.

QC for SPECT Systems with External Sealed AC Source

1. When no patient imaging is performed, the shielded container must be shut. The mechanics of the shutter must be checked regularly.
2. To assure that transmission images (and scatter images, if applicable) are acquired in the appropriate energy windows, daily energy peaking should be performed using the pulse height energy analyzer.
3. A blank transmission scan should be acquired at least weekly according to the manufacturer's specifications. The blank scan should be inspected for cold spots and bands of missing data.
4. Transmission to crosstalk ratio (TCR) should be monitored at least monthly using a cylinder phantom as outlined in the ASNC instrumentation guidelines. The TCR should be trended over time, and substantial decrease in ration should serve as a guide when the source needs replacement.

QC for Systems with X-Ray-Based AC

1. During the acquisition of the X-ray CT, a sign indicating "X-ray in Use" must be illuminated above the entrance of the imaging room.
2. A moveable lead-shielded screen must be placed between the X-ray tube and the technologist at all times.
3. The accuracy of CT numbers must be checked daily by acquiring a CT image of a water-filled cylinder and by determining the Hounsfield units. If the error is greater than five Hounsfield units (i.e., different than the expected 0 Hounsfield units) service must be called.
4. Field uniformity of the reconstructed CT image of the cylinder must be checked daily by comparing CT numbers in different areas of the cylinder image.
5. Coregistration of transmission and emission images may be verified by acquiring SPECT and CT images of an anthropomorphic cardiac phantom. This should be done at least as part of acceptance testing.
6. AC accuracy testing can be performed using an anthropomorphic cardiac phantom. A normal homogeneous cardiac phantom demonstrates mild inferior attenuation, which should be corrected by applying AC.

The ASNC published a position statement on SPECT AC, emphasizing many of the above mentioned QC issues *(3)*.

Preventive Maintenance

It is usually recommended that service be scheduled every 6 months for preventive maintenance of the camera and computer system. Depending on the gamma camera and whether any defaults have to be corrected, this usually takes 4–8 h to complete. Having imaging equipment inoperable for any length of time is a burden on the daily operation of the imaging facility; but *scheduled* maintenance is easier to tolerate than unexpected breakdown of a gamma camera. Not infrequently, preventive maintenance detects technical problems before they become a clinical problem.

NONIMAGING EQUIPMENT QC

Table 19-3 lists some important items for nonimaging equipment QC. The following subsections discuss the individual items.

Dose Calibrator Constancy

The constancy of the dose calibrator must be checked each working day prior to use. A cesium-137 (Cs-137) source is normally used for this purpose. The standard known source is measured daily in the dose calibrator. The daily measurements should be recorded in a logbook. The RSO usually provides a table with ranges of measured activities for any given day. Because the Cs-137 source decays, the range will change continually. The measurements of Cs-137 activity must fall within the daily predefined range and thus confirm that the dose calibrator functions properly.

Table 19-3
Nonimaging Equipment QC

QC	Frequency
Dose calibrator	
Constancy	Daily
Accuracy	Quarterly
Linearity	Quarterly
Survey meter	
Source check	Daily
Calibration	Yearly
Treadmills and ECG equipment	
Electrical safety	Yearly
Glucose meter	Daily
Defibrillator	Monthly

Dose Calibrator Accuracy

In addition to the daily QC check, the dose calibrator should undergo quarterly QC requirements. To perform the accuracy test of the dose calibrator, one needs four known standard sources. Co-57, Co-60, Cs-137, and Ba-133 are commonly used for this test. Each source is measured in the dose calibrator, and the activity is recorded. The radio safety officer (RSO) should set acceptable measured ranges of activities for each radioisotope.

Dose Calibrator Linearity

The second quarterly required QC test of the dose calibrator is a linearity test. One draws a known amount of Tc-99m (usually around = 100 mCi) in a vial and periodically measures and records the measured activity of the vial as it decays. Typically, two to three measurements per day are taken until the source has decayed to 30 μCi. The RSO can again be of assistance in determining whether the measurements are within acceptable limits.

Glucose Meter

A capillary blood glucose meter is required when glucose loading is performed for F-18 FDG viability studies. However, it is also useful to have a glucose meter in the laboratory to check blood glucose levels in patients with diabetes. The glucose meter should be checked daily using an aqueous glucose test solution.

QA AND CQI

QA is a program for the systematic monitoring and evaluation of various aspects of a project, service, or facility to insure that standards of quality are being met. It is an important process that allows for timely identification of problems or areas of improvement, and it facilitates the initiation of necessary changes in policies or procedures and improves efficiency. Documentation of internal laboratory QA and CQI activities is a requirement for accreditation by the ICANL. Table 19-4 lists some QA terminology

---

To begin a QA program.

- Support of the medical director or manager is required
- Decide what area needs QA
  - Problem area
  - Uncertain of status in an area

Table 19-4
Quality Assurance Terminology

Indicator	Predefined item that is being assessed
Threshold	Limit tolerated before action is needed and beyond which the situation is unacceptable
Corrective action	Measure used to correct the problem and return to within the threshold

Table 19-5
Possible Suggested Areas for Quality Assurance

Technical issues
  Reproducibility
  Poor quality studies
  Service call response times
  Camera downtime
  Camera QC
  Quality ECG tracings
Safety
  Misadministrations
  Radioisotope spills
  Inadvertent needle sticks (staff)
  Patient incidents
  Staff incidents
Efficiency
  Patient waiting times
  Exam backlog
  Camera usage
Satisfaction
  Patient satisfaction
  Referring physician satisfaction
Interpretation
  Reviewer reproducibility
  Comparison to another modality
Reporting
  Timeliness of report generation
  Timeliness of signing
  Timeliness of mailing
  Transcription errors
  Errors with entering in database
  Quantity of errors

– What information or data concerning quality are needed
- Determine limits or thresholds
- Determine corrective action to be taken to fix the problem
- Write a protocol including thresholds and corrective actions
- Create a form or worksheet for the collection of data
- Make data collection part of laboratory routine (for future re-evalua-tions)
- Take the corrective action and fix the problem

Table 19-5 lists only some suggested areas. There are numerous other aspects of the operation of a laboratory that can be submitted to QA. It is important to remember that a QA program should be an individualized process. Those aspects addressed by a QA program in one laboratory may not necessarily be relevant for another laboratory. Ultimately, a QA program should result in an improvement of services. Every individual laboratory may have specific needs. For instance, detailed documentation of downtime of an old camera may be used as a persuasive argument for replacing old equipment. As was mentioned before, a laboratory must be able to provide evidence of periodic internal QA activity for accreditation by ICANL.

REFERENCES

1. DePuey EG (2006). *Imaging Guidelines for Nuclear Cardiology Procedures.* Available at http://www.asnc.org/imageuploads/Imaging%20Guidelines%20Instrumentation.pdf (accessed May, 2007).
2. DiFilippo FP, Abreu SH, Majmundar H (2006). *Collimator Integrity. ASNC Clinical Update.* Available at http://www.asnc.org/imageuploads/Collimator IntegrityClinicalUpdate.pdf (accessed May, 2007).
3. Heller GV, Links J, Bateman TM, Ziffer JA, Ficaro E, Cohen MC, Hendel RC (2004). *Attenuation Correction for Myocardial Perfusion SPECT Scintigraphy.* Available at http://www.asnc.org/imageuploads/AttenuationCorrectionPosition Statement.pdf (accessed May, 2007).

20 Miscellaneous Additional Laboratory Protocols and Policies

> Every nuclear cardiology imaging facility should have written, up-to-date, and dated protocols for all procedures. In addition, written protocols and policies should be in place for all other medical and non-medical procedures and anticipated incidents. Such written protocols are an important requirement for laboratory accreditation by the ICANL (see also Chapter 22).

Key Words: Written policies.

Protocols and policies should be easily available to the staff for consultation, i.e., copies should be present in the imaging rooms and stress laboratory. In many hospitals, protocols and policies also are posted on the hospital's website.

These policies not only help to run a laboratory more efficiently but also prepare them for dealing with potential problems. Safety should be a major concern for any laboratory. The policies listed in this chapter, and other not listed, are also required by the ICANL for accreditation as a nuclear cardiology laboratory (see also http://www.icanl.org—Menu: "The Standards" for the requirements of protocols and policies).

A nuclear cardiology imaging facility should have at the minimum written detailed protocols and policies for the following:

- Radiation safety and handling of radiopharmaceuticals
- Clinical indications of procedures
- Medical emergencies
- Patient identification
- Patient pregnancy assessment, policy concerning breast-feeding
- Patient confidentiality
- Diagnostic imaging procedures

From: *Contemporary Cardiology: Nuclear Cardiology, The Basics*
By: F. J. Th. Wackers, W. Bruni, and B. L. Zaret © Humana Press Inc., Totowa, NJ

- Stress procedures
- Equipment QA (imaging and no imaging)
- Infection control
- Electrical equipment safety
- Fire safety

Protocols should be reviewed regularly, dated, and signed by the medical and/or technical director.

RADIATION SAFETY AND HANDLING OF RADIOPHARMACEUTICALS

Written radiation safety protocols are extremely important. Radiation safety must be taken seriously. A good source to consult is the *Guide of Diagnostic Nuclear Medicine* by JA Siegel *(1)* and the ICANL website http://www.icanl: "Standards." The medical director, and preferably also other interpreting medical staff, must be an authorized user(s). Every imaging facility should have a designated RSO. There should be written policies on the receipt, handling and storage of radioisotopes/radiopharmaceuticals, as well as the proper preparation and calibration of radiopharmaceutical, proper administration of radiopharmaceuticals, disposal of the radioactive trash, and how to handle spilling of radioactivity. The policies should also discuss the pregnancy and breast-feeding, proper use and quality control of radiation safety equipment, and techniques/measures to reduce radiation exposure of patients and technological staff.

PATIENT IDENTIFICATION

Every laboratory should have a policy on how to properly identify or confirm a patient's identity. In a hospital laboratory, in-patients usually wear ID bracelets that should be used to verify identity. For outpatients, it is not sufficient to just call a patient's name in the waiting area. There have been many instances where a patient misunderstood the name called and answered to the wrong name. The written protocol should specify that a patient's identity should also be checked by verifying data of birth or social security number.

PATIENT PREGNANCY ASSESSMENT

All women of childbearing years should be asked whether or not they might be pregnant prior to beginning the stress or imaging procedure. The protocol should include under what age a women should be asked if she is pregnant, what to do if she answers "may be, or I don't know," and what to do if she indicates that she ispregnant. The type of pregnancy test must be specified. There should also be a written protocol concerning breast-feeding patients and fetus exposure and protection.

PATIENT CONFIDENTIALITY

All patient records and information must be kept confidential, and each laboratory should have a written policy in place on how this issue is assured. Patient confidentiality has become extremely important with the new HIPAA regulations (see Chapter 18, pg. 333–334).

CLINICAL INDICATIONS

Each clinical procedure protocol should contain a brief summary of the clinical indications for stress testing and radionuclide imaging. The indications should be in compliance with the published AHA/ACC guidelines and Guidelines for Appropriateness that can be found online at http://www.acc.org and http://www.asnc.org.

STRESS PROCEDURES

The various stress procedures must be described in detail, such as indication for procedure, performance of procedure (treadmill, pharmacologic), evaluation of patient during test, defined stress endpoints, criteria for radiopharmaceutical injection, non-radioactive pharmaceuticals, post-stress monitoring, and treatment of adverse effects.

DIAGNOSTIC IMAGING PROCEDURES

The protocols must describe indication for procedure, patient preparation and education, radiopharmaceutical dose, weight limitations for 1-day versus 2-day protocols for males and females, detailed camera setup, camera-specific acquisition and processing protocol, and display and labeling and saving of image data. In addition, the imaging protocol should include effective dose and critical organ dose.

CARDIAC EMERGENCY

A written protocol should be in place for cardiac emergencies.

In general, exercise testing is very safe. Using the Bruce, modified Bruce protocol, or other standardized graded protocols, cardiac emergencies (persistent severe ischemia, acute infarction, and cardiac death) occur infrequently (1:10,000 exercise tests). However, with an increasingly sicker patient population and greater number of patients with known coronary artery disease referred for study, cardiac emergencies may occur more frequently. Consequently, laboratory personnel should be well prepared to deal with cardiac emergencies.

A qualified health care provider, certified in cardiopulmonary resuscitation (CPR) or ACLS, should supervise and be responsible for stress testing. As a rule, two people are needed to administer an exercise test. Defibrillation equipment and "crash cart" must be present in the immediate vicinity of the stress laboratory. Laboratory personnel (including technologists and administrative personnel) should know what to do when a "code" is called.

In order to deal adequately with emergencies, all exercise staff and preferably also imaging staff should know the following:

1. Emergency phone number(s),
2. Where emergency equipment and medications, i.e., crash cart, are located,
3. How to assemble the Ambu bag and hook up to oxygen,
4. How to turn on the defibrillator and place chest leads,
5. How to start and perform CPR,
6. How to assist physician(s) and nurse(s) during CPR.

ELECTRICAL EQUIPMENT SAFETY

All electrical equipment should be checked annually to ensure that it is safe to use. A written policy on what to do if unsafe electrical equipment is found and how to use electrical equipment properly is recommended.

Fire Safety

A written policy on what to do in the case of a fire is highly recommended. The policy should include information such as how to use a fire extinguisher, whom to contact in case fire or smoke is detected, what steps to take to contain the fire, and what is the best evacuation route.

INFECTION CONTROL

Control of infection is an important concern in hospitals and in outpatient facilities. A written policy on how to use properly universal precautions should be in place. The policy should discuss the use of gloves, aseptic techniques, and proper disposal of biohazardous trash.

The following are illustrative examples of written policies.

They are examples to give an idea about the degree of detail that is required. For a complete list of required written protocols, go online and download "The Standards" for accreditation at http://www.icanl.org.

Example 1. Dose Calibration and Administration

- Every radioactive kit prepared must have a Dose Log Sheet.
- The log sheet must contain the radiopharmaceutical, date, total activity in kit in mCi, total volume used in kit, concentration (activity in mCi/volume in mL), and time the kit was prepared.
- Every patient dose must be logged in on the Dose Log Sheet with patient name, procedure (Stress or Rest), and time.
- To calculate the concentration at the time of injection:
  - Take the original concentration and multiply by the decay factor (Tc-99m decay chart hanging on bulletin board).
- To calculate how much isotope to draw up:

$$- \frac{\text{Dose desired (mCi)}}{\text{New concentration (mCi/mL)}} = \text{volume to draw up (mL)}$$

- Assay the dose in the dose calibrator
- Adjust the dose as necessary to get the desired dose
- Label the dose with the patient name, activity, time, and isotope
- Record actual dose drawn up on Dose Log Sheet
- Important: A patient can only be injected with $\pm10\%$ of the desired dose. If the dose is adjusted for the patients weight, note on the log sheet and refer to the Tc-99m Adjusted Dose Chart.
- Pediatric patients (< 18 years old) must have their dose adjusted for their weight using the following formula:

$$- \frac{\text{Weight (lb)}}{150 \text{ (lb)}} \times \text{adult dose}$$

  - Example: child of 50 lbs, usual adult dose $= 25\,\text{mCi}$
  - Thus,
    $50\,\text{lb} / 150\,\text{lb} \times 25\,\text{mCi} = 8.33\,\text{mCi}$ to be given to this child

  Note: Nonstandard dosing should be given only after consultation with the nuclear cardiologist.
- All doses should be carried in a lead carrying case or lead pig. All doses should be in a lead syringe shield during injection
- All injections are done through a three-way tubing for rest and exercise tests, or a Y-connector for adenosine and dobutamine tests
- The port should be swabbed with an alcohol pad prior to injection
- Rest and exercise injections should be flushed with 10 cc of normal saline

- Adenosine and dobutamine injections should be flushed with 4 cc of normal saline
- All needles, syringes, and gloves must be placed in appropriate hot trash receptacles

Revised: October 2002
Reviewed: February 2007
(signature)

Example 2. Hot Trash Policy

- Hot trash is to be collected, boxed, stored, and discarded every week. All needle boxes should have tops on and all red bags should be tied closed. Wear gloves when dealing with any potential radioactive material or trash. Please review the following checklist when storing and/or discarding hot trash.
- Place all needle boxes and red bags in black biohazard boxes.
- Survey the decay room and hallway and record measurements in the appropriate section of the decay log book (located in the inner decay room on the shelf).
- Label the boxes with the date and the next available log number (ex: C###). Boxes containing needle boxes must be labeled SHARPS.
- Record the date and log number of each box in the decay log book.
- Record the potential discard date of the boxes (2 months from the storage date!).
- See if any previously stored boxes can be discarded.
- Survey the boxes to be discarded and record the measurements and the date in the decay book (if they are not equal to background or less, they cannot be discarded!).
- Take the boxes to be discarded to (...location...) and label as "trash."

Revised: 10/06
(signature)

Example 3. Patient Pregnancy Assessment

- Nuclear Technologists will ask all female patients under 50 years of age if they are or might be pregnant or are breast-feeding.

- If the patient answers No, it MUST be recorded in the computerized hospital information system or worksheet for documentation. For example: *Patient states not pregnant/breast-feeding*. Initial and date the statement.
- A pregnancy test will be administered if a patient states they do not know or might be pregnant. Negative results will be recorded on the worksheet for documentation. For example: *Patient given urine pregnancy test and a negative result was obtained*. Initial and date the statement.

Urine Pregnancy Test:

- Have the patient urinate into a paper cup.
- Open a pregnancy test kit and fill the dropper with urine.
- Fill the corner hole on the kit from the dropper with urine until the paper is saturated.
- Wait approximately 60 s or until the display hole turns completely pink.
  - If a "−" sign appears, the patient is NOT pregnant.
  - If a "+" sign appears, the patient IS pregnant.
- The technologist will inform the physician if a patient is pregnant.
- The physician will contact the referring physician to consult in the decision to proceed with the exam, limit the exam, or cancel the exam.
- If a decision is made to proceed, the physician will discuss with the patient the risk versus benefits so that an informed decision can be made.
- All exams performed on pregnant patients will be documented on the requisition and in the report by the nuclear cardiologist.

Revised: 5/2001
Reviewed: 2/2007
(signature)

Example 4. Patient Identification Policy

In-patients:

- All in-patients must have a formal hospital information system request in their nuclear cardiology procedure folder.
- Check hospital information system request to verify type of study you will be doing on the patient.

- Ask patient their first and last name, *do not* call them by name as a confused patient may answer yes incorrectly.
- Verify the patient's name by checking their ID bracelet. No exam should be performed on a patient without an ID bracelet.
- Have the Fellow or Nurse check the patient's hospital chart if any discrepancies arise.

Outpatients:

- All outpatients should have a written request with them or have a faxed copy in their nuclear cardiology procedure folder.
- Verify patients *first* and *last* name.
- Ask the patient's birth date to verify the patient's identity.

If patients with similar names have procedures, take extra precaution for proper identification and attach colored notes to the chart to alert the physician who will be interpreting the study.

Revised: December 2001
Reviewed: February 2007
(signature)

Example 5. Nuclear Cardiology Daily Survey Protocol

- Area surveys must be performed each day that patients are examined in the laboratory.
- On weekends and holidays, only surveys of the rooms actually used are necessary.
- All trash bins, linen hampers, and cold needle boxes must be surveyed in each imaging and stress room.
- Log the survey results in the Daily Room Survey Log book.
- Remember to record background activity and to check the battery of the survey meter.
- If any trash, linen, or needle boxes are found to be hot (twice background), they must be stored in the lead cabinet in the hot lab for decay. The box or bag is to be labeled with the date of storage.
- Any surface found to be contaminated or hot (twice background) must be cleaned and resurveyed. All cleaning should be done using gloves and blue absorbent pads to prevent further contamination. Collect all absorbent pads and gloves in trash bags to be held for decay in the lead cabinet in the hot lab. If the area still measures greater than 2 mR/h at 1 inch, the area must be closed until sufficient decay occurs to bring the area into

specifications. See Radioactive Spill Procedure or contact the RSO for more details.

- Hot trash or contaminated areas should be brought to the attention of the chief technologist.
- The technologist performing the surveys must initial the logbook.

Revised: October 2006
(signature)

Example 6. Nuclear Cardiology Weekly Wipe Test Procedure

Tube number	Room number	Survey area
1		Background
2		Background
3		Background
4	Imaging room 1	Imaging room 1 Floor
5	Imaging room 1	Imaging room 1 Work Area
6	Imaging room 2	Imaging room 2 Floor
7	Imaging room 2	Imaging room 2 Work Area
8	Prep room 3	Prep room Floor
9	Prep room 3	Prep room Work Area
10	Imaging room 4	Imaging room 4 Floor
11	Imaging room 4	Imaging room 4 Work Area
12	Imaging room 5	Imaging room 5 Floor
13	Imaging room 5	Imaging room 5 Work Area
14	Imaging room 6	Imaging room 6 Floor
15	Imaging room 6	Imaging room 6 Work Area
16	Radiopharmacy	Radiopharmacy Floor
17	Radiopharmacy	Radiopharmacy Work Area (shield)
18	Radiopharmacy	Radiopharmacy Work Area (sink)
19	Stress lab 1	Stress lab 1 Floor
20	Stress lab 1	Stress lab 1 Treadmill
21	Stress lab 2	Stress lab 2 Left Floor
22	Stress lab 2	Stress lab 2 Left Treadmill
23	Emergency	Chest Pain Center Floor
24	Emergency	Chest Pain Center Work Area
25	Emergency	Chest Pain Center Treadmill
26		Cs-137 Test Source
27		Co-57 Test Source

Wipe tests of all of the above areas must be done weekly. The assigned technologist is responsible for doing the weekly wipes.

- Wipe the specified areas with Q-tips and insert them into the test tubes. Make sure the tube holder has the Protocol 20 clip on it and take to the Research lab to be counted in the well counter.
- Place the holder on the conveyer belt of the counter and hit F5 key to begin counting. The Protocol 20 clip will initiate the counter to run the Wipe test protocol automatically.
- When the counting is complete, take the printout and check for contamination.
- Any areas found to be contaminated are to be cleaned following the steps in the radiation spill policy and re-wipe tested. If the wipe test is found to be clear, place it in the Weekly Wipe Test Manual located in the hot lab. If the area is still contaminated, the area must be closed off and re-tested in the morning prior to use.

Revised: 10/02
   Reviewed: 2/2007
   (signature)

Example 7. Tc-99m Tetrofosmin Gated SPECT Acquisition

Indication: Assessment of myocardial perfusion at rest and exercise
Patient Setup:
Get patient on table with arms up over his/her head
Place three ECG leads on the patient's chest and check that you have a good R-R trigger
Computer Setup:
On acquisition terminal click on Acquisition card
Click on Add, slide to Patient, and under user protocol select H-mode Tetrofosmin/Sestamibi
Select appropriate protocol for stress or rest
Acquisition parameters are as follows: Parallel-hole LEHR collimator, 140 keV (20%), 64 × 64 matrix, 1.33 zoom, 180°, 32 stops, 16 bins, start angle 0°, feet first, supine, trigger 100% center and 150% width
Adjust frame time if necessary: 25 s/frame high dose
                                    30 s/frame low dose

Click on Gantry icon
Select Home position and click OK to message
Click on Gantry icon
Select wheelchair height to load patient onto table and click OK to message
Click camera on
Move to cardiac tomo click Yes
Slide table in, so heart is in FOV
Pop-up window says Detectors will move out—Yes
Pop-up window says Center patient in FOV, move both detectors close to patient—OK to store position. *You must move detectors in, you cannot leave them at the limit or you will get an error.*
Click OK to move the detectors out
Myosight H-mode Gated SPECT Acquisition (continued)
Heads will rotate to A/P position
Move detectors close to patient and click OK
Click OK to move to start position
Written: 7/05
Reviewed: 1/07
(signature)

Example 8. Exercise Protocol

Indication

1. Diagnosis of obstructive coronary artery disease
2. Risk assessment and prognosis in patients with symptoms or known coronary artery disease.

Pre-Exercise Assessment

- Explanation of procedures
- Obtain IV access using aseptic technique
- Obtain patient history and medication
- Obtain baseline ECG (limb leads and trunk), heart rate, blood pressure
- Evaluate heart and lung sounds

During Exercise

- Select Bruce protocol (see chart)
- Print two ECGs per stage per protocol in use
- Continuous monitoring of ECGs during exercise

- Print two ECGs at the end of each stage
- Continuous monitoring of symptoms (chest pain, lightheadedness, nausea, etc.)
- Make reference to the Borg Scale (patient's perception of workload)

Radioisotope Injection

The radiopharmaceutical is injected at the moment one of the test termination endpoints is reached. The patient must continue to exercise for 2 min after injection. The time is recorded on the worksheet. If needed the incline of the treadmill may be decreased or/and the speed lowered.

Test Termination Endpoints

- Severe fatigue
- ST segment depression > 2 mm (horizontal or downsloping)
- Severe angina
- Severe shortness of breath/severe wheezing
- Significant drop (20 mmHg) in blood pressure
- Significant elevation of blood pressure:
  - Systolic: > 220 mmHg
  - Diastolic: > 110 mmHg

- Signs of severe peripheral circulatory insufficiency: lightheadedness, nausea, and pallor
- Onset of second or third-degree AV block
- Ventricular tachycardia, supraventricular tachycardia
- Subject requests to stop
- For imaging study, patient should reach or exceed target heart rate prior to the injection of radioisotope (220-age × 0.85)
- Patient may not reach target heart rate if they are on β-blocker therapy. The test is then symptom-limited

Note: Patient should be able to complete at least stage 2 (7 METS). If not, switch to pharmacological stress

Post Exercise

Monitor patient's blood pressure and heart rate every 1 min for 6 min post exercise
Monitor ECG continuously for 6 minutes post exercise
Continue to monitor further if chest pain or significant EGC changes continue

Post imaging ECG and further monitoring throughout imaging
are recommended if changes occur late into recovery
Written: 7/03

Revised: 7/06
(signature)

REFERENCES

1. Siegel JA. Guide for diagnostic nuclear medicine (2002) available at
http://www.nrc.gov/ materials/miau/miau-reg-initiatives/guide_2002.pdf (accessed
June 2007).

21 Emergency Department Imaging

In recent years, many hospitals have instituted chest pain centers (CPCs) in hospital emergency departments (EDs) for the purpose of efficient triage of patients with chest pain and normal or non-ischemic rest ECG. The American Society of Nuclear Cardiology published a position paper on the use of radionuclide imaging in the ED *(1)* (online at http://www.asnc.org—Menu: "Manage Your Practice": Guidelines & Standards").

Key Words: Acute rest imaging, Chest pain center.

PROTOCOL

The evaluation of patients with chest pain in a CPC typically involves two parts:

1. Rule out acute coronary syndrome (ACS) by acute rest SPECT imaging or serial assessment of biomarkers for myocardial injury (CK, CK-MB, and troponin-I).
2. If ACS has been excluded, perform stress test with or without SPECT imaging.

Acute resting Tc-99m sestamibi or Tc-99m tetrofosmin imaging has high (99%) negative predictive value to exclude ACS *(1,2)*. In a randomized controlled trial, resting Tc-99m sestamibi perfusion imaging improved ED triage decision making and reduced unnecessary hospitalizations *(3)*.

LOCATION OF IMAGING

Although it is convenient, and perhaps preferable, to have a dedicated satellite stress/imaging laboratory on the ED premises (**Figs 21-1 and 21-2**), this is not a necessity. By design, patients evaluated in a CPC are low-risk patients. Higher-risk patients should

From: *Contemporary Cardiology: Nuclear Cardiology, The Basics*
By: F. J. Th. Wackers, W. Bruni, and B. L. Zaret © Humana Press Inc., Totowa, NJ

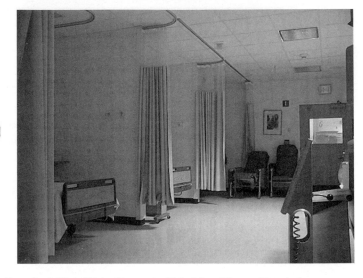

Fig. 21-1. Four-bed Chest Pain Center in Yale-New Haven Hospital.

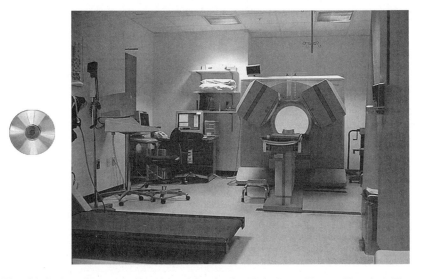

Fig. 21-2. Imaging and procedure room in the Yale-New Haven Hospital Chest Pain Center.

be hospitalized. Thus, there is no serious patient safety concern with regard to transporting patients from the ED to a remote nuclear medicine laboratory in the hospital.

The most important difference between imaging in a CPC and imaging in the regular laboratory is that ED patients are unscheduled and present themselves 24 h a day, 7 days a week. This brings different logistic challenges into play.

CHALLENGES FACED IN CHEST PAIN CENTERS

The following are challenges faced in chest pain centers:

Staffing
   On-call 24/7
Radiation safety
   Storage
   Injection, spill
Patient safety
   Selection
   Emergencies
Imaging protocol
   Acute rest imaging
   Optional stress imaging
Timely interpretation
   Attending-on-call
   Communication with ED

Staffing

A nuclear cardiologist and technologist should be on call during off-hours and weekends. These studies can be read by tele-nuclear cardiology (see Chapter 18).

For rest imaging, the injection of radiopharmaceutical is preferably performed while the patient is still having pain or < 2h after pain has abated.

Although some centers have arrangements for acute resting injection at any time, many centers have reached compromises with the ED and agreed on blackout periods during the late evening and night when no imaging is performed.

Patients in whom an ACS has been excluded are eligible for stress testing.

We found that "batch processing" of patients who are ready for stress testing works well for both patients and staff.

In our CPC, we perform stress tests with or without imaging in three periods:

- Morning (around 9:00 am)
- Late afternoon (around 5:00 pm)
- Evening (around 9:00 pm)

Radiation Safety

In order to perform acute rest imaging 24 h per day in the ED, two options can be considered:

1. Preparation and radiolabeling of radiopharmaceutical kit in the ED facility. A dose can be drawn up when needed.
2. Ready-to-use unit doses delivered by commercial radiopharmacy.

Furthermore, the area used for radiotracer storage should have the following:

- Lead brick shielding and lead shield with glass for safe handling of radioactive material (**Fig. 21-3**).
- Dose calibrator for assaying and adjusting dose prior to injection.

Because the nuclear cardiology technologists on call generally are not on site during the off hours, it is useful if selected ED medical staff ("injectors") have received appropriate radiation safety training for injection of radiopharmaceutical in patients with acute chest pain. This will enable patients to be injected *during pain*, instead of waiting for a technologist to arrive. When the technologist arrives, the patient will be ready to be imaged.

Radioactive spills are always a concern in a nuclear imaging facility. However, if the "injectors" are appropriately trained by the RSO,

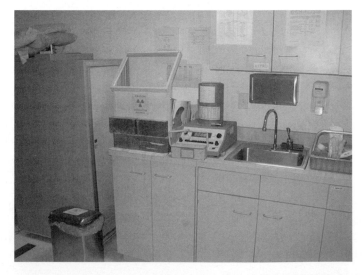

Fig. 21-3. Hot-lab area in Chest Pain Center. The lead-shielded working area and the dose calibrator fit on the counter top next to the zinc. Note wastebasket for radioactive waste.

spills should not occur more frequently. The "injector" should have been trained in how to handling radioisotopes and containing and decontaminating spills in the event that occurs.

Acute Rest Imaging Protocol

Activity (dose)	15 mCi, weight < 200lbs
	25 mCi, weight > 200lbs
Time interval after injection	30–45 min
Patient position	Supine
Imaging	Standard protocol (ECG gated)
Prone imaging	If inferior attenuation suspected

Disposition after acute rest imaging in CPC:

Normal: Discharge home
            Optional stress testing
Abnormal: Hospitalization

Although studies have clearly shown that patients with normal acute rest SPECT images have an excellent short-term outcome, and thus can be discharged when images are normal, some centers nevertheless perform stress testing prior to discharge.

Even when rest imaging (or biomarkers of myocardial injury) excludes ACS, patients may nevertheless have significant underlying coronary artery disease. A stress test prior to discharge is therefore useful to complete the cardiology work-up of patients with acute chest pain.

Radionuclide imaging plays an important role in this setting because approximately one-half of CPC patients cannot be evaluated by exercise ECG, because of inability to exercise, baseline ECG abnormalities that may preclude interpretation of ECG during exercise, or high pretest likelihood of coronary artery disease (4).

Stress Testing

Protocol	Standard Bruce Exercise ECG
	Standard Bruce Exercise Tc-99m-agent SPECT
	Adenosine vasodilation Tc-99m-agent SPECT
Dose	25 mCi [if second dose after first low (15 mCi) dose, or next day in obese patients who had first high (25 mCi) dose]

> **Disposition after stress testing in a CPC:**
>
> Normal: Discharge home
> Abnormal: Hospitalization
> *If only mildly abnormal consider:*
>   Discharge home with arrangements for follow-up as
> outpatient

Timely Interpretation

Because the CPC is a 24/7 operation, rest imaging results and the results of stress tests must be communicated as soon as possible to the attending ED physicians. The nuclear cardiology attending serves as a consultant to the ED attending.

Tele-nuclear cardiology (see Chapter 18) allows for remote reading of ECGs and nuclear images and is essential for the efficient operation of a CPC.

CT Coronary Angiography and SPECT Imaging in the ED

Recently, the results of a randomized controlled trial in the ED in patients with acute chest pain using the combined approach of CT coronary angiography and stress SPECT imaging were published *(5)*. Although CT coronary angiography was able to identify immediately those patients with no or minimal coronary disease and those with severe coronary artery disease, about 25% of patients did require additional stress SPECT imaging to elucidate the pathophysiologic significance of intermediate severity coronary lesions. Future studies are necessary to determine how to best use such combined approach.

REFERENCES

1. Wackers FJTh, Brown KA, Heller GV, Kontos MC, Tatum JL, Udelson JE, Ziffer JA (2002). American Society of Nuclear Cardiology position statement on radionuclide imaging in patients with suspected acute ischemic syndromes in the emergency department or chest pain center. *J Nucl Cardiol* 9:246–250.
2. Heller GV, Stowers SA, Hendel RC, Herman SD, Daher E, Ahlberg AW, Baron JM, Mendes-deLeon CF, Rizzo JA, Wackers FJTh (1998). Clinical value of acute rest technetium-99m-tetrofosmin tomographic myocardial perfusion imaging in patients with acute chest pain and nondiagnostic electrocardiograms. *J Am Coll Cardiol* 31:1011–1017.
3. Udelson JE, Beshansky JR, Ballin DS, Feldman JA, Griffith JL, Handler J, Heller GV, Hendel RC, Pope JH, Ruthazer R, Spiegler EJ, Woolard RH, Selker HP (2002). Myocardial perfusion imaging for evaluation and triage of patients with suspected acute cardiac ischemia. *JAMA* 288:2693–2700.

4. Abbott BG, Abdel-Aziz I, Nagula S, Monico EP, Schriver JA, Wackers FJTh (2001). Selective use of SPECT myocardial perfusion imaging in a chest pain center. *Am J Cardiol* 87:1351–1355.

5. Goldstein JA, Gallagher MJ, O'Neill WW, Ross MA, O'Neil BJ, Raff GL (2007). A ramdomized controlled trial of multislice coronary computed tomography for evaluation of acute chest pain. *J Am Coll Cardiol* 49:863–871.

22 Laboratory Accreditation

Continuing QA is an integral part of the present-day practice of medicine. Compliance by health care providers with quality standards set by organizations such as the Joint Commission on the Accreditation of Healthcare Organizations (JCAHO) is a matter of public record that can be carefully examined by the public as well as Health Maintenance Organizations (HMOs) and other health insurance providers. Throughout this book, references have been made to standards of quality set by the ICANL. In this chapter laboratory accreditation for nuclear cardiology is discussed in further detail.

Key Words: Laboratory accreditation, ICANL, Common reasons for delayed accreditation.

The ICANL was created in 1997 by experts in the field of nuclear cardiology to provide a mechanism for voluntary peer review of nuclear cardiology imaging facilities *(1)*. Subsequently, several Insurance Carriers and Health Maintenance Organizations (HMOs) in several states have adopted payment policies for reimbursement for nuclear cardiology services, requiring accreditation of the laboratory by ICANL (**Fig. 22-1**). One of the largest HMOs in the country, UnitedHealthCare Group, effective March 1, 2008, requires that all freestanding facilities and physician offices performing outpatient imaging studies that bill on CMS-1500 claim form obtain accreditation as a condition for reimbursement (see also for up to date information regarding payment policies http://www.icanl.org under: "Reimbursement").

From: *Contemporary Cardiology: Nuclear Cardiology, The Basics*
By: F. J. Th. Wackers, W. Bruni, and B. L. Zaret © Humana Press Inc., Totowa, NJ

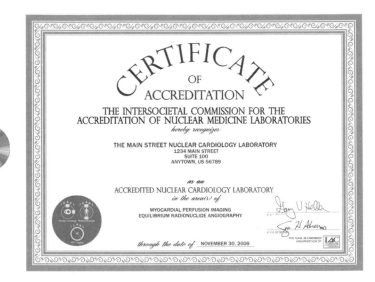

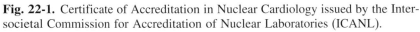

Fig. 22-1. Certificate of Accreditation in Nuclear Cardiology issued by the Intersocietal Commission for Accreditation of Nuclear Laboratories (ICANL).

PURPOSE OF ACCREDITATION

The purpose of accreditation is twofold:

1. To set and provide realistic and well-defined objective standards of quality for nuclear laboratories.
2. To educate and assist laboratories in achieving this goal.

TIME COMMITMENT

For a well-organized and well-run laboratory, it should not be difficult to obtain ICANL accreditation. This book contains a good deal of information about the material that is requested in an accreditation application. Well-written and detailed procedure protocols, evidence of QC and QA, good-quality images, and clear reports are key elements that characterize a successful application for ICANL accreditation *(2)*. However, one should be willing to make the time commitment to put all the material together for a complete application. On an average, this work may take between 3–5 months.

COMPONENTS OF THE ICANL ACCREDITATION APPLICATION

The *ICANL Standards* form the basis of the accreditation program. This comprehensive document provides standards for all aspects of patient testing and care and was created following the classical triad of quality assessment: structure, process, and outcome.

Part I, Structure of Imaging Facility

In this part of the application, the education, training, and credentials of the medical, technical, and other staff members are evaluated. In addition, the physical facilities, workload, equipment, and instrumentation must be described and listed. In order to be eligible for accreditation, one should have an imaging facility that has been in existence for at least 6 months and/or performed at least 300 studies.

Part II, Process of Nuclear Cardiology

In this part of the application, the degree of standardization of procedures in the applicant laboratory is evaluated. Standardization is an important means to maintain quality overtime regardless of personnel or equipment changes. Written protocols for all imaging and non-imaging procedures must be in place (see also Chapter 20). The following are key protocols:

1. General policies and protocols
2. Clinical procedures
3. Equipment QC
4. Radiation safety
5. Administrative protocols
6. Interpretation and reporting

As an example, of the clinical procedures, the acquisition, processing, and display of radionuclide images must be described in great detail, step-by-step, as it is performed actually in the applicant laboratory using the specific imaging equipment. The procedure protocol should contain sufficient detail that, for example, a newly hired technologist can start to work immediately from the written protocol and deliver the usual quality of work. Similar detailed protocols should be in place for the performance of stress testing, with details about the stress procedure, patient monitoring, timing of radiopharmaceutical injection, and treatment of adverse effects.

The ICANL adheres to, and requires laboratories to follow, the updated ASNC Imaging guidelines *(3)*, as published online at http://www.asnc.org.

Part III, Outcome and QA

In this part of the application, the quality of nuclear cardiology services and procedures is examined. The so-called "end product". This includes QA of imaging and non-imaging equipment and QA of imaging procedures and imaging results (see also http://www.icanl.org) *(4)*. The most important evaluation for accreditation involves peer review of randomly selected patient **images** and **reports** to referring physicians.

REVIEW PROCESS

Two trained reviewers independently review each application. The reviewers objectively evaluate whether the submitted written material is in substantial compliance with the *ICANL Standards*. An important component involves judging the quality of images and final reports. The reviewers each make an independent decision on the basis of the submitted material. The ICANL also conducts a *site visit* of every facility that applies for accreditation. These site visits primarily concentrate on the review of camera(s) and equipment, nuclear images, quality control procedures, radiation safety protocols, and observation of the laboratory in operation and of patient care. Both the application reviewers and the site visitor provide a report of significant findings and a recommendation to the ICANL Board of Directors, who review the submitted information and decide on the accreditation status of the laboratory.

ACCREDITATION

After review of a laboratory's application, the ICANL Board of Directors will make one of four decisions:

1. *Accreditation* granted for laboratories found to be in substantial compliance with the *ICANL Standards*. Accreditation is granted for a 3-year period. Accredited laboratory has the right to carry the ICANL logo on their letterhead.
2. *Provisional accreditation* for 1 year pending correction of minor deficiencies and/or submission of additional documents. After deficiencies have been corrected, the provisional status is converted to full accreditation for a 3-year period starting at the date of Board of Directors decision.
3. *Delayed accreditation* for up to 1 year, during which significant deficiencies and/or lack of adherence to the ICANL Standards need to be corrected. After 1 year, the deficiencies must have been corrected before accreditation can be granted for a 3-year period starting at the date of Board of Directors decision.
4. *Denied accreditation*. Any laboratory that has been denied accreditation has the right to appeal against the decision and may be re-evaluated by a new review ICANL panel. Denial occurs rarely and indicates that the laboratory functions significantly below ICANL Standards.

The laboratories will receive notice in writing about the Board of Director's decision within 2–3 weeks after the Board meeting.

COMMON REASONS FOR DELAYED ACCREDITATION

1. Inadequate quality of reports, i.e., missing components or elements, use of non-standard nomenclature, lack of integration of stress and imaging data, and failure to render a clear and concise conclusion.
2. Inadequate procedure protocols, i.e., laboratory-specific protocols that describe step-by-step imaging, processing, and stress procedures.
3. Insufficient documentation of quality control procedures and radiation safety measures and protocols.

Extensive further and updated information concerning the ICANL Standards and help with submitting an application is available online at http://www.icanl.org.

REFERENCES

1. Wackers FJTh (1999). Blueprint of the Accreditation Program of the Intersocietal Commission for the Accreditation of Nuclear Medicine Laboratories. *J Nucl Cardiol* 6:372–374.
2. Wackers FJTh (2003). Accreditation of nuclear cardiology laboratories: an educational process. *J Nucl Cardiol* 10:205–207.
3. DePuey EG (2006). *Imaging Guidelines for Nuclear Cardiology Procedures*, available at http://www.asnc.org—Menu: "Manage Your Practice": "Guidelines & Standards". (accessed May 2007)
4. Intersocietal Commission for Accrediation of Nuclear Laboratories. Access on line http://www.icanl.org. (accessed May 2007)

23   Coding and Billing

Accurate coding and billing of procedures performed in the laboratory are extremely important. The following serves as a brief introduction to correct coding. However, it is not the intention, nor is it possible, to provide definitive guidelines for any specific laboratory. While coverage rules may differ from state to state as well as across different health insurance carriers, there are basic coding tenets that have been established by the Medicare program, which are generally followed across the country. As always, nuclear cardiology practices should seek advice and check with local billing experts for accuracy.

Key Words: Coding and billing, Fraud awareness, ICD-9 codes, CPT codes, Reimbursement.

RECOMMENDED STEPS FOR CORRECT CODING AND BILLING

1. Credentialing process
    a. Providers
        Providers must have current medical licenses, up-to-date curriculum vitae, records of CME credit hours, specialty board certifications (Certification Board of Nuclear Cardiology [CBNC], American Board of Radiology [ABR], or American Board of Nuclear Medicine [ABNM]), malpractice insurance, and, if a foreign medical school graduate, a Educational Commission for Foreign Medical School Graduate (ECFMG) certificate.
        To be eligible for reimbursement, more payers are now requiring CBNC certification for nuclear cardiologists as well as ICANL accreditation for laboratories.
    b. Payer participation
        If not familiar with contracts, employ someone who can contact insurers to find out if there are special requirements for billing for nuclear cardiology procedures. One should look to negotiate

From: *Contemporary Cardiology: Nuclear Cardiology, The Basics*
By: F. J. Th. Wackers, W. Bruni, and B. L. Zaret © Humana Press Inc., Totowa, NJ

reimbursements and clearly understand the restrictions. A payer can have several plans and all will have separate rules so it is important to create an index or guide for each payer to help alleviate questions at the time of patient appointment booking.

2. Patient eligibility
   a. Referrals
      Verification that the patient belongs to a participating health insurance carrier.
   b. Payer authorizations
      Some payers require pre-approval of a test. For Medicare patients, no pre-approval is needed.
3. Patient visit
   Documentation: The nuclear cardiology report serves as documentation for visit.
4. Billing requirements
   a. Valid International Classification of Diseases, Ninth Edition (ICD-9) code(s)
   b. Appropriate Current Procedural Terminology (CPT) code(s)
   c. Appropriate modifiers
   d. Timely reporting
   e. Timely filing

Fraud Awareness

Providers must recognize their responsibility in complying with Medicare regulations. Medicare compliance requires that providers determine whether services they are furnishing are covered under the Medicare program. If services are not covered, providers should not submit a bill to Medicare without a signed Advanced Beneficiary Notice (ABN) form and added modifiers GA or GZ. The ABN form indicates that the patient is aware that he/she is responsible for payment. The modifier GA indicates that a waver of liability on file, whereas the modifier GZ indicates that the item or service is expected to be denied, not reasonable and necessary.

General Principles

In order to receive reimbursement for diagnostic procedures, practices must correctly code for the specific procedure performed as well as an appropriate corresponding ICD-9 code. Be sure that the hard copy reports, which are maintained by the practice, document all of these critical details and that the correct component of the global procedural code is documented (e.g., professional or technical component).The diagnosis code(s) must fit the procedure code(s).

A complete list of CPT codes can be found in CPT reference books, i.e., CPT® Professional, which can be ordered online: http://www.ingenixonline.com or by calling 1-800-Ingenix (464.3649). CPT codes are updated at regular time intervals. One should always use the most recent codes. The codes shown below were valid in the years 2006–2007.

Reimbursement may occur under two distinctly different scenarios:

1. The provider is the sole owner of all equipment, e.g., physicians' office: technical, procedural, and interpretative billing are bundled in one (global fee).
2. The provider of services is not the owner of the equipment, e.g., within hospital setting: technical billing is separate from procedural and interpretative billing.

ICD-9 codes are used to justify the performance of a particular procedure.

A complete list of ICD-9 codes can be found in the ICD-9-CM reference book, i.e., ICD-9-CM for Physicians; volumes 1 & 2, which can be ordered online at http://www.ingenixonline.com.

ICD-9 codes are updated at regular time intervals. One should always use most recent codes. The following codes were valid in 2006–2007.

Tables 23-1 and 23-2 list examples of ICD-9 and CPT codes.

Table 23-1
A Few Examples of Useful ICD-9 Codes in Nuclear Cardiology

ICD-9 codes	Item
786.50	Chest pain unspecified
413.0–413.9	Angina decubitus, other and unspecified angina pectoris
786.05	Shortness of breath
794.31	Abnormal ECG
414.00–414.05	Coronary atherosclerosis of unspecified type of vessel native or coronary atherosclerosis of unspecified bypass graft
V72.81	Pre-operative cardiovascular examination
412	Old myocardial infarction
410.0–410.82	Acute myocardial infarction of anterolateral wall, episode of care unspecified – acute myocardial infarction of other specified sites, subsequent episode of care

(Continued)

Table 23-1
(*Continued*)

ICD-9 codes	Item
411.0–411.89	Postmyocardial infarction syndrome – other acute and subacute forms of ischemic heart disease other
428.0–428.1	Congestive heart failure (CHF) unspecified, left heart failure
428.9	CHF unspecified
780.2	Syncope
426.0–426.9	Atrioventricular block complete – conduction disorder unspecified
V42.1	Heart replaced by transplant
V42.2	Heart valve replaced by transplant
996.03	Mechanical complications due to coronary bypass graft

Table 23-2
CPT Codes for Nuclear Cardiology Procedures

CPT codes	Item
78464	Myocardial perfusion imaging SPECT: single study (i.e., stress or rest), including attenuation correction when performed, with or without quantification
78465	Myocardial perfusion imaging SPECT: multiple studies (i.e., stress–rest, same day or 2 days), including attenuation correction when performed, with or without quantification
78478 add-on code, must be used with either 78464 or 78465	Myocardial perfusion imaging (SPECT) with wall motion analysis
78480 add-on code, must be used with either 78464 or 78465	Myocardial perfusion imaging (SPECT) with EF assessment
93015 (global)	Cardiovascular stress test, MD supervision, ECG tracing and report and interpretation
93016 (not global)	Cardiovascular stress test (MD supervision)
93017 (not global)	Cardiovascular stress test (for obtaining ECG tracing only)

93018 (not global)	Cardiovascular stress test (for interpretation only)
78481	First-pass angiocardiography: single study
78483	First-pass angiocardiography : multiple studies
78472	Cardiac blood pool imaging : single study, gated equilibrium, planar wall motion study plus EF
78473	Cardiac blood pool imaging : multiple studies
78496 add-on code, must be used with 78472	Cardiac blood pool imaging : single study with RVEF
78494	Cardiac blood pool imaging : single study SPECT, at rest wall motion plus EF

Tables 23-3 to 23-7 summarize examples of appropriate coding for technical, professional, and supply components for ungated Tl stress SPECT imaging. Note that for appropriate reimbursement, the physician's report *must* state why pharmacological stress was used instead of treadmill exercise.

Table 23-3
Tl-201 Stress SPECT Imaging

CPT codes for technical component	Item	CPT codes for professional component	Item
78465-TC	Myocardial perfusion imaging SPECT: multiple studies	78465-26	Myocardial perfusion imaging SPECT: multiple studies
93016	Cardiovascular stress test, MD supervision	93018	Cardiovascular stress test: interpretation/report
A9505	TI-201 thallous chloride, per mCi		NP: Nurse practitioner code PA: Physician assistant code

Table 23-4
ECG-gated Stress Sestamibi SPECT Imaging *(example of total coding)*

CPT codes for technical component	Item	CPT code for professional component	Item
78465-TC	Myocardial perfusion imaging SPECT scan: multiple studies	78465-26	Myocardial perfusion imaging SPECT scan: multiple studies
93016	Cardiovascular stress test, MD supervision	93018	Cardiovascular stress test: interpretation/report
78478-TC	Myocardial perfusion with wall motion	78478-26	Myocardial perfusion with wall motion
78480-TC	Myocardial perfusion with EF	78480-26	Myocardial perfusion with EF
A9500	Tc-99m sestamibi: dose up to 40 mCi		

Table 23-5
ECG-gated Rest Equilibrium radionuclide Angiocardiography *(example of total coding)*

CPT codes for technical component	Item	CPT code for professional component	Item
78472-TC	Gated blood pool imaging single study at rest	78472	Gated blood pool imaging single study at rest
A4641	Supply of Tc-99m pyrophosphate *or*		Red blood cell labeling (in vivo) *or*
A9560	Tc-99m Ultratag, labeled red blood cells, diagnostic, per study dose up to 30 mCi		Red blood cell labeling (in vitro)

Table 23-6
Codes for Supply of Radiopharmaceuticals

CPT codes	Item
A9505	TI-201: thallous chloride per mCi
A9500	Tc-99m sestamibi: per dose up to 40 mCi
A9502	Tc-99m tetrofosmin: per dose up to 40 mCi
A4641	Supply of radiopharmaceutical diagnostic imaging agent, not otherwise specified (unlisted code)
78990	If provider does not accept "A" codes: provision of radiopharmaceutical

Table 23-7
Codes for Administering Pharmaceuticals

HCPCS codes	
J1245	Dipyridamole: per 10 mg
J0152	Adenosine: per 30 mg unit (Adenoscan®)
J0150	Adenosine: per 6 mg unit (Adenocard®)
J0280	Aminophylline: up to 250 mg
J1250	Dobutamine: per 250 mg
99070	If provider does not accept "J" codes: provision of pharmaceutical

Coding Compliance

It is important to create an internal coding compliance program that monitors appropriateness of coding and billing of the stress testing and imaging facility. When errors and possible violations are detected, they should be documented and appropriate course of action should be taken to avoid repetition.

Warning: The following codes should *NEVER* be used in combination, e.g., for dual isotope imaging, in attempt to bill separately for the Tl-201 part.
    78465 (SPECT MPI multiple studies) and:
    78460 (Tl planar MPI single study), or
    78461 (Tl planar MPI multiple studies), or
    78464 (SPECT MPI single study)
This represents double billing, which is fraudulent.

Communication between physicians and billing staff is essential.
There should be a voluntary compliance program with checks
and balances. The physicians are responsible to ensure that provided
services are reasonable and necessary. The coding and billing should
match services provided and there should be proper documentation
(i.e., request for services and detailed reports about services and
results). Inappropriate coding and billing could result in decreased
reimbursements and possibly expose the facility to the risk of audits.

We suggest that billing and compliance personnel acquire and
reference the National Correct Coding Primer with CorrectCodeChek,
published by Part B News Group. This useful reference book may serve
as a guide for how to avoid denials for bundled codes and how to select
correct coding combinations. One can obtain a copy of this manual,
which is updated quarterly, by calling customer service at 1-877-397-
1496, or online at http://www.partbnews.com/pbnweb/resources.htm.

Questions About Reimbursement

For Medicare reimbursement, your local Medicare carrier should
be able to answer most questions. In the case of third party payers,
one may consult professionals at the payers' local or regional office.
One can also call the ASNC Health Policy Director Chris Gallagher
at 301-215-7575 or e-mail at gallagher@asnc.org.

On the ASNC website, one will find some very useful case studies,
examples, and tips for correct coding (http://www.asnc.org—Menu:
"Manage Your Practice" : "Practice Tips") (Accessed June 2007).

24 Appropriateness Criteria for Nuclear Cardiology Procedures

> In addition to performing high-quality nuclear cardiology studies and interpreting them correctly, it is highly relevant to assist referring physicians with respect to ordering studies that are most appropriate for the clinical question posed in an individual patient.

Key Words: Appropriateness of procedures, Framingham risk estimates, Pretest probability of disease.

In an attempt to address this question, the ASNC and American College of Cardiology formed a panel charged with assessing the risk and benefits of various nuclear cardiology procedures for several specific clinical indications or clinical scenarios *(1)*.

The panel consisted of 12 members with diverse backgrounds, including nuclear cardiologists, referring physicians, health services researchers, and a payer representative. Only 58% of the panel were nuclear cardiologists.

The panel defined 52 indications that were felt to cover the clinical spectrum of the patients seen in nuclear cardiology testing. Although this is not a totally comprehensive listing, it was felt to cover those indications routinely encountered in clinical practice.

With only a few exceptions, all indications refer to ECG-gated SPECT myocardial perfusion imaging. In all perfusion studies, it is also assumed that left ventricular function and regional wall motion are evaluated as part of the same study. For stress imaging, it is assumed that all patients able to exercise would do so, and those unable to exercise would undergo pharmaologic stress.

Each of 52 indications were graded by the panel and placed into one of three categories listed in Table 24-1.

From: *Contemporary Cardiology: Nuclear Cardiology, The Basics*
By: F. J. Th. Wackers, W. Bruni, and B. L. Zaret © Humana Press Inc., Totowa, NJ

The classification was based upon the following:

1. Review of the literature
2. Published guidelines *(2–9)*
3. Pretest likelihood of coronary artery disease for symptomatic patients (Table 24-2).
4. Framingham risk criteria for risk determination in asymptomatic patients (Table 24-3 and Figs. 24-1 and 24-2).
5. Expert opinion of the panel members

Table 24-1
Appropriateness Categories

Appropriate: The specific study is generally acceptable and is a reasonable approach for the indication.

Inappropriate: The specific study is generally not acceptable and not a reasonable approach for the indication

Uncertain: The specific study *may* be a reasonable approach for the indication. However, it was felt that at the present time more research and/or patient information is needed for a more definitive classification.

Age (Low-risk level)*	30-34 (2%)	35-39 (3%)	40-44 (3%)	45-49 (4%)	50-54 (5%)	55-59 (7%)	60-64 (8%)	65-69 (10%)	70-74 (13%)	Absolute Risk	Absolute Risk‡
Points †										Total CHD‡	Hard CHD¶
0	1.0									2%	2%
1	1.5	1.0	1.0							3%	2%
2	2.0	1.3	1.3	1.0						4%	3%
3	2.5	1.7	1.7	1.3	1.0					5%	4%
4	3.5	2.3	2.3	1.8	1.4	1.0				7%	5%
5	4.0	2.6	2.6	2.0	1.6	1.1	1.0			8%	6%
6	5.0	3.3	3.3	2.5	2.0	1.4	1.3	1.0		10%	7%
7	6.5	4.3	4.3	3.3	2.6	1.9	1.6	1.3	1.0	13%	9%
8	8.0	5.3	5.3	4.0	3.2	2.3	2.0	1.6	1.2	16%	13%
9	10.0	6.7	6.7	5.0	4.0	2.9	2.5	2.0	1.5	20%	16%
10	12.5	8.3	8.3	6.3	5.0	3.6	3.1	2.5	1.9	25%	20%
11	15.5	10.3	10.3	7.8	6.1	4.4	3.9	3.1	2.3	31%	25%
12	18.5	12.3	12.3	9.3	7.4	5.2	4.6	3.7	2.8	37%	30%
13	22.5	15.0	15.0	11.3	9.0	6.4	5.6	4.5	3.5	45%	35%
>14	26.5	>17.7	>17.7	>13.3	>10.6	>7.6	>6.6	>5.3	>4.1	>53%	>45%

* Low absolute risk level= 10-year risk for total CHD endpoints for a person the same age, blood pressure <120/<80 mmHg, total cholesterol 160-199 mg/dl, HDL-C ≥45 mg/dl, non smoker, no diabetes. Percentage show 10-year absolute risk for total CHD end points

† Points = number of points from Table 21-3

‡ 10-year absolute risk for total CHD endpoints estimated from Framingham data corresponding to Framingham points (Table 21-3)

¶ 10-year absolute risk for total CHD endpoints approximated from Framingham data corresponding to Framingham points (Table 21-3)

Color Key for Relative Risk

Green	Violet	Yellow	Red
Below Average risk	Average risk	Moderately above average risk	High risk

Men

Fig. 24-1. Relative and absolute risk estimates for coronary heart disease in men as determined from Framingham scoring (modified from ref 10).

Table 24-2
Pretest Probability of Coronary Artery Disease by Age, Gender, and Symptoms

Age (years)	Gender	Typical/definite angina pectoris	Atypical/probable angina pectoris	Nonanginal chest pain	Asymptomatic
30–39	Men	Intermediate	Intermediate	Low	Very low
	Women	Intermediate	Very low	Very low	Very low
40–49	Men	High	Intermediate	Intermediate	Low
	Women	Intermediate	Low	Very low	Very low
50–59	Men	High	Intermediate	Intermediate	Low
	Women	Intermediate	Intermediate	Low	Very Low
60–69	Men	High	Intermediate	Intermediate	Low
	Women	High	Intermediate	Intermediate	Low

High, > 90% pre-test probability; intermediate, 10–90% pre-test probability; low, 5–10% pre-test probability; very low, < 5% pre-test probability. Typical/definite angina pectoris: substernal chest pain or discomfort that is provoked by exertion or emotional stress and relieved by rest and/or nitroglycerin. Atypical/probable angina pectoris: chest pain or discomfort that lacks one of the characteristics of typical or definite angina pectoris. Nonanginal chest pain: chest pain or discomfort that meets one or none of the typical angina characteristics (modified from ref. (8))

Table 24-3
Global Risk Assessment in Asymptomatic Individuals (Framingham Score)

Risk factor	Risk points	
	Men	Women
Age (years)		
<34	−1	−9
35–39	0	−4
40–44	1	0
45–49	2	3
50–54	3	6
55–59	4	7
60–64	5	8
65–69	6	8
70–74	7	8
Total cholesterol (mg/dl)		
<160	−3	−2
169–199	0	0
200–239	1	1
240–279	2	2
≥280	3	3
HDL-C (mg/dl)		
<35	2	5
35–44	1	2
45–49	0	1
50–59	0	0
≥60	−2	−3
Systolic blood pressure (mm Hg)		
< 120	0	−3
120–129	0	0
130–139	1	1
140–159	2	2
≥160	3	3
Diabetes		
No	0	0
Yes	2	4
Smoker		
No	0	0
Yes	2	2

Add up the points:
Age _____
Cholesterol _____
HDL-C _____
Blood pressure _____
Diabetes _____
Smoking _____
Total points _____

HDL-C, high-density lipoprotein cholesterol. Ten-year absolute coronary heart disease risk (Framingham Risk): low, < 10% risk, score < 5; Moderate, 10–20% risk, score 5–8; High, > 20% risk, score > 9.

Age (Low-risk level)*	40-44 (2%)	45-49 (3%)	50-54 (5%)	55-59 (7%)	60-64 (8%)	65-69 (8%)	70-74 (8%)	Absolute Risk Total CHD‡	Absolute Risk Hard CHD¶
Points ↑									
0	1.0							2%	1%
1	1.0							2%	1%
2	1.5	1.0						3%	2%
3	1.5	1.0						3%	2%
4	2.0	1.3						4%	2%
5	2.0	1.3						4%	2%
6	2.5	1.7	1.0					5%	2%
7	3.0	2.0	1.2					6%	3%
8	3.5	2.3	1.4	1.0				7%	3%
9	4.0	2.7	1.6	1.1	1.0	1.0	1.0	8%	3%
10	5.0	3.3	2.0	1.4	1.3	1.3	1.3	10%	4%
11	5.5	3.7	2.2	1.6	1.4	1.4	1.4	11%	7%
12	6.5	4.3	2.6	1.9	1.6	1.6	1.6	13%	8%
13	7.5	5.0	3.0	2.1	1.9	1.9	1.9	15%	11%
14	9.0	6.0	3.6	2.6	2.3	2.3	2.3	18%	13%
15	10.0	6.7	4.0	2.9	2.5	2.5	2.5	20%	15%
16	12.0	8.0	4.8	3.4	3.0	3.0	3.0	24%	18%
≥17	>13.5	>9.0	>5.4	>3.9	5.4	5.4	5.4	>27%	>20%

* Low absolute risk level= 10-year risk for total CHD endpoints for a person the same age, blood pressure <120/<80 mmHg, total cholesterol 160-199 mg/dl, HDL-C ≥45 mg/dl, non smoker, no diabetes. Percentage show 10-year absolute risk for total CHD end points

† Points = number of points from Table 21-3

‡ 10-year absolute risk for total CHD endpoints estimated from Framingham data corresponding to Framingham points (Table 21-3)

¶ 10-year absolute risk for total CHD endpoints approximated from Framingham data corresponding to Framingham points (Table 21-3)

Key for Relative Risk

Green	Violet	Yellow	Red
Below average risk	Average risk	Moderately above average risk	High risk

Women

Fig. 24-2. Relative and absolute risk estimates for coronary heart disease in women as determined from Framingham scoring (modified from ref 10).

The appropriateness of nuclear cardiology studies for the 52 indications evaluated by the panel are outlined in Tables 24-4 to 24-13. Each table deals with a broad clinical scenario or indication. Within each table there are further subdivisions. Each indication has been rated either as appropriate, inappropriate, or uncertain.

The panel viewed 52% of the indications as appropriate, 25% as inappropriate, and 23% as uncertain.

This assessment by the panel should be viewed as a basis for considering when and in what situation a specific test should be done. These criteria may ultimately become a basis for reimbursement. However, as is stated in the report, these criteria are not substitutes for "sound clinical judgment and practice experience with each patient and clinical presentation." Clearly, there may be both medical and non-medical situations that would impact on the application of these criteria to a specific patient. As always, clinical judgment must be employed in criteria implementation. Finally, it is also stated in the report that "the local availability or quality of equipment or personnel may influence the selection of appropriate imaging procedures."

Table 24-4
Detection of Symptomatic Cad

Indication	Appropriateness recommendation
Evaluation of chest pain syndrome	
1. Low pre-test probability of coronary artery disease. ECG interpretable AND able to exercise	Inappropriate
2. Low pre-test probability of coronary artery disease. ECG uninterpretable OR unable to exercise	Uncertain
3. Intermediate pre-test probability of coronary artery disease. ECG interpretable AND able to exercise	Appropriate
4. Intermediate pre-test probability of coronary artery disease. ECG uninterpretable OR unable to exercise	Appropriate
5. High pre-test probability of coronary artery disease. ECG interpretable AND able to exercise	Appropriate
6. High pre-test probability of coronary artery disease. ECG uninterpretable OR unable to exercise	Appropriate
Acute chest pain (in reference to rest perfusion imaging)	
7. Intermediate pre-test probability of coronary artery disease. ECG—no ST elevation AND initial cardiac enzymes negative	Appropriate
8. High pre-test probability of coronary artery disease. ECG—ST elevation	Inappropriate
New-onset/diagnosed heart failure with chest pain syndrome	
9. Intermediate pre-test probability of coronary artery disease	Appropriate

Table 24-5
Detection of Asymptomatic Cad (Without Chest Pain Syndrome)

Indication	Appropriateness recommendation
Asymptomatic	
10. Low coronary heart disease risk (Framingham risk criteria)	Inappropriate
11. Moderate CHD risk (Framingham)	Uncertain
New-onset *or* diagnosed heart failure *or* LV systolic dysfunction without chest pain syndrome	
12. Moderate coronary heart disease risk (Framingham). No prior coronary artery disease evaluation AND no planned cardiac catheterization	Appropriate
Valvular heart disease without chest pain syndrome	
13. Moderate coronary heart disease risk (Framingham). To help guide decision for invasive studies	Uncertain
New-onset atrial fibrillation	
14. Low coronary heart disease risk (Framingham). Part of the evaluation	Uncertain
15. High coronary heart disease risk (Framingham). Part of the evaluation	Appropriate
Ventricular Tachycardia	
16. Moderate to high coronary heart disease risk (Framingham)	Appropriate

Table 24-6
Risk Assessment: General and Specific Patient Populations

Indication	Appropriateness recommendation
Asymptomatic	
17. Low coronary heart disease risk (Framingham)	Inappropriate
18. Moderate coronary heart disease risk (Framingham)	Uncertain
19. Moderate to high coronary heart disease risk (Framingham). High-risk occupation (e.g., airline pilot)	Appropriate
20. High coronary heart disease risk (Framingham)	Appropriate

Table 24-7
Risk Assessment with Prior Test Results

Indication	Appropriateness recommendation
Asymptomatic _or_ stable symptoms. Normal prior SPECT study	
21. Normal initial SPECT perfusion study. High coronary heart disease risk (Framingham). Annual SPECT MPI study	Inappropriate
22. Normal initial SPECT perfusion study. High coronary heart disease risk (Framingham). Repeat SPECT MPI study after 2 years or greater	Appropriate
Asymptomatic _or_ Stable Symptoms. Abnormal catheterization _or prior SPECT study_	
23. Known coronary artery disease on catheterization _or_ prior SPECT perfusion study in patients who have not had revascularization procedure. Asymptomatic _or_ stable symptoms. Less than 1 year to evaluate worsening disease	Inappropriate
24. Known coronary artery disease on catheterization _or_ prior SPECT perfusion study in patients who have not had revascularization procedure.	Appropriate
Worsening symptoms. Abnormal catheterization _or prior SPECT study_	
25. Known coronary artery disease on catheterization _or_ prior SPECT study	Appropriate
Asymptomatic: CT coronary angiography	
26. Stenosis of unclear significance	Uncertain
Asymptomatic: prior coronary calcium agatston score	
27. Agatston score ≥ 400	Appropriate
28. Agatston score < 100	Inappropriate
UA/NSTEMI, STEMI, _or_ chest pain syndrome. Coronary angiogram	
29. Stenosis of unclear significance	Appropriate
Duke treadmill score	
30. Intermediate Duke treadmill score. Intermediate coronary heart disease risk (Framingham)	Appropriate

UA, unstable angina.
NSTEMI, non ST elevation myocardial infarction.
STEMI, ST elevation myocardial infarction.

Table 24-8
Risk Assessment: Preoperative Evaluation for Non-Cardiac Surgery

Indication	Appropriateness recommendation
Low-risk surgery	
31. Preoperative evaluation for non-cardiac surgery risk assessment	Inappropriate
Intermediate-risk surgery	
32. Minor to intermediate perioperative risk predictor. Normal exercise tolerance (greater than or equal to 4 METS)	Inappropriate
33. Intermediate perioperative risk predictor *OR* poor exercise tolerance (less than 4 METS)	Appropriate
High-risk surgery	
34. Minor perioperative risk predictor. Normal exercise tolerance (greater than or equal to 4 METS)	Uncertain
35. Minor perioperative risk predictor. Poor exercise tolerance (less than 4 METS)	Appropriate
36. Asymptomatic up to 1 year post normal catheterization, noninvasive test, or previous revascularization	Inappropriate

Table 24-9
Risk Assessment: Following Acute Coronary Syndrome

Indication	Appropriateness recommendation
STEMI-hemodynamically stable	
37. Thrombolytic therapy administered. Not planning to undergo catheterization	Appropriate
STEMI-hemodynamically unstable, signs of cardiogenic shock *or* mechanical complications	
38. Thrombolytic therapy administered	Inappropriate
UA/NSTEMI—no recurrent ischemia *or* no signs of heart failure	
39. Not planning to undergo early catheterization	Appropriate
ACS-asymptomatic post-revascularization (PCI *or* CABG)	
40. Routine evaluation prior to hospital discharge	Inappropriate

UA, unstable angina.
NSTEMI, non ST elevation myocardial infarction.
STEMI, ST elevation myocardial infarction.
ACS, acute coronary syndrome.

Table 24-10
Risk Assessment: Post-Revascularization (PCI or CABG)

Indication	Appropriateness recommendation
Symptomatic	
41. Evaluation of chest pain syndrome	Appropriate
Asymptomatic	
42. Asymptomatic prior to previous revascularization. Less than 5 years after coronary artery bypass surgery	Uncertain
43. Symptomatic prior to previous revascularization. Less than 5 years after CABG	Uncertain
44. Asymptomatic prior to previous revascularization. Greater than or equal to 5 years after CABG	Appropriate
45. Symptomatic prior to previous revascularization. Greater than or equal to 5 years after CABG	Appropriate
46. Asymptomatic prior to previous revascularization. Less than 1 year after PCI	Uncertain
47. Symptomatic prior to previous revascularization. Less than 1 year after PCI	Inappropriate
48. Asymptomatic prior to previous revascularization. Greater than or equal to 2 years after PCI	Uncertain
49. Symptomatic prior to previous revascularization. Greater than or equal to 2 years after PCI	Uncertain

CABG, coronary artery bypass graft surgery.
PCI, percutaneous coronary intervention.

Table 24-11
Assessment of Viability/Ischemia

Indication	Appropriateness recommendation
Ischemic cardiomyopathy assessment of viability/ischemia (includes SPECT imaging for wall motion and ventricular function)	
50. Known coronary artery disease on catheterization. Patient eligible for revascularization	Appropriate

Table 24-12
Evaluation of Ventricular Function

Indication	Appropriateness recommendation
Evaluation of left ventricular function	
51. Non-diagnostic echocardiogram	Appropriate
Use of potentially cardiotoxic therapy (e.g., doxorubicin)	
52. Baseline and serial measurements	Appropriate

REFERENCES

1. ACCF/ASNC (2005). Appropriateness criteria for single photon computerized tomography myocardial perfusion imaging (SPECT MPI). *J Am Coll Cardiol* 46:1587–1605.
2. Klocke FJ, Baird MG, Lorrell BH, et al. (2003). ACC/AHA/ASNC Guidelines for the clinical use of cardiac radionuclide imaging. *Circulation* 108:1404–1418.
3. Gibbons RJ, Balady GJ, Bricker JT, et al (2002). Summary article. ACC/AHA Guideline update for exercise testing. *Circulation* 106:1883–1892.
4. Hunt SA, Abraham WT, Chin MH, et al. (2005). ACC/AHA Guideline update for the diagnosis and management of chronic heart failure in the adult. *J Am Coll Cardiol* 46:e1–e82.
5. Eagle KA, Berger PB, Calkins H, et al. (2002). ACC/AHA guideline update for perioperative cardiovascular evaluation for non-cardiac surgery. *Circulation* 105:1257–1267.
6. Antman EM, Anbe AT, Armstrong PW, et al. (2004). ACC/AHA guidelines for the management of patients with ST-elevation myocardial infarction. J Am Coll Cardiol 44;671–719.
7. Gibbons RJ, Abrams J, Chatterjee K, et al. (2002). ACC/AHA guideline update for the management of patients with chronic stable angina. *Circulation* 107:149–158.
8. Braunwald E, Antman E, Beasley JW, et al. (2002). ACC/AHA guideline updates in the management of unstable angina and non-ST-segment elevation myocardial infarction. *J Am Coll Cardiol* 40:1366–1374.
9. Bonow RO, Carabello B, de Leon AC Jr, et al. (1998). ACC/AHA practice guidelines for the management of patients with valvular heart disease. *J Am Coll Cardiol* 32:1486–1588.
10. Grundy SM, Pasternak R, Greenland P, Smith S, Fuster V (1999). Assessment of cardiovascular risk by the use of multiple risk factor assessment equations. A statement for healthcare professionals from the American Heart Association and the American College of Cardiology. *Circulation* 100:1481–1492.

Index

Printed in the United States of America.